DR. EARL
MINDELL'S
SECRETS OF
NATURAL
HEALTH

ALSO BY EARL MINDELL AND VIRGINIA HOPKINS:

PRESCRIPTION ALTERNATIVES: HUNDREDS OF SAFE, NATURAL PRESCRIPTION-FREE REMEDIES TO RESTORE AND MAINTAIN YOUR HEALTH

DR. EARL MINDELL'S SECRETS OF NATURAL HEALTH

~

A Complete Program for Vibrant Well-Being

EARL L. MINDELL, R.PH., PH.D.
and VIRGINIA HOPKINS, M.A.

KEATS PUBLISHING

LOS ANGELES

NTC/Contemporary Publishing Group

The purpose of this book is to educate. It is sold with the understanding that the publisher and author shall have neither liability nor responsibility for any injury caused or alleged to be caused directly or indirectly by the information contained in this book. While every effort has been made to ensure its accuracy, the book's contents should not be construed as medical advice. Each person's health needs are unique. To obtain recommendations appropriate to your particular situation, please consult a qualified health care provider.

Library of Congress Cataloging-in-Publication Data
Mindell, Earl
  [Secrets of natural health]
  Dr. Earl Mindell's secrets of natural health : a complete program for vibrant well-being
/Earl L. Mindell and Virginia Hopkins.
        p. cm
  Includes bibliographical references and index
  ISBN 0-87983-985-6
   1. Alternative medicine. 2. Herbs-Therapeutic use. 3. Nutrition. 4. Health. I. Title:
   Secrets of natural health. II. Hopkins, Virginia. III. Title.

   R733 .M565 2000   00-028733
   613-dc21

Published by Keats Publishing
A division of NTC/Contemporary Publishing Group, Inc.
4255 West Touhy Avenue, Lincolnwood, Illinois 60646-1975 U.S.A.

Interior design: Andrea Reider

Printed in the United States of America

International Standard Book Number: 0-87983-985-6

00 01 02 03 04 VH 18 17 16 15 14 13 12 11 10 9 8 7 6 5 4 3 2 1

CONTENTS ~

INTRODUCTION ~

Because I am a pharmacist as well as a nutritionist and herbalist, I have a unique point of view on natural health and alternative medicine. I have first-hand knowledge of how drugs work in the body, how they are prescribed, and why doctors prescribe the drugs they do. I am not going to do too much "doctor bashing" in this book, and I acknowledge that by and large, medical doctors are well meaning, if misguided, in their approach to health care.

THE "PILL FOR EVERY ILL" MIND-SET

The information you are exposed to in the media and from your doctor tends to be shamefully awash in misleading drug company advertising and marketing fictions that can be harmful to your health and even increase your risk of death. In this book, I'm going to tell you about some of these misconceptions and dangers and give you some safe, effective, natural solutions for many health problems.

I want you to understand, for the sake of your health, that nearly all doctors are unduly influenced by drug companies from the time they're in medical school until the day they retire. Even medical school curriculums are extremely biased toward the disease/drug approach to health care. In medical school, doctors are first taught anatomy and physiology, then how to diagnose disease, and then what drug to prescribe to treat a disease. Their approach to medicine and healing is very limited and narrow, with a primary focus on symptoms.

Also starting in medical school, doctors are courted, cajoled, and bribed with expensive meals, gifts, equipment, vacations, and free drugs by the pharmaceutical company sales reps. Doctors in prac-

tice may be given the "incentive" of a free vacation or expensive gift if they sell a certain amount of a drug.

Once a doctor is in practice, most of his or her information about drugs is going to come from drug company sales reps—the average doctor just doesn't have time to keep up with the latest medical journals. This is why doctors practice medicine under seemingly incredible misconceptions and fallacies that a simple glance at a biochemistry textbook could correct.

To make matters worse, insurance companies have gotten into the business of practicing medicine and may refuse to cover a patient's treatment if the doctor doesn't prescribe the drug approved by the insurance company for treating that disease. This problem is even more exaggerated in an HMO, which may itself dictate the standards of care. If the doctors don't follow those so-called "standards," they run the risk of losing their jobs, their medical licenses, or their hospital privileges. For a doctor fresh out of medical school, half a million dollars in debt and probably with a family to support, these are potent incentives to toe the line and forget the facts.

There is very little genuine care and concern for your health and well-being among the drug companies. The closest you'll come to concern from the typical health care organization is a desire not to be involved in a lawsuit.

With this knowledge, it's easy to understand how a doctor may be unduly influenced to prescribe drugs. In the past century, our medical system has created a very powerful MD mind-set that says that there's a pill for every ill. But the first vow of a new doctor is to "do no harm," and buying into drug company hype and handing out pills for every ill is a sure way to inflict damage on patients. My fervent hope is that as patients become increasingly disenchanted with a medical system that's not working, they'll turn to alternative sources of healing and medicine, and the MDs will be forced to change their ways or become extinct.

Many important health matters, such as the causes and prevention of illness, the role of nutrition in illness, and the role of the mind and emotions in illness, are either completely ignored in medical school or given a few token hours. Ironically, it's difficult or impossible to help people stay healthy without taking these factors into account. The good news is that there's a change in the wind. Some insurance companies and HMOs are coming to the realization that they could save millions of dollars a year in health care costs by simply paying attention to preventive care practices such as educating patients about nutrition and a healthy lifestyle. Nearly all of our common chronic diseases, including heart disease, diabetes, and arthritis, are completely preventable.

THE PSYCHOLOGY OF GOING TO THE DOCTOR

Something else you should be aware of is the psychology of going to the doctor. All too often, the real reason people go to the doctor is because they're having problems in their personal lives, and they don't know where else to turn. They go to the doctor with some minor complaint, hoping in some vague way that the doctor will fix their problem, or at least give them some comfort and attention. But going to the doctor is likely to make you sick! Patients don't like to walk away from a doctor's office without a prescription, and doctors like to please their patients, and that can be the start of a long battle with ill health. You'll take the prescription for, say, an allergy drug, antacid, H2 blocker, antibiotic, painkiller, or sleeping pill, and your symptoms will go away for a while. But pretty soon you're noticing other symptoms, which are caused by the first prescription, so you go to the doctor again, and you get another prescription, which causes a new round of side effects. Pretty soon you're spending hundreds of dollars a month on drugs and you feel terrible, and it

never occurs to you that the symptoms could be caused by all the drugs. And all you went in for in the first place was a chronically stuffy nose or heartburn, symptoms that might have easily been handled by keeping the cat off the bed or giving up on those greasy french fries!

My advice to you is to avoid going to the doctor as much as possible. All illness is caused by an imbalance of some kind in the body. Most of those imbalances can be corrected with lifestyle changes and nutritional healing. We are far more intelligent and knowledgeable about our bodies than we give ourselves credit for. Developing an awareness of what you're doing to create that ache or pain is a key to good health.

Unless you are acutely ill or have acutely serious symptoms, before calling for a doctor's appointment, ask yourself: Am I doing everything I can to keep my life balanced and whole? Am I eating well, getting some exercise, taking some vitamins, and spending time with loved ones or helping others? Am I living a life of moderation and balance? Am I drinking too much alcohol or too many sodas? Could I give up that third or fourth cup of coffee? Am I eating plenty of fresh vegetables? Am I avoiding pesticides indoors and outdoors? Could I give up that doughnut I have for breakfast? Do I need to spend more time taking care of myself and less time worrying about the health of my loved ones? Could I reduce the stress in my life? Would I feel better if I had a heart-to-heart talk with my spouse? If you have moderate symptoms that have been bothering you for a while, you can probably track down the cause yourself.

If you're unable to track down the cause of your ill health, or if you're looking for a tune-up for optimal health, I suggest that you see a naturopathic doctor, a chiropractor (many of them use nutrition and herbs for healing and balancing the body), or an MD specializing in alternative medicine. They are more likely to work with you in a balanced way that addresses more than symptoms and drugs. I will certainly go to an MD if I have a broken bone, and I'll certainly use antibiotics if I have pneumonia, but these are very much the exceptions. Most of us are only suffering from the consequences of our bad habits, and that can be fixed!

1 CREATING YOUR PERSONAL SUPPLEMENT PLAN ~

THE ABCs OF SUPPLEMENTS

Entering a store that specializes in supplements can be an overwhelming experience for someone who doesn't known their ABCs—that's vitamin A, vitamin B, and vitamin C! This chapter is designed to give you a basic overview of what I consider your essential daily supplements, including vitamins, minerals, amino acids, and antioxidants. You'll also find individual vitamin plans for your age, sex, and lifestyle, as well as plenty of information about treating specific health concerns with nutritional supplements.

You'll notice that all the supplement amounts I recommend are higher than the RDA (recommended dietary allowance) set by the government. This is because the RDA is the amount of the vitamin you need to take to keep from getting a vitamin deficiency disease. This is a long way from the amount you need to keep you in good health for the rest of your life. If you start with my basic vitamin plan and adapt it to your own personal needs, you'll be well on your way to a life of optimum health and energy. This chapter will introduce you to the basics. Throughout the rest of the book, you'll find more in-depth information on most of the vitamins and minerals as they relate to specific health concerns.

Do You Really Need to Take Supplements?

If you were to eat the best possible diet of nutrient-rich organic foods and live a stress-free life, and assuming also that your environment was free of pollutants and toxins, you would not need to take supplements. But the reality of our lives is much different. It is virtually impossible to escape the pervasive pollution of our environment. Our soil is depleted of many essential minerals, and by the time once-fresh fruits and vegetables reach us in the supermarket, they have lost much of their nutritional value. We eat processed foods and junk foods with little or no nutritional value, and we eat much more sugar and salt per year than is good for us. Add to that the stresses of daily life, prescription drugs, exposure to estrogenic hormones in meat, and all the other factors in our daily lives that pull our biochemistry out of balance, and the need for vitamins and other supplements becomes apparent. In today's world, we need to take supplements just to maintain our health and prevent the onset of chronic diseases.

Taking vitamins and other supplements is health insurance that makes up for what you're not getting in your diet and for the added nutritional demands made on the body by stressful lifestyles. Illness, aging, and genetic weaknesses add to your individual nutritional needs. If there is a lot of cancer in your immediate family, you should be taking the supplements that are known to help prevent cancer, such as vitamin E and selenium. If your family has a history of heart disease, you need to create a heart-healthy lifestyle that includes a low-fat diet, plenty of exercise, and plenty of antioxidants and magnesium.

The key to creating your own individual supplement plan is paying attention to your body's needs. If you find that you're getting colds a lot, there are lifestyle factors you'll want to evaluate, such as whether you're getting enough sleep, whether you're allergic to something in your diet or something in your home or office, or maybe simply whether you're dressing warmly enough in cold weather. But you'll also want to increase your vitamin C and E consumption and possibly your zinc (and you may want to take the useful herb echinacea) at the first sign of the sniffles.

Taking vitamins and minerals is not a substitute for a good diet or a healthy lifestyle. A vitamin can never reproduce all the nutrition packed into a fresh vegetable or an egg, for example. The single biggest factor that shows up in studies of heart disease, cancer, and aging over and over again is that those who eat the most fresh vegetables live the longest and healthiest lives. And no amount of antioxidants will substitute for drinking plenty of clean water and doing moderate exercise. Nonetheless, taking supplements is your backup plan for good health, providing the extra support you need to go beyond simply maintaining your health to having lots of energy and a clear mind.

For Best Results . . .

Most vitamins and minerals are best absorbed when taken with food, spaced out as evenly as possible during the day. The best time to take supplements is after meals. The amino acids are an exception to this. If you are taking a separate amino acid supplement, it is usually best to take it between meals.

Because some vitamins can be excreted in the urine, taking your vitamins after breakfast, after lunch, and after dinner will give you the highest body level of nutrients. If you must take your vitamins all at one time, taking them after the largest meal of the day will usually give the best results.

Minerals and vitamins are mutually dependent on each other for proper absorption. For example, vitamin C aids in the absorption of iron; calcium aids in the absorption of vitamin D; and zinc aids in the absorption of vitamin A. So take your minerals and vitamins together.

Tablets, Capsules, and Liquids

Supplements come in many forms, but the most common are tablets, capsules, and liquids. Multivitamins generally come in tablet form, but be sure they aren't so large that you can't swallow them, and be sure they actually dissolve once they get into your digestive system. One way to find out how well vitamin tablets dissolve is to drop one in a little bit of vinegar, which approximates the acidity of your stomach. Depending on its size, the tablet should be nearly completely dissolved within an hour. If it isn't, you can bet you're not getting the full value from it. Some supplements work best in the small intestine, and these may be put into a tablet with a special coating that doesn't allow it to dissolve until it is out of the stomach.

Capsules are usually gelatin shells filled with the powdered form of the supplement. The gelatin dissolves quickly in the stomach, allowing the supplement to begin its work right away.

If you have trouble absorbing nutrients, you may want to consider some of the powdered or liquid vitamins, which don't have to be broken down as much in the gut.

VITAMINS YOU SHOULD TAKE EVERY DAY

There are some vitamins that everyone, regardless of age or lifestyle, should take every day. These vitamins are essential for good health and peak energy, as they have a great many jobs to do in the body.

Vitamin A/Beta-Carotene

Vitamin A is a fat-soluble vitamin that is stored in your body and doesn't need to be supplemented daily except in relatively small amounts. In fact, taking vitamin A in large doses over a long period of time can cause a toxic reaction because it accumulates in the body.

Vitamin A promotes growth, strong bones, and healthy skin and is essential to the production of sex hormones. Vitamin A works closely with zinc. People with acne can often eradicate it just by taking vitamin A supplements for a few months. Vitamin A is also known as an anti-infective because it can help fight infections. In fact, if you have any type of lung infection, taking an extra vitamin A supplement for a week or two can help knock it out. Vitamin A is also called the ophthalmic vitamin because it helps improve eyesight.

Vitamin A is found in many vegetables, especially the orange and yellow vegetables, such as carrots, squash, yams, and cantaloupe. It's also found in liver, fish oil, and eggs. One carrot can deliver up to 15,000 IU of beta-carotene. Add a carrot a day to your apple a day!

Beta-carotene is a precursor to vitamin A, meaning that the body can make vitamin A from beta-carotene. That's the best way to get your vitamin A in a supplement, because it doesn't accumulate in the body the way vitamin A does. Beta-carotene is a potent antioxidant. Many recent studies have shown that people who have plenty of beta-carotene in their diet have a lower rate of cancer and coronary artery disease.

The B-Complex Vitamins

The B-complex family are water-soluble vitamins involved in nearly every function of the body, from the manufacture of sex hormones and the health of brain neurons to breaking down food and forming healthy red blood cells. The B vitamins play a key role in converting carbohydrate foods into glucose, or simple sugars, for use as energy.

The B-complex vitamins I'm going to cover here include vitamin B_1 (thiamine), vitamin B_2 (riboflavin), vitamin B_3 (niacin), vitamin B_6 (pyridoxine), vitamin B_{12} (cobalamin), biotin, choline, folic acid, inositol, and vitamin B_5 (pantothenic acid). It's best to take the B-complex vitamins together, because too much or too little of one can throw the others out of balance.

The B vitamins are found in whole grains, many nuts and root vegetables, meat, poultry, fish, eggs, dairy products, and fruit.

Vitamin B_1/Thiamine

Vitamin B_1 promotes growth, aids in the digestion of carbohydrates, can improve your mental attitude, can help fight sea- and airsickness, relieves dental postoperative pain, and aids in the treatment of shingles and other herpesviruses. Vitamin B_1 is also essential for the normal functioning of nerve tissues, muscles, and the heart. Taking vitamin B_1 as a supplement can create an odor on the skin that humans can't smell but that repels insects, especially mosquitoes.

Smokers, drinkers, heavy sugar consumers, antacid users, and those on birth control pills need more B_1.

Vitamin B_1 can cause high blood pressure in excess.

Vitamin B_2/Riboflavin

Vitamin B_2 aids in growth and reproduction, promotes healthy hair, skin, and nails, alleviates eye fatigue, eliminates sore mouth and lips, and helps your body burn carbohydrates, fats, and proteins. A deficiency of vitamin B_2 may cause a decreased ability to generate the antibodies that help the body resist disease. A deficiency may also result in itching and burning of the eyes, cracking of the corners of the lips, and inflammation of the mouth. If you are a heavy coffee or alcohol drinker, are on the pill, are under a lot of stress, or eat lots of processed foods (please don't!), you may need extra vitamin B_2. Natural sources of vitamin B_2 include liver, kidney, milk, cheese, and most B_1 sources.

Vitamin B_3/Niacin/Niacinamide

Niacin is the most potent and effective cholesterol-lowering substance known. The only reason it isn't the best-selling cholesterol-lowering medicine is because it's an inexpensive, natural substance that can't be patented by the drug companies. If they can't patent it, they can't charge you high prices, so they aren't interested in promoting it. Niacin not only lowers LDL, or "bad," cholesterol but also raises HDL, or "good," cholesterol. (If your physician has you on cholesterol-lowering drugs, don't stop taking them without supervision.)

Niacin has gotten some bad press. Some forms of it can cause flushing and itching, and high, prolonged doses of timed-release niacin can cause liver problems. If you begin with a small dose and gradually work your way up to a higher dose, you should be able to minimize these problems. Niacinamide is used more often than niacin, since it minimizes the burning, flushing, and itching of the skin that frequently occurs with nicotinic acid. More recently, some vitamin manufacturers have developed "no-flush" niacin formulas that deliver all the benefits of niacin without the unpleasant side effects. These formulas are made by combining niacin with inositol hexanicotinate, an ester involved in sending messages within the nervous system. In any case, niacin is still safer and more effective than any of the pharmaceutical cholesterol-lowering drugs.

Niacin also aids in promoting a healthy digestive system, gives you healthy skin, can prevent or ease the severity of migraine headaches, increases circulation, especially in the upper body, can reduce high blood pressure, is an antidiarrheal, increases your energy through proper food utilization, helps fight canker sores, helps fight bad breath, is a possible cancer inhibitor, and is necessary for the metabolism of sugar.

Niacin is found naturally in lean meat, whole grains, green vegetables, and beans.

Vitamin B_6/Pyridoxine

This vitamin is actually a group of vitamins called pyridoxine, pyridoxal, and pyridoxamine, but B_6 is often just called pyridoxine. This important vitamin is crucial to the formation of all the steroid hormones, including the sex hormones and the cortisones. Women can often correct PMS and menopause problems simply by taking a vitamin B_6 supplement. It also helps protect against osteoporosis. This B vitamin also plays an essential role in maintaining a healthy nervous system and a healthy cardiovascular system. Researchers have recently recognized that a high level of homocysteine, a by-product of amino acid metabolism, is at least as important a risk factor in heart disease as high cholesterol or high blood pressure, and vitamin B_6, together with the B vitamins folic acid and vitamin B_{12}, reduces the level of homocysteine in the body.

Vitamin B_6 also helps assimilate protein and fat, aids in converting tryptophan to niacin, is an anti-nauseant (effective for morning sickness), can help with PMS and menopause symptoms, helps synthesize antiaging nucleic acids, reduces "cotton mouth" and urination problems caused by tricyclic antidepressant drugs, reduces night muscle spasms, leg cramps, and hand numbness, and works as a natural diuretic.

Vitamin B_6 occurs naturally in meat, fish, egg yolk, cantaloupe, cabbage, milk, soy products, peanuts, and brown rice.

A deficiency of vitamin B_6 may result in nervousness, insomnia, skin eruptions, and loss of muscular control.

Vitamin B_6 can be toxic in high doses, so do not take over 500 mg a day.

Vitamin B_{12}/Cobalamin

Vitamin B_{12} is commonly known as the "red vitamin," cobalamin. Because it is so effective in small doses, it is one of the few vitamins generally recommended in microgram (mcg) doses. Vitamin B_{12} is not well absorbed in the digestive tract, so the best ways to take it are intranasally or sublingually (under the tongue).

I believe that a very high percentage of senility symptoms in older people are caused by a simple vitamin B_{12} and folic acid deficiency. As we age, we don't produce as much stomach acid, and as a result, we don't absorb our food as well. This is particularly true of the B vitamins, and especially B_{12}. Many older people tend to have poor nutrition anyway, but even with good nutrition, if there is an absorption problem, a vitamin B_{12} deficiency may result. Anyone over the age of fifty who is experiencing problems such as memory loss, forgetfulness, depression, loss of appetite, and fatigue should try a few weeks of B_{12} shots (given by doctors and other health care professionals) to see if the symptoms clear up. Supplements of folic acid and vitamin B_6 should be given along with the B_{12}, as they work best together.

Vitamin B_{12} forms and regenerates red blood cells, which carry oxygen to the tissues, giving you more energy and preventing anemia. It also promotes growth in children and gives them an increased appetite. Moreover, this vitamin helps maintain a healthy nervous system, can relieve irritability, improves circulation, memory, and balance, and can enhance immunity in the elderly. Vitamin B_{12} also plays an important role, along with folic acid and vitamin B_6, in keeping homocysteine levels low. As mentioned earlier, homocysteine raises the risk of heart disease.

Vitamin B_{12} is found naturally in liver, beef, pork, eggs, milk, and cheese. Vitamin B_{12} is found in significant amounts only in animal foods, so if you are a vegetarian, it is important to take a B_{12} supplement.

Biotin

Biotin is one of the more recently discovered B vitamins, but it is a key vitamin in maintaining healthy hair and skin. It can keep your hair from turning gray, prevent baldness, and ease muscle pains, and it is important for healthy skin.

Biotin is found naturally in whole grains, milk, vegetables, and nuts. It is present in minute quantities in every living cell and is also synthesized by intestinal bacteria.

A deficiency of biotin may lead to hair loss, extreme exhaustion, drowsiness, muscle pains, and loss of appetite.

Choline

Choline is an ingredient in lecithin, a naturally occurring fat emulsifier found in eggs, soy and other legumes, nuts, and some meats such as liver. Choline is one of the few substances able to penetrate the blood-brain barrier, going directly to brain cells, where it plays a role in transmitting nerve impulses. For this reason, taking lecithin may help with memory, the ability to learn, and symptoms of senility and Alzheimer's.

Because of its effects on fats, choline lowers cholesterol, aids the liver in removing poisons and drugs from your bloodstream, is necessary for normal fat metabolism, and minimizes excessive deposits of fat in the liver.

Lecithin and choline are found naturally in egg yolks, green leafy vegetables, and legumes.

A deficiency of choline may result in cirrhosis and fatty degeneration of the liver and hardening of the arteries.

Folic Acid

Folic acid has recently been recognized as a key vitamin in preventing a type of birth defect called neural tube defects, such as spina bifida. It is important that all sexually active women at any risk whatsoever for getting pregnant get at least 200 mcg of folic acid every day, and preferably 400 mcg.

Folic acid works hand in hand with vitamins B_6 and B_{12} to reduce the levels of harmful homocysteine in the blood. A deficiency of folic acid, vitamin B_6, and vitamin B_{12} significantly raises your risk of heart disease by raising homocysteine levels.

Folic acid improves lactation in nursing women, can act as a pain reliever, delays gray hair (along with PABA and pantothenic acid), prevents canker sores, helps against anemia (along with iron, copper, and vitamin C), is essential to the formation of red blood cells by its action on the bone marrow, aids in protein metabolism, and contributes to normal growth.

Too much folic acid can cause problems for epileptics and people with allergies.

Folic acid is found naturally in dark green leafy vegetables and in meat.

Inositol

Inositol combines with choline to form lecithin, and it has many of the same benefits. It can be very helpful in treating eczema. It also lowers cholesterol, is important for healthy hair, helps metabolize body fat, is a relaxant, and can help relieve diabetic peripheral neuropathy.

Inositol is found naturally in fruits, nuts, whole grains, milk, and meat. Cantaloupe and citrus fruits are especially good sources.

Vitamin B_5/Pantothenic Acid

Vitamin B_5 is also called pantothenic acid. It aids in the growth of cells, helps maintain normal skin, is crucial to the development of the central nervous system, is required for the synthesis of antibodies, is necessary for normal digestive processes, helps heal wounds, prevents fatigue, is an antiallergy and anti-stress supplement, and fights infections. In some people, vitamin B_5 helps relieve arthritis symptoms, but in other people, it can aggravate them.

Pantothenic acid is found naturally in organ meats, eggs, whole grains, bran, and peas.

Vitamin C

Vitamin C, also called ascorbic acid, is water-soluble and one of the superstars of the vitamin world. It is a powerful antioxidant that slows the aging process and helps prevent heart disease and cancer. It also plays an important role in healing wounds, helps prevent fatigue, is an antihistamine, helping to reduce allergy symptoms, helps fight infections by building antibodies, can stop bleeding gums, lowers cholesterol, is an anticancer agent, prevents the production of nitrosamines (cancer-causing agents), is a natural laxative, lowers the incidence of blood clots in the veins, therefore decreasing the risk of heart attack and stroke, decreases the severity and length of the common cold, and increases the absorption of iron. Vitamin C works as a team with other vitamins, minerals, and enzymes to strengthen the collagen in connective tissue and promote capillary integrity.

Vitamin C is found naturally in nearly all fresh food and meat. It is especially high in citrus fruits, berries, greens, cabbages, and peppers. Vitamin C is destroyed by cooking, which is one of the many reasons to eat plenty of fresh raw fruits and vegetables.

Vitamin C in large doses can cause mild diarrhea. Either buy an esterified form of vitamin C or back off the dose until the diarrhea stops.

Bioflavonoids

Bioflavonoids are organic compounds found in plants. These powerful substances reduce inflammation and pain, strengthen blood vessels, improve circulation, fight bacteria and viruses, improve liver function, lower cholesterol levels, and improve vision. Bioflavonoids help prevent bruising by strengthening capillary walls. For this reason, they are also helpful for diabetics in improving circulation and can help prevent eye problems such as cataracts and macular degeneration. Bioflavonoids are also beneficial in hypertension and help build resistance to infections and colds.

Vitamin C is found combined with bioflavonoids in nature, and in supplements it works much more effectively when combined with bioflavonoids.

Bioflavonoids are found in a wide variety of plants. Some of the best food sources are the white material underneath citrus fruit peels as well as peppers and berries. Although bioflavonoids are not considered essential to life, and therefore are not classified as vitamins, it is becoming clear that they *are* essential to good health.

Whatever vitamin C you are taking should be combined with a bioflavonoid complex. Each works best when combined with the other.

Vitamin D

Vitamin D is also called calciferol, ergosterol, and the "sunshine vitamin." This hormonelike vitamin regulates the use of calcium and phosphorus in the body and is therefore necessary for the proper formation of teeth and bones. It is especially important in infancy and childhood. Most of our vitamin D is manufactured in the body when our skin is exposed to sunlight. This is why it's important to get regular exposure to sun. Taken with vitamins A and C, vitamin D can help prevent colds. It is also used to treat conjunctivitis.

Vitamin D is found naturally in fish oil, fats, and dairy products. Vitamin D should not be taken in high doses long-term because it accumulates in the body and can be toxic at high doses. However, it can be an essential vitamin for people who aren't getting enough sun.

Vitamin E

Vitamin E is also called tocopherol. It is available in several different forms, both liquid and solid. Vitamin E is another superstar in the vitamin world, able to help us fend off heart disease and important to hundreds of biochemical processes in the body. Vitamin E is a powerful antioxidant that slows the aging process and also helps prevent cancer. It works with beta-carotene to protect the lungs from pollution, prevents and dissolves blood clots, helps prevent scarring when used externally on the skin, accelerates burn healing, can lower blood pressure by its diuretic action, prevents night cramps, lazy leg, and leg cramps, helps prevent cataracts, and enhances the immune system.

Vitamin E is found naturally in whole grains, green leafy vegetables, vegetable oils, meat, eggs, and avocados.

Today, many cardiologists recommend 400 IU of vitamin E daily. The dry (succinate) form of vitamin E is preferred for people over forty because it is more easily absorbed by the digestive system.

MINERALS YOU SHOULD TAKE EVERY DAY

Minerals work in partnership with hormones, enzymes, amino acids, and vitamins. They are required to build and maintain the structure of the body. They are involved in the breakdown of food during digestion, and some are instrumental in maintaining fluid balance inside cells. Those that are currently considered essential for human nutrition are calcium, phosphorus, iron, potassium, selenium, magnesium, and zinc. In reality, however, many more minerals are needed to maintain optimal health. Chromium, cobalt, copper, manganese, and potassium are important in their own right, even though we only require them in very small amounts.

Processed or refined foods (for example, white flour and white sugar) are almost devoid of minerals, which is one reason I strongly recommend eating whole foods, such as grains, fruits, and vegetables, which are very rich in minerals in their unrefined state.

Another reason we tend to be deficient in minerals is that our soil is depleted. Modern agricultural methods using commercial fertilizers do not replace the rich array of minerals found naturally in soil, so vegetables grown in those soils do not have the minerals we need for good health. This is one of the best reasons I know of to eat organic fruits and vegetables (besides reducing your exposure to pesticides).

An excess of minerals can cause just as many problems as a deficiency, so be cautious about taking any mineral beyond recommended doses. Certain nutritional deficiencies may require high doses of specific minerals, which should be prescribed by a health care professional.

Let's take a closer look at the minerals you should be getting daily.

Calcium

Calcium is the most abundant mineral in the body. It builds and maintains bones and teeth, helps blood to clot, aids vitality and endurance, regulates heart rhythm, and helps muscles relax. Calcium also plays a role in maintaining fluid balance within the cells. Calcium can't do its work maintaining strong bones without its partners magnesium and phosphorus. Most of us get plenty of phosphorus in our diets, but many North Americans are deficient in magnesium, and calcium should always be taken with magnesium. There is some disagreement about what the ratio of calcium to magnesium should be, but most supplements provide a 3:1 ratio of calcium to magnesium, which is fine. Because of their relaxing effect on the muscles, calcium and magnesium can be taken just before bed to aid in sleeping and to prevent leg cramps.

Contrary to popular opinion, milk is not a good source of calcium because it has a poor calcium-to-magnesium ratio, so the body can't put it to work. I believe that dairy products cause more health problems than they solve, and I recommend that you get the majority of your calcium from fresh vegetables, especially green leafy vegetables, and from soy foods, sardines, salmon, and nuts. A high-protein diet and excessive consumption of phosphorus-containing sodas can deplete calcium from the bones.

Boron, Chromium, and Cobalt

Boron is a trace mineral that works with calcium, magnesium, and vitamin D to help prevent osteoporosis. Boron is abundant in apples and grapes.

Chromium helps the body utilize protein and fats, and helps the body burn fat more efficiently during exercise. Use the chromium picolinate form. Chromium also helps prevent and lower high blood pressure.

Cobalt is a stimulant to the production of red blood cells, is a component of vitamin B_{12}, and is necessary for normal growth. A deficiency of cobalt can cause anemia.

Iron

Iron is required in the manufacture of hemoglobin, a component of blood, and helps carry oxygen in the blood. To work efficiently, there must also be sufficient copper, cobalt, manganese, and vitamin C.

Iron is not efficiently excreted from the body and can accumulate in tissues. Recent research has shown that excessive amounts of iron in the tissues raise the risk of heart disease. Some researchers theorize that part of the reason a woman's risk of heart disease increases after menopause is that she is not losing iron every month during menstruation. Although iron is an essential mineral, it is important not to take too much iron in supplemental form. A deficiency can cause a specific disease called iron deficiency anemia.

Magnesium

Magnesium is one of the superstars of the mineral world. It is necessary for calcium and vitamin C metabolism and literally hundreds of enzyme reactions in the body. It plays a key role in regulating fluid balance in the cells and is essential for normal functioning of the nervous, muscular, and cardiovascular systems. Magnesium deficiency is very common in North America, and I believe that it is a more common and important risk factor for heart disease than mainstream medicine acknowledges. I recommend that anyone with heart disease or at risk for heart disease take an extra supplement of 300–400 mg of magnesium daily. Fatigue and muscle weakness can also be signs of magnesium deficiency.

Magnesium is found naturally in whole grains, figs, nuts and seeds, bananas and other fruits, and green vegetables.

Potassium

Potassium is a key mineral in regulating the pH balance and fluid balance in the body. It balances sodium in the cells and, along with calcium and magnesium, regulates heart rhythm. Potassium can be depleted by any type of abnormally large fluid loss, such as strenuous exercise, diarrhea, hypoglycemia, and the use of diuretics, such as those used to lower blood pressure. When potassium is deficient, it can cause nerve and muscle dysfunction, bloating due to water retention, ringing in the ears, and insomnia. Potassium is naturally found in citrus fruits, cantaloupe, tomatoes, watercress, all green leafy vegetables, the mints, sun-flower seeds, bananas, and potatoes. Most people can easily get enough potassium in their daily diet, but many multivitamins contain potassium. Don't take potassium supplements in addition to your multivitamin without the supervision of a health care professional, as an excess can throw other minerals out of balance and affect fluid balance in the cells.

Manganese and Selenium

Manganese is an important trace mineral that activates various enzymes and other minerals. Without it, our bodies can't utilize vitamins B_1 and E properly. The central nervous and digestive systems use manganese, and it is also needed for proper thyroid gland function.

Selenium could be called the anticancer mineral. Over and over again, population studies have shown that people living in geographical areas with selenium-depleted soil have a higher rate of cancer, especially colon cancer. Selenium is an antioxidant that also stimulates the immune system. It works synergistically with vitamin E, each enhancing the actions of the other. Selenium is found in high concentrations in semen, and men seem to need more of this mineral than women. A selenium deficiency can cause dandruff, dry skin, and fatigue.

Copper and Zinc

Copper and zinc balance each other in the body, and a deficiency of one can cause an excess of the other. Copper is necessary for absorption and utilization of iron and the formation of red blood cells.

An essential mineral, zinc plays multiple roles. It controls muscle contractions along with magnesium and calcium, helps normal tissue function, and is essential in protein and carbohydrate metabolism and the functioning of the immune system. A lack of zinc in your diet can increase fatigue and cause a susceptibility to infection and injury, as well as a reduction in alertness. When you exercise vigorously, you lose a lot of zinc, so it's important for athletes to take a zinc supplement. Zinc is found in many foods, including most vegetables, whole grains, dairy products, many nuts and seeds, fish, and meat.

Zinc should be present in all good multivitamin formulas. But as with all minerals, don't take zinc in excess, as it will cause other imbalances in your body. Zinc works best in combination with vitamin A, calcium, and phosphorus.

THE AMAZING AMINO ACIDS

Protein is made up of amino acids. Although there are dozens of amino acids, only some amino acids are produced in the body. All eight of the essential amino acids are made in very small amounts by the bacteria found in the intestines, but they must also be supplied from food intake.

The Essential Amino Acids

- Lysine
- Leucine
- Isoleucine
- Methionine
- Phenylalanine
- Threonine
- Tryptophan
- Valine

The following amino acids are essential for pregnant women (for the developing fetus), and for infants: histidine, taurine, and cysteine. Eric R. Braverman and Carl C. Pfeiffer, in their book *The Healing Nutrients Within* (Keats Publishing, 1997), argue that the following amino acids are conditionally essential and necessary for anyone under stress: alanine, arginine, aspartic acid, carnitine, cystine, GABA, glutamic acid, glutamine, glycine, homocysteine (toxic in high doses), hydroxyproline, proline, and serine.

Amino acids play a variety of important roles in every part of the body, including the immune system, the digestive system, metabolism, detoxification, and glucose balance. In the brain, some of the amino acids taken as supplements work very well to combat depression, enhance mood, and improve sleep, while others improve memory and cognitive abilities.

When we eat proteins, they are broken down into peptides, which are proteins made up of only a few amino acids, and then absorbed into the body.

How to Take Amino Acids

All amino acids should be taken between meals with juice or water, and not with protein, unless they are included in a multivitamin. Because individual amino acids can have such a powerful effect on the body, I recommend that if you're taking them to treat a specific chronic problem, such as heart disease or depression, you work with a health care professional.

Many amino acids serve as precursors for others. For example, cysteine is a precursor to glutathione, and since glutathione is somewhat unstable in supplement form, you can take cysteine or *N*-acetylcysteine as a supplement to boost your glutathione levels.

If you're taking amino acids, taking a B vitamin complex at the same time will enhance their absorption and metabolism.

If you want to know more about amino acids, I highly recommend Braverman and Pfeiffer's book.

Important Amino Acids You Should Take

Here are some of the amino acids that should be included in your supplement regimen, especially if you are a vegetarian, aren't absorbing nutrients well, have problems with depression, or simply need a high-powered regimen.

Alanine

Alanine is a nonessential amino acid that enhances the immune system, lowers the risk of kidney stones, and aids in alleviating hypoglycemia by regulating sugar. Alanine is released by the muscles for energy, and athletes may enhance their performance by taking alanine supplements. In very high doses, alanine suppresses taurine. Alanine has also been used successfully to treat epilepsy, high cholesterol, and liver disease in alcoholics.

Arginine

Arginine is a conditionally essential amino acid that increases sperm count in men, accelerates wound healing, tones muscle tissue, helps metabolize stored body fat, and promotes physical and mental alertness. Arginine is important in estrogen production, and a deficiency may contribute to an estrogen deficiency. Research with rodents has demonstrated that arginine can reduce the growth of tumors. Arginine can aggravate herpes and bring on an outbreak. Those who suffer from herpes outbreaks should avoid arginine supplements and arginine-containing foods such as nuts, chocolate, and coffee. Arginine also should not be taken by growing children.

Aspartic Acid

Aspartic acid is a nonessential amino acid that is highly concentrated in the body. It can enhance the immune system as well as increase stamina and endurance. Aspartic acid should be used as a supplement with great care because it is one of the major excitatory neurotransmitters in the brain and can be toxic in excess. The artificial sweetener aspartame breaks down in the stomach to aspartic acid and phenylalanine (among other things), and consuming an excessive amount of these amino acids is related to the widespread health problems among people who are sensitive to aspartame, including headaches, dizziness, and seizures.

Carnitine

Although carnitine is not an essential amino acid, a deficiency can cause fatigue, muscle weakness, heart disease, acidic blood, high triglyceride levels, and brain degeneration. Taking carnitine as a supplement can enhance the body's ability to burn fat, prevent heart disease, and minimize brain deterioration as we age.

Lysine is a precursor to carnitine, and to manufacture carnitine, the body also needs vitamin B_6, niacin, iron, and vitamin C.

If you're at risk for heart disease or already have heart disease, carnitine is an essential supplement for you. Carnitine supplements can lower triglyceride levels, raise HDL ("good") cholesterol, lower LDL ("bad") cholesterol, and improve irregular heartbeats, reduce angina attacks, and have an overall strengthening effect on the heart.

Carnitine is an especially important supplement to take when you're losing weight, because it cleans up substances called ketones in the blood, formed when the body is breaking down fat.

Although carnitine is being used successfully to treat the symptoms of Alzheimer's and senility, you don't need to have a failing memory to benefit from it. Studies have shown that carnitine supplementation improves long-term memory, increases alertness, improves learning ability, and can improve mood.

Carnitine's ability to protect brain neurons and enhance their responsiveness also makes it one of our most important antiaging supplements. Carnitine essentially acts as an antioxidant in the brain.

The forms of carnitine I recommend are either L-carnitine, acetyl-L-carnitine, or L-acetylcarnitine. Do not take the synthetic D or DL forms of carnitine, as they can have negative side effects.

Cystine and Cysteine

Cysteine is another conditionally essential amino acid and an important antiaging nutrient. Cystine and cysteine can be readily converted by the body into one another. Cysteine's most important role in the body is detoxification. In addition, it is an antioxidant. Cysteine is a precursor to the important amino acids taurine and glutathione.

When given as a supplement, cysteine raises glutathione levels in the body. Because of this, it is used routinely in hospital emergency rooms to prevent liver damage when people overdose on drugs or alcohol. It is also used to detoxify in cases of heavy-metal poisoning and to protect against the harmful side effects of chemotherapy and radiation. Cysteine is currently being used successfully to raise T cell levels in AIDS patients. Cysteine is also important in preventing eye problems such as cataracts and macular degeneration.

Foods that contain high levels of cysteine include onions, garlic, yogurt, wheat germ, and red meat.

A form of cysteine called *N*-acetylcysteine is widely used in Europe for coughs, asthma prevention, and chronic bronchitis, because it is very effective at breaking up mucus in the lungs. If you have a tendency to get winter coughs, take it at the first sign of lung troubles.

Don't take more than the recommended dosage of cysteine, as an excess can upset the balance of your body's chemistry just as much as a deficiency can.

Gamma-Aminobutyric Acid (GABA)

One of the best-known neurotransmitters (substances that transmit nerve impulses to the brain), GABA has a calming effect. In the brain, GABA balances glutamic acid, an excitatory amino acid. The three amino acids GABA, glutamic acid, and glutamine are constantly being transformed into one another as needed by the body.

GABA plays a major role in brain function. The benzodiazepine drugs, such as Valium, work because they stimulate GABA receptors in the brain.

GABA optimizes the body's use of vitamin C. It can lower blood pressure, and it may be involved with the release of growth hormone.

Glutamic Acid

Glutamic acid works closely with GABA, particularly in the brain. However, while GABA is calming, glutamic acid is the opposite. In people who are deficient in it, glutamic acid can help improve brain function, alleviate fatigue, and elevate mood. However, in excess, glutamic acid can become an excitotoxin, overstimulating brain cells and killing them. I recommend that you work with a health care professional when using glutamic acid as a supplement.

Glutamine

Glutamine is the third in the trio, working with GABA and glutamic acid. It is abundant in the brain and also in the intestines, where it plays an important role in maintaining a healthy mucous lining. Taking glutamine before and after surgery can significantly reduce healing time. Manganese is a mineral that is essential to the synthesis of glutamine, and glutamine is essential to the synthesis of niacin, as is tryptophan. Glutamine has been used successfully to help alco-

holics in the withdrawal process; it can greatly decrease the craving for alcohol.

Glutamine seems to be a food for cancer tumors, so do not take this as a supplement if you have cancer. Because it plays a role in regulating brain neurotransmitters, it can be toxic in high doses.

Glutathione

I call glutathione (known as GSH) the "triple threat" amino acid because it is a tripeptide made from the amino acids cysteine, glycine, and glutamic acid. It is found in the cells of nearly all living organisms on earth, and its primary job is waste disposal. Glutathione is a powerful antioxidant. It also binds to toxins in the liver, the body's primary cleansing organ, and allows them to be flushed efficiently.

If you have heart disease, are at a high risk for it, or have high LDL cholesterol levels, try raising your glutathione levels. Glutathione is too big a molecule to digest, so we can't take it as a supplement. We can, however, take the amino acid cysteine, one of its major building blocks. (See chapter 2 for more information on how to raise glutathione levels and its health benefits.)

Glycine

Glycine is a conditionally essential amino acid that produces glycogen, which mobilizes glucose (blood sugar) from the liver. It also bolsters the immune system. Like GABA and taurine, glycine has a calming effect on the brain. A deficiency is thought to be linked to Parkinson's disease, and glycine may increase acetylcholine in the brain, improving memory and cognitive function.

Glycine has a sweet taste that can mask bitterness, and it is sometimes used as a sweetener. It is also used as a food additive to prevent the rancidity of fats and to act as an antioxidant. Glycine can lower cholesterol, heal gout, and speed up wound healing. It stimulates growth hormone and can aid in the healing of a swollen and infected prostate.

Histidine

Although histidine is not an essential amino acid for adults, it is essential to fetal and infant growth. It is a precursor of histamine, which stimulates inflammation in allergies. A histidine deficiency is found in many arthritis patients, and supplementation sometimes helps. Histidine can help keep people from biting their nails, dilate blood vessels, alleviate symptoms of rheumatoid arthritis, alleviate stress, and help increase libido. A histidine deficiency contributes to the development of cataracts. Because elevated histidine levels can cause mental problems, it is not recommended as a daily supplement for adults.

Isoleucine, Leucine, and Valine

Isoleucine, leucine, and valine are essential amino acids known as branched-chain amino acids. They are key ingredients in the body's ability to handle stress and produce energy. They are used by the muscles for energy and are needed in hemoglobin formation. Taking these branched-chain amino acids as a supplement can speed healing after surgery and may help build muscle. These three amino acids may also work as neurotransmitters and have some ability to relieve pain. Alcoholics and drug addicts tend to be deficient in leucine, glutamine, GABA, and citrulline.

Lysine

Lysine is an essential amino acid involved in metabolism, muscle tissue, the immune system, and growth. A deficiency may cause nausea, dizziness, and anemia. Taking it as a supplement helps improve concentration, enhances fertility, aids in preventing fever blisters or cold sores (herpes simplex), and shortens the healing period for herpes. Lysine is found in meat, eggs, fish, milk, and cheese. When treating a herpes outbreak, up to 5 g (5,000 mg) a day may be taken.

Methionine

Methionine is an essential amino acid that plays an important role in metabolism. It is a lipotropic agent, meaning it reduces fat, particularly in the liver. It also protects the kidneys, aids in lowering cholesterol, is a natural chelating agent for heavy metals, and aids in maintaining beautiful skin. It

also builds new bony tissue. A deficiency of methionine may lead to heart disease, fatty degeneration, and cirrhosis of the liver. Methionine has been used to treat schizophrenia, Parkinson's, and depression. It can be found in sunflower seeds, meat, eggs, fish, milk, and cheese.

Phenylalanine

Phenylalanine is an essential amino acid that plays a key part in brain function and is a major precursor to many brain chemicals, including the amino acid tyrosine and catecholamines such as dopamine and epinephrine. Other brain chemicals, including vasopressin, somatostatin, and ACTH, contain phenylalanine. Morphine and codeine also contain phenylalanine.

Like the other amino acids that affect brain function, phenylalanine can be very helpful as a supplement if there is a deficiency but can be harmful in excess. The artificial sweetener aspartame breaks down in the stomach to form aspartic acid and phenylalanine. The phenylalanine accounts for some of the adverse reactions to the sweetener. Some people are born with a sensitivity to phenylalanine called phenylketonuria (PKU). If not caught in infancy, whereupon foods containing phenylalanine can be avoided, PKU can cause serious retardation.

In people who are deficient in phenylalanine, it can improve memory and mental alertness, act as an antidepressant, and help suppress appetite, reduce pain, and increase sexual interest. It can also raise blood pressure, so be cautious in its use if you have high blood pressure. It cannot be metabolized if a person is deficient in vitamin C.

I recommend taking phenylalanine in the D or DL-phenylalanine form.

Proline and Hydroxyproline

Proline and hydroxyproline are conditionally essential amino acids that aid in wound healing and can help increase learning ability. These two amino acids are found in the highest amounts in the body's collagen tissue. Hydroxyproline is most important in bone and connective tissue. Proline is one of the amino acids that seems to stimulate tumor development, and people with cancer should not take it as a supplement. In fact, it is probably not necessary to supplement proline or hydroxyproline at all, as they tend to be in the body in abundance, and an excess can cause imbalances in other amino acids.

Serine

Serine is a conditionally essential amino acid that is made from glycine and can also be made into glycine and cystine. It can help alleviate pain, and it produces cellular energy. An excess in the body or very high supplemental doses can cause psychosis. Serine is another amino acid that promotes tumor growth and so should not be taken by anyone who has cancer. There is no need to supplement serine, as our bodies tend to make what we need in abundance.

Taurine

Taurine is an amino acid that is essential to infants but nonessential to adults. It is a very useful amino acid in treating some forms of epilepsy. It plays an important role in the heart, eyes, brain, gallbladder, and blood vessels, particularly keeping fluids and mineral balance in cells stable and stabilizing cell membranes. Taurine is an important supplement for anyone who has heart disease, but should be taken under the guidance of a health care professional if you are on heart disease drugs. Taurine is also important in stabilizing cell membranes in the brain; as a neurotransmitter, it can have a calming effect. It can also improve memory and has been used to treat insomnia, anxiety, and high blood pressure. The food additive MSG can reduce taurine levels. Because taurine can enhance the action of insulin, diabetics and hypoglycemics should use it with care.

Threonine

Threonine is an essential amino acid that can be deficient in vegetarian diets. It is a precursor to the important amino acid glycine, which acts as a brain sedative. Threonine is essential to normal growth, helps prevent fatty buildup in the liver, is necessary for utilization of protein in the diet, stimulates the immune system, and has been used to treat manic depression and multiple sclerosis. A deficiency results in negative hydrogen balance in the body. Threonine levels decline with age, making them valuable antiaging supplements.

Tryptophan

Tryptophan is an essential amino acid with many valuable uses. It is a precursor to niacin, which prevents pellagra and mental deficiency. It plays a role in regulating sleep and is closely tied to the production of serotonin in the brain. A deficiency causes insomnia. It is useful as a relaxant and antianxiety agent as well.

Tryptophan was widely used as a sleep aid until a contaminated batch made in Japan reportedly killed eleven people. In spite of the fact that uncontaminated tryptophan is entirely safe and is used in baby foods and in nutritional powders for senior citizens, the FDA has pulled it off the market as a nutritional supplement as of this writing. Tryptophan was pulled off the market within weeks before the drug Prozac was approved by the FDA. It is interesting that the inexpensive, safe, and effective tryptophan does essentially the same thing in the brain that Prozac does, without the side effects. The fact that tryptophan is not available in the United States is purely political and has no basis in a lack of safety.

Tyrosine

Tyrosine is a nonessential amino acid that acts as a precursor to many other amino acids and brain chemicals. It is important in times of stress and plays a part in maintaining a healthy thyroid gland. It also yields L-dopa, making it useful in the treatment of Parkinson's disease. It has an important role in stimulating and modifying brain activity, helps control drug-resistant depression and anxiety, and helps amphetamine users to reduce their dosage to minimal levels in a few weeks. It can also help cocaine addicts kick their habit by helping to avert the depression, fatigue, and extreme irritability that accompany withdrawal. It can worsen the symptoms of schizophrenia.

The artificial sweetener aspartame raises tyrosine levels in the brain, which may cause toxicity in sensitive people.

A FEW IMPORTANT ANTIOXIDANTS

Antioxidants are one of your best forms of health insurance, both against the modern maladies that plague so many of us, such as heart disease, cancer, and diabetes, and against the diseases of aging, such as arthritis and digestive difficulties. There are hundreds and probably even thousands of antioxidants, most of them found naturally in plants, particularly fresh fruits and vegetables, but also in herbs. Antioxidants are also present to some degree in seafood and in some animal foods.

Antioxidants neutralize the damage of oxidation by squelching free radicals. What does that mean? We can think of oxidation as similar to what happens to metal when it rusts or what happens to an apple when it turns brown. Have you ever prevented a cut-up apple from turning brown by squeezing some lemon juice on it? The vitamin C in the lemon juice is an antioxidant that stops the oxidation process. When meat spoils or oil goes rancid, oxidation is to blame.

An unstable oxygen molecule has a missing electron, creating what is called a free radical. These unstable oxygen molecules go to war in the body, grabbing onto other cells in their attempt to find another electron and stabilize. Every time a free radical stabilizes itself by attacking another cell, it leaves the cell it attacked damaged. That cell becomes unstable and in turn goes after another, creating a chain reaction. This is the process known as oxidation.

The damage that free radicals do includes cell mutation, cardiovascular disease, cataracts, macular degeneration, arthritis, and diseases affecting the brain, kidneys, lungs, digestive system, and immune system. Free radicals are involved in the damage done by alcoholism, aging, radiation injury, iron overload, and diseases that affect the blood, such as strokes. Once the process of oxidation begins, it can be hard to stop, so your best health plan is to prevent it in the first place.

Free-radical production is a natural part of our complex interaction with oxygen. In fact, free radicals act as enzymes and chemical messengers, and we couldn't live without them. It is when they become excessive that we begin to get sick. Environmental pollution and poor dietary choices have pushed our free radical burden beyond what our bodies can handle. This is why we need antioxidant supplements.

Let's take a quick look at some of my favorite antioxidants. (For more on these miracle nutrients, refer to chapter 2.)

Coenzyme Q10 (Ubiquinone)

A versatile and powerful antioxidant, coenzyme Q10 (CoQ10) is the superstar when it comes to fighting "bad" LDL cholesterol. It works well in combination with vitamin E.

CoQ10 exists in every living cell—in other words, it is ubiquitous. Its chemical name, in fact, is *ubiquinone*. Without this enzyme, our cells cease to function. Heart and liver cells have the most CoQ10. Stress, illness, and aging decrease the body's CoQ10 levels.

CoQ10 helps regulate heart function. Many older people whose heart function has degenerated and who try CoQ10 report an almost immediate boost in their energy levels. People who suffer from angina report that the pain disappears and they can do some exercise. Studies have shown that people on heart medication can greatly reduce their dosage of medicine if it is combined with CoQ10.

CoQ10 can work powerfully to heal gum disease.

Food sources are mackerel, sardines, soybeans, peanuts, and walnuts.

All CoQ10 is not created equal. The powder inside the capsules should be dark yellow.

Superoxide Dismutase (SOD)

Superoxide dismutase (SOD) is an enzyme that acts as a potent antioxidant, especially with skin tissue, and may be able to slow the aging process. SOD is destroyed in the stomach, so it needs to be used either as a cream or taken in an enteric-coated capsule, which passes through the stomach intact and dissolves in the intestines. SOD injections have been used successfully to treat scleroderma, a hardening of the skin. SOD with liposome is expensive, but if you have a stubborn skin problem, it might be worth a try.

The Bioflavonoid Antioxidants

Quercetin

You should get to know this antioxidant, anticancer, and antiallergy agent. This bioflavonoid may also have antiviral properties. Red and yellow onions are the best food sources of quercetin, although most fruits and vegetables contain some. You can also get it as a supplement.

Proanthocyanidins/PCOs/Grapeseed Extract

PCOs are another powerful free-radical neutralizer that, like quercetin, are bioflavonoids. Because PCOs are water-soluble, the body is able to quickly and easily use them as an antioxidant. They also reduce inflammation, improve circulation, and improve the flexibility of connective tissues. Although proanthocyanidins are found in many fruits and vegetables, much of the supply is depleted by the time it gets to us. Most fruits and vegetables are grown in depleted soil, picked before they are ripened, sprayed with pesticides and fungicides, and stored for long periods of time.

Grapeseed extract is a good source of PCOs.

PCOs can also be very effective in relieving allergy symptoms, because they inhibit the release of histamines.

Ginkgo Biloba

Ginkgo biloba has been used by the Chinese medicinally for at least five thousand years. The leaves of this ancient tree provide a powerful antiaging aid, particularly in regard to improving brain function. It improves memory, learning, and communication ability, as well as other symptoms of senility. It can also cure dizziness and improve balance.

Ginkgo is one of the best-selling medicines in Europe, sold to an estimated ten million people every year. It has been the subject of over three hundred scientific studies.

Ginkgo improves circulation throughout the body and improves oxygen flow to the brain. It is also useful for treating vision problems such as cataracts and macular degeneration, varicose veins, cold or numb feet and hands, ringing of the ears (tinnitus), leg cramps, and headaches. It improves cholesterol levels and circulation to the heart. (You'll find more information on ginkgo in chapter 2.)

Green Tea

Green tea contains bioflavonoids called polyphenols, which are potent antioxidants. These polyphenols neutralize free radicals, preventing the oxidation of fats. Green tea polyphenols lower blood pressure and cholesterol levels, improve digestion, and help prevent ulcers and strokes. The polyphenols in green tea also block the formation of cancer cells and inhibit viral and bacterial growth.

You can simply drink green tea to reap its benefits, or you can take a green tea polyphenol supplement. (See chapter 2 for more information.)

THE WONDER OF ENZYMES

There isn't a cell in the body that functions without the help of enzymes. Enzymes are the magic ingredients that make all the other ingredients in the body work together. It is estimated that enzymes are facilitating thirty-six million biochemical reactions in the human body every minute. There are thousands of different enzymes at work, each with its own individual assignment.

Without the appropriate enzyme to bind to, vitamins and minerals are just so much organic matter, and even oxygen itself is just another molecule. Enzymes regulate all living matter, plants and animals alike. Take away enzymes and you no longer have something that is living.

Enzymes speed up processes that might take much longer without their help. They build proteins that create tissue, remove toxins, help prevent the aging process within cells, and change nutrients into useful energy.

We are born with enzymes already in our body, and we get some from food. However, enzymes are very sensitive to heat and processing (including microwaving and pasteurizing), so they are not found in cooked or processed food. This means that you need to get your enzymes from fresh, uncooked food, such as raw fruits and vegetables, or from enzyme supplements.

Some enzyme experts believe that factors such as stress, malnutrition, junk food, alcohol, and cigarettes destroy and thus deplete enzymes. They theorize that many digestive problems and immune disorders occur when we are deficient in enzymes.

The enzymes that we know about are classified according to their purpose in the body. There are oxidoreductases, transferases, hydrolases, lyases, isomerases, and ligases. The digestive enzymes are the hydrolases, and these will be examined more closely in chapter 5, Fiber and Digestion.

Some of the best food sources of enzymes are avocados, bananas, papayas, mangoes, pineapples, sprouts, and the aspergillus plant.

How to Take Digestive Enzymes

When you take a digestive enzyme, be sure to take one that includes the three major types of enzymes: amylase, protease (or proteolytic enzymes), and lipase. If you eat dairy products and want some help digesting the lactose in them, get an enzyme supplement that contains lactase. Take enzyme supplements just before or with meals.

HOW DRUGS CAN DEPLETE NUTRIENTS

In North America, we are addicted to drugs, and I don't mean the street drugs. It would probably be more accurate to say that our doctors and our mainstream medical system are addicted to drugs. The medical mind-set is to diagnose a disease and then prescribe a pill for it. Very little thought is given to what caused the disease in the first place or whether lifestyle changes and nutrition could correct the disease. As a result, Americans, and particularly older Americans, are, on the average, taking from three to eight drugs regularly.

I call this the drug treadmill. You go to get a physical checkup with your doctor after the age of fifty, and if you have slightly high cholesterol or blood pressure, if your joints hurt, or if your blood sugar is a bit off balance, you're likely to be put on a drug, with no suggestion that dietary changes or exercise might help. That drug will cause side effects. When you complain of these side effects to your doctor, you will be prescribed another drug, which in turn will cause a new set of side effects, for which you will be prescribed yet another drug, and so on. Pretty soon you're feeling tired all the time—and you're depressed. Moreover, you're gaining weight, can't sleep, have a chronic cough, and have no sex drive. You're not exercising anymore and you're drinking twice as much coffee and eating twice as much sugar to try to bring your energy up. If you complain to your doctor about all the drugs and all the side effects, you will be threatened with the dire consequences of going off the drugs and told that the side effects are simply part of old age. Hogwash!

Nearly all diseases of old age can be very well managed naturally with herbs and supplements that have few or no side effects. And most of these ailments can be prevented or reversed simply by lifestyle changes that include drinking plenty of fresh, clean water, getting some moderate exercise, cutting down on fat (particularly the hydrogenated oils) and sugar, eating plenty of fresh vegetables, and taking some supplements. There is no reason why the vast majority of us can't enjoy a relatively pain-free old age with energy and vigor.

Nearly all the prescription and over-the-counter drugs prescribed by your doctor will have side effects. What's more, important nutrients are depleted by some of the more common drugs. It is therefore imperative that you educate yourself. There are many books available on prescription drugs that can be understood by the average person. Read up on the drugs you're taking to find out if they are really safe and effective and what the side effects are. And even more important, take the steps to get off the drugs (with your doctor's guidance) and take care of yourself.

Many prescription drugs cause depletion of the body's essential vitamins and minerals. A recent scientific study shows that ingredients found in common over-the-counter (OTC) cold, pain, and allergy remedies actually lower the blood level of vitamin A in animals. Because vitamin A protects and strengthens the mucous membranes lining the nose, throat, and lungs, a deficiency of vitamin A could actually break down these membranes, giving bacteria a cozy home to multiply in. Therefore, the drugs that are supposed to alleviate the cold may actually be prolonging it!

The effects of drugs on nutrient levels will be discussed throughout the book, but here's a brief introduction.

Aspirin

Aspirin is often touted as the wonder drug to take for everything from heart disease to colon cancer. These claims are very flimsy and based more on advertising than on reality. You should know that four thousand people die from the side effects of aspirin every year, and an additional sixty thousand are hospitalized. Aspirin is well known for causing gastrointestinal bleeding, and even a small amount of aspirin can *triple* the excretion rate of vitamin C from the body. In addition, aspirin can contribute to a deficiency in folic acid, one of the B vitamins. A deficiency of folic acid can lead to anemia, digestive disturbances, graying hair, and growth problems. Taking aspirin at night will reduce the production of the hormone melatonin and may result in insomnia.

Corticosteroids

In spite of their horrendous side effects if used long-term, including bone loss and fragile skin, millions of people are dependent on corticosteroids such as prednisone. These belong to a class of drugs called cortisones, used to ease the pain of arthritis, relieve lung congestion, and treat autoimmune diseases. They are also prescribed for skin problems and blood and eye disorders. Researchers conducted a study of twenty-four asthmatics using cortisone-type drugs and found that the zinc levels were 42 percent lower than in patients not treated with corticosteroids. A zinc deficiency can lead to loss of taste and smell as well as a loss in sexual desire. Zinc is necessary for male potency and the health of the prostate gland.

Zinc also enhances wound healing and is essential for a clear complexion.

Birth Control Pills

Oral contraceptives are made from a synthetic hormone that can lead to a deficiency in zinc, folic acid, and vitamins C, B_6, and B_{12}. A deficiency of B_{12} can lead to emotional mood swings. A B_6 deficiency can cause depression (and indeed, many women on the pill are depressed). Women taking oral contraceptives (birth control pills) should take at least an extra 25–50 mg of B_6, 1,000 mcg of B_{12}, 400 mg of folic acid, and 1,000 mg of vitamin C. Low vitamin C levels may account for increased susceptibility to blood clotting. I would recommend that you use another method of birth control, as the pill raises your risk of strokes and cancer and causes many unpleasant side effects.

Antacids and Diuretics

Antacids are routinely prescribed for digestive complaints such as heartburn or ulcers. In truth, what most people need is to cut back on the coffee, sugar, and fatty, greasy, and spicy foods and to eat less and exercise more. Antacids interfere with the proper absorption of nutrients. Antacids that contain aluminum disturb calcium and phosphorus metabolism. Phosphorus deficiency, which is very rare (except in antacid users), can cause fatigue, loss of appetite, and fragile bones.

Diuretics, which are commonly prescribed for high blood pressure, also flush potassium and other minerals out of the body. Even potassium-sparing diuretics do not spare other minerals. You should be doubling your intake of minerals if you're taking diuretics.

CHOOSING A SUPPLEMENT PLAN THAT WORKS FOR YOU

Basic Supplement Program for Adults

Not everyone requires the same vitamins and minerals. But here is my basic program, which you can then adapt according to the guidelines in the following pages for specific ages and problems. There are many multivitamins available that will give you the doses listed here. Look for one that dissolves easily, that is small enough to swallow easily, that uses natural (not synthetic) vitamins, and that doesn't use binders, fillers, or colorings.

Ideally you'll take a high-potency two- or three-a-day multivitamin that gives you the following nutrients:

- Beta-carotene or carotenoids, 10,000–15,000 IU
- The B vitamins, including:
  B_1 (thiamine), 25–50 mg
  B_2 (riboflavin), 25–100 mg
  B_3 (niacin), 25–100 mg
  B_5 (pantothenic acid), 25–100 mg
  B_6 (pyridoxine), 50–100 mg
  B_{12} (cobalamin), 100–1,000 mcg
  Biotin, 100–300 mcg
  Choline, 25–100 mg
  Folic acid, 200–400 mcg
  Inositol, 100–300 mg
- Vitamin C, 1,000–3,000 mg
- Vitamin D, 100–500 IU
- Vitamin E, at least 400 IU
- Minerals:
  Boron, 1–5 mg
  Calcium (citrate, lactate, or gluconate), 100–500 mg (women should take a total of 600–1,200 mg daily)
  Chromium (picolinate), 200–400 mcg
  Copper, 1–5 mg
  Magnesium (citrate or gluconate), 100–500 mg (women should take a total of 300–600 mg daily)
  Manganese (citrate or chelate), 10 mg
  Selenium, 25–50 mcg
  Vanadium (vanadyl sulfate), 25–200 mcg
  Zinc, 10–15 mg

Because vitamin C, vitamin E, calcium, and magnesium tend to make a multivitamin pill larger, you can take a multivitamin with small amounts of those vitamins and then take the others separately. A calcium/magnesium combination works well at bedtime, when it will help you relax and prevent leg cramps.

Supplements for Children

Children's nutritional needs are different from adults', not only because they're growing, but also because they're smaller.

Your doctor can recommend liquid vitamins for infants and toddlers. If your household is vegetarian, I recommend an additional amino acid supplement that includes all the essential amino acids plus histidine, taurine, and cysteine, which are essential for growing children.

Here are recommendations for children from the age of four to prepuberty (around the age of eleven to thirteen):

- Vitamin A/beta-carotene, 5,000–10,000 IU
- The B vitamins, including:
  B_1 (thiamine), 0.9–1.3 mg
  B_2 (riboflavin), 1.1–1.5 mg
  B_3 (niacin), 12–17 mg
  B_5 (pantothenic acid), 4–50 mg
  B_6 (pyridoxine), 1.1–2 mg
  B_{12} (cobalamin), 3–5 mcg
  Biotin, 50–150 mcg
  Folic acid, 150–350 mcg
- Vitamin D, 100 IU
- Vitamin C, 150–500 mg
- Vitamin E, 15–25 IU
- Minerals:
  Calcium (citrate, lactate, or gluconate), 800 mg
  Chromium (picolinate), 80–200 mcg
  Iron, 10–12 mg
  Magnesium (citrate or gluconate), 200–300 mg
  Selenium, 100–200 mcg
  Zinc, 10 mg
- Bioflavonoids (amount varies with the type, but they will enhance the action of the other nutrients)

Supplements for Teens

Minimizing the consumption of junk food, maximizing the consumption of vegetables, and enjoying daily aerobic exercise is the best health program a teen can follow.

Be sure your teens are getting enough calcium, as good bone growth in the teens can prevent osteoporosis later in life. A diet with too much protein (more than 2 ounces per day) and too many sodas containing phosphorus will leach calcium from the bones and can increase the risk of osteoporosis later in life. Milk is not a very good source of calcium, because it has a poor calcium-to-magnesium ratio, and the bone building doesn't happen without magnesium. If your teens are milk drinkers, have them take a magnesium tablet with their milk. Fresh vegetables are a much better source of calcium. Exercise is also one of the best ways to build strong bones and will help balance the surges of hormones teens have to cope with.

Plenty of clean water will play a major role in preventing acne and clearing the body of toxins. If your teens are having problems with acne, you can add a vitamin A supplement (5,000 IU), an additional 400 IU of vitamin E, and a B-complex vitamin until the problem clears up. Avoiding refined carbohydrates such as cakes and cookies as well as fried foods will help tremendously. Yogurt is the best acne prevention food a teen can eat, and it will also supply calcium. Buy plain yogurt and sweeten it with fruit.

If your teen is suffering from depression, try a B-complex vitamin and some exercise.

Here are my recommendations for teens:

- Vitamin A/beta-carotene, 5,000 IU
- The B vitamins, including:
  B_1 (thiamine), 1.5 mg
  B_2 (riboflavin), 2 mg
  B_3 (niacin), 18 mg
  B_5 (pantothenic acid), 50 mg
  B_6 (pyridoxine), 2.5 mg
  B_{12} (cobalamin), 5 mcg
  Biotin, 75–150 mcg
  Folic acid, 200 mcg
- Vitamin C, 300–500 mg
- Vitamin D, 100 IU
- Vitamin E, 50–100 IU
- Minerals:
  Calcium (citrate, lactate, or gluconate), 1,200 mg
  Chromium (picolinate), 200 mcg
  Iron, 18 mg
  Magnesium (citrate or gluconate), 350–400 mg
  Selenium, 200 mcg
  Zinc, 10–15 mg

Supplements for Pregnant Women

Pregnant women have special supplement needs, both to support the growing fetus and to support themselves. There are also supplements to avoid when you are pregnant. The best rule of thumb when considering whether to take any type of supplement, pill, or potion when you are pregnant is: When in doubt, don't.

And remember, no vitamin regimen is a substitute for a balanced diet of wholesome foods, including whole grains, fresh fruits and vegetables, legumes, and moderate amounts of protein.

The Basic Supplement Program for Adults will work well with pregnancy, with the following changes and cautions:

Folic acid is an extremely important vitamin in preventing birth defects such as neural tube defects (spina bifida). Women of childbearing age who are at any risk of getting pregnant should be taking 400 mcg of folic acid daily.

Women experiencing morning sickness can take 30–50 mg of vitamin B_6, which should solve the problem.

If you are suffering from varicose veins or other signs of poor circulation in the extremities, you can take the recommended dose of a standardized ginkgo biloba extract.

Vitamins to be avoided during pregnancy include vitamin A (use beta-carotene), and don't overdo the iron—no more than 30 mg daily.

Pregnant women should take extra calcium and magnesium, 600 mg of calcium and 300 mg of magnesium, and extra zinc for a total of 25 mg. The calcium and magnesium should be taken separately from the iron, because they can interfere with iron absorption.

The problem of preeclampsia, also called toxemia, or pregnancy-induced high blood pressure is nearly always caused by a magnesium deficiency. Your best bet is to prevent it by taking magnesium from day one.

A pregnancy multivitamin should contain all the essential minerals and the trace minerals chromium, manganese, and molybdenum.

Supplements for Seniors

As we age, we have special vitamin needs for a variety of reasons. One is that the signals from the

pituitary that regulate hormones
⁀hat digestion and absorption of
s efficient, vastly decreasing the
ᵤ taken in by the body, even with
ᵤiet. This makes supplements especially
important as part of an antiaging program.

Over and over again, studies have shown that eating plenty of fresh vegetables and moderate exercise are two keys to a healthy and energetic old age.

For more information on the foods, herbs, and supplements that help slow the aging process, I recommend *Earl Mindell's Anti-Aging Bible* (Simon & Schuster, 1996).

Here are the extra supplements I recommend for seniors in addition to the Basic Supplement Program for Adults:

- Glucosamine sulfate for stiff joints (follow directions on bottle)

- Betaine hydrochloride to aid digestion (follow directions on bottle)
- Digestive enzymes (follow directions on bottle)
- Vitamin B$_{12}$, 1,000 mg every three days, sublingually or intranasally
- Vitamin B$_6$, 50 mg daily
- Folic acid, 100 mcg daily
- Bioflavonoid antioxidant formula (for example, rutin, hesperidin, PCOs as grapeseed extract, green tea extract, quercetin)
- Ginkgo biloba (follow directions on bottle)
- Melatonin if you're having trouble sleeping, 1.5 mg 1 hour before bed
- Magnesium, 300 mg daily
- Glutathione (take *N*-acetylcysteine, a precursor, and follow directions on bottle)
- Coenzyme Q10, 30–90 mg daily
- L-carnitine, 500–1,000 mg daily
- Ginseng when recovering from illness or for stamina

2 THE SUPER ANTIOXIDANT MIRACLE ~

NATURE'S NEUTRALIZERS: THE ANTIOXIDANTS

Vitamins and minerals are nutrients that are essential to life and to good health, and yet less than 10 percent of Americans meet even the RDA (recommended dietary allowance) of vitamin intake. This leaves more than 90 percent of the population short of essential nutrients. In fact, even the RDA is far short of what you need to stay healthy, indicating only the amount of a nutrient you need to keep from getting sick. The amounts of nutrients you need for vibrant good health and energy are much higher than the RDA.

Taking antioxidants not only optimizes your health and energy levels but is a form of health insurance. These miraculous substances also give us a way to protect our bodies from air pollution, pesticides, food additives, and radiation, not to mention the effects of aging, stress, and illness.

You've probably heard a lot about the best-known antioxidants, vitamins C and E and beta-carotene, but there are other lesser-known antioxidants with actions that are even more potent. I call these the *super antioxidants*. These substances, while not called vitamins because they aren't essential to life, are powerful weapons in your arsenal of nutritional healing supplements.

Although some, like grapeseed extract, seem to be beneficial for virtually all parts of the body, others, like ginkgo biloba, specifically enhance memory. There are literally hundreds of scientific studies showing that these super antioxidants can do everything from preventing heart disease and cancer to improving vision and enhancing brain function.

What are these new miracle supplements? Actually, they aren't new; we just know more than we used to about them and how they work in helping to protect our bodies. Let's begin by finding out what's behind antioxidant power. There are hundreds and probably even thousands of antioxidants, most of them found naturally in plants, particularly fresh fruits and vegetables, but also in herbs. Antioxidants are also present to some degree in seafood and in some animal foods. Other antioxidants, such as coenzyme Q10 and glutathione, the body can manufacture itself.

Oxidation and Free Radicals

The word *oxidation* takes its name from oxygen, an element that is essential to life but that can be harmful in some forms inside the body. A "good" oxygen molecule has its electrons paired up, making it stable. An unstable, or "bad," oxygen molecule has a missing electron, creating what is called a free radical. These unstable oxygen molecules go to war in the body, grabbing onto other cells in their attempt to find another electron and stabilize. This electron can be captured from DNA, cell wall membranes, lipids, proteins, or almost any other tissue component. Every time a free radical stabilizes itself by attacking another cell, it leaves the cell it attacked damaged. That cell becomes unstable and in turn goes after another, creating a chain reaction. This is the process known as oxidation.

Free-radical damage is thought to be an initiating factor in cancer because it can cause healthy cells to mutate into cancerous ones. Cardiovascular disease, arthritis, premature aging, macular degeneration, and cataracts can also be traced back to oxidative damage. Diseases affecting the brain, immune system, digestive tract, lungs, and kidneys involve free radicals. Alcoholism, iron overload, stroke, and radiation injury all produce huge quantities of free radicals. An oxidation chain reaction is difficult to stop once it gets started. Supplying your body with sufficient antioxidant nutrients is the best way to prevent free radicals from making you sick.

What creates free radicals? First, our bodies naturally produce free radicals as part of our complex interaction with oxygen. Our bodies convert much of the food we eat to sugars. Tiny cellular power plants called mitochondria, which are present in every cell, use these sugars plus oxygen to produce energy. By-products of this energy production are free radicals, which if not neutralized by antioxidants create cellular damage.

Free radicals also play a positive role in the body. They act as chemical messengers, helping in the production of hormones and activating enzymes, which are necessary to nearly every system in the body. Free radicals are used by the immune system to fight off invading bacteria and viruses. They have become a problem largely because of the polluted environment we live in and our poor diets.

It is excessive free radicals, not balanced properly with antioxidants, that do damage. The ideal body with ideal nutrition in an ideal environment would have the ability to counteract the free radicals it produces with the antioxidants it takes in and produces, keeping the free radicals under control. Heavy exercise produces free radicals, but it also has beneficial effects on the body that help counteract them.

Put On Your Antioxidant Armor

There are dozens of environmental causes of free-radical production. The biggest culprits we know of are pollutants, such as smog; toxins, such as chlorine; herbicides and pesticides; radiation; some food additives; cigarette smoke; many prescription drugs; and rancid oil. Furthermore, most Americans eat relatively few fresh fruits and vegetables, our main natural sources of antioxidants.

What we have in today's world is a situation where we end up with more free radicals than our bodies can handle. These excess free radicals cause oxidation damage in our bodies. This is where supplements come in.

One of the facts of modern life is that nearly all of us are exposed to pollutants and toxins every day. From the moment we get up in the morning and shower with chlorinated water (I hope you aren't drinking it!), eat pesticide- and additive-laden food, drive to work breathing in car exhaust and toxic fumes from the interior of our cars, work in a building that's most likely toxic from the chemicals put in paneling and carpets, use machines that emit fumes and radiation, and then return home, where we use pesticides, herbicides, spray cans, and cleaning products with toxic fumes—whew! Enough already! But don't despair. There are ways to fight back.

Consume Plenty of Free-Radical Neutralizers

The very best way to get your antioxidants and other vitamins is to eat plenty of whole, preferably organic foods. Fresh fruits and vegetables are your primary dietary source of antioxidants. Those highest in antioxidant power are:

- Fresh or frozen broccoli, cauliflower, and cabbage. Don't boil your vegetables and lose most of the nutrients in the water. Steam them or eat them raw. If you don't have a steamer, buy one for a few dollars that fits in most pots. You'll find them in your supermarket or kitchen supply store.
- Dark green leafy vegetables, such as spinach and kale
- Onions and garlic
- The "yellow" vegetables, such as carrots, sweet potatoes, and pumpkins
- Fresh, whole fruits rather than canned fruits and juices

Eat Some Seafood for Omega-3 Fatty Acids

Seafood is very high in the omega-3 fatty acids, which can actually *reduce* the damage caused by oxidation. However, since much of our fish is contaminated with pollutants, follow these safe fish-eating rules:

- Rotate the kinds of fish you eat, and don't eat any one kind of fish more than once a week.
- Don't eat fish caught close to shore or in rivers and lakes, which are more likely to be polluted.
- Avoid the skin, which has a higher concentration of toxins.

Although all seafood contains omega-3 fatty acids, the highest concentrations are found in mackerel, salmon, tuna (packed in water, please), herring, and sardines. One of my favorite fishes is sea bass. Although it's not quite as high in omega-3 fatty acids as the other fishes I've listed, it is caught in deep offshore waters, so it's relatively pollutant free.

Other foods high in omega-3 fatty acids are avocados and almonds.

Steer Clear of Rancid Oils

One of the biggest sources of free radicals in the Western diet is rancid oil. Unfortunately, the processed vegetable oils (corn, safflower, sunflower, soy, and so on) so heavily promoted for good health for the past thirty years have probably been major contributors to disease in this country. They are high in omega-6 fatty acids, which are very unstable and go rancid almost instantly when they are processed. These rancid fats wreak havoc in the body, setting loose a chain reaction of oxidation. Meat also contains omega-6 fatty acids, but if you eat it in moderation, the benefits of the nutrients you receive from it will outweigh the damage of the omega-6.

Avoid corn, safflower, sunflower, cottonseed, and other vegetable oils that are "hydrogenated," "polyunsaturated," or otherwise processed. The hydrogenated oils are synthetic, not-found-in-nature pseudosaturated oils that are worse for you than the real thing. Even "cold-pressed" vegetable oils are suspect because they go rancid so quickly (most within hours after you open the container). To prevent rancidity, add the contents of a 400 IU vitamin E oil capsule to the bottle of vegetable oil when you open it. Some brands already have vitamin E added.

Olive oil is the only vegetable oil that is low in omega-6 fatty acids and doesn't go rancid quickly. Canola oil is better than most at 60 percent omega-3 fatty acids, but still goes rancid fairly quickly. Look for canola oil with vitamin E added, or add it yourself as suggested above.

Coconut oil is a good oil because it is high in stearic acid, which has a neutral effect on cholesterol, doesn't go rancid quickly, and is excellent for baking. I would much rather have you use coconut oil than hydrogenated oils such as Crisco and margarine. I know this flies in the face of mainstream dietary advice, but tropical oils were drummed out of the American diet for political reasons within the food-manufacturing industry, not for sound nutritional reasons.

Minimize Pollutants to Keep Free Radicals at Bay

Here are some guidelines to help you minimize your exposure to free radical–producing pollutants.

- Drink clean water (filtered), six to eight glasses daily.
- Wash, peel, or even scrub fruits and vegetables well, and eat organic produce whenever possible.
- As much as possible, eat whole, unprocessed foods without additives and preservatives.
- Read food labels.
- Stand up for your right to work in a pollution-free environment. If you think something at work is making you sick, pursue it. It could be mold or fungus in the heating or cooling system, fumes from wall paneling or carpets, or a coworker's cigarette smoke.
- Minimize your use of spray cans, herbicides, and pesticides.
- Avoid processed vegetable oils, eat meat in moderation, eat more seafood, and consume more olive oil.

Antioxidants and Aging

Scientists who study aging are increasingly focusing on the cumulative damage done to cellular DNA over time by oxidation. Many believe that taking antioxidant supplements can slow the aging process by preventing free-radical damage. There are plenty of studies to back up this point of view. Every indication is that the typical diseases of aging can largely be avoided by leading a healthy lifestyle and taking anti-oxidants. For example, in a study from the Harvard School of Public Health, more than 130,000 healthy middle-aged and older adults who consumed at least 100 IU of vitamin E every day for two or more years had a reduced risk of cardiovascular disease.

As we age, our digestive system becomes less efficient and doesn't absorb nutrients as well. Taking vitamins, and particularly antioxidants, is an important key to preventing age-related diseases caused by nutritional deficiencies.

A Canadian study of ninety-six healthy people over age sixty-five found that those who took a multivitamin containing the RDA of vitamins and minerals plus slightly higher levels of vitamin E and beta-carotene had stronger immune systems and half as many infections as those taking placebos. I hope that in the future we have RDAs for children, teenagers, adults, and senior citizens that will specifically address the needs of each age-group.

Antioxidants and Cardiovascular Disease

Staying free of heart disease involves more than just taking care of your heart. You need to take care of your entire cardiovascular system, including your arteries, veins, and capillaries, as well as the blood that runs through them.

Antioxidants go to work in all these areas of the body to prevent aging and disease. There are literally dozens of studies showing these protective effects. For example, the Scottish Heart Health Study, which is tracking over ten thousand middle-aged men, evaluated the intake of vitamins C and E and beta-carotene and found that there was a protective effect for all three antioxidants. High vitamin E levels proved to be specifically protective against angina.

In a smaller study that actually measured vitamin levels in 152 people ranging in age from twenty-six to sixty-five, there was a significantly lower rate of coronary heart disease in those who had higher levels of vitamins A, C, and E and beta-carotene.

One of the primary roles of antioxidants in the cardiovascular system is to prevent LDL, or "bad," cholesterol from oxidation. According to a report out of the University of Texas Southwestern Medical Center, animal and human studies have shown that antioxidant supplementation with vitamin E reduces the extent of LDL oxidation. Their work also underscores the importance of eating monounsaturated fatty acids, such as olive oil and canola oil, as well as the tropical oils, such as coconut oil, rather than polyunsaturated fatty acids, such as corn oil and other vegetable oils.

Other nutrients that reduce LDL oxidation include beta-carotene and vitamin C. A study published by the NIH (National Institutes of Health) set out to measure the power of antioxidants to reduce oxidation of LDL cholesterol. They evaluated nineteen middle-aged people with high cholesterol (an average total cholesterol of 283 mg/dl and an LDL of 197 mg/dl), along with fourteen control subjects of similar age and normal cholesterol. The high-cholesterol group received a daily dose of 30 mg of beta-carotene, 1,000 mg of vitamin C, and 800 IU of vitamin E. After one month of the vitamin therapy, the onset of LDL oxidation was prolonged by 71 percent, and the rate of oxidation was decreased by 26 percent. This study showed that after one month of antioxidant supplementation, people with high cholesterol significantly reduced their susceptibility to LDL oxidation.

Many large epidemiological (population) studies have been done comparing diet, cholesterol levels, and rates of heart disease. There are population groups in Europe that eat just as much if not more saturated fat than Americans, yet have less heart disease. Some of this difference may be due to their consumption of red wine, which is high in bioflavonoids, but there is increasing evidence that it is also due to their higher consumption of fresh fruits and vegetables.

Antioxidants and Cancer

Free radicals in tissues and cells damage essential body chemicals and can harm DNA, the very building blocks of life. DNA damage can begin the process of cancer. Antioxidants are part of the body's natural cancer prevention mechanism, and supplements are a useful way to boost them. A major study in China showed that over five years, a group that took 15 mg of beta-carotene, 30 mg of vitamin E, and 50 mg of selenium per day showed a 21 percent lower risk of dying from stomach cancer.

Another study, comparing cancer-afflicted and cancer-free patients, showed that vitamin supplementation was associated with significantly reduced risk of basal cell cancer. In fact, the cost of supplementing the diet of the general population with antioxidants like selenium and vitamin E would be much less expensive and more appropriate than the treatment of the disease.

Several population studies have linked consumption of soy foods to a lower risk of certain cancers, including cancers of the breast, prostate, stomach, and lung. Soybeans contain many compounds generating great interest in the medical community, including the isoflavones, some of which act as antioxidants.

Antioxidants and Arthritis Pain

Antioxidants have a profound influence on diseases of the connective tissue, such as arthritis. They can often play a large part in reducing the pain of arthritis and can greatly cut down on the need for medications such as aspirin or acetaminophen, which are used frequently to treat pain.

This was confirmed by a German study using the antioxidant selenium. The group using the selenium had far healthier joints than those who used a placebo. People with arthritis tend to be deficient in selenium.

The antioxidant vitamins E and C can also be deficient in connective tissue diseases, and both are extremely important in the development and maintenance of cartilage.

Antioxidants and Exercise

There's no doubt about it. Exercise is definitely good for you. Less fat, increased bone density, and reduced heart disease and cancer risks are a few of its benefits. However, exercise does generate free radicals. This is a normal result of increased oxygen consumption and is not normally a problem because the body's natural antioxidant systems are designed to handle the extra load. Unfortunately, the high level of pollutants in our environment and the nutritional deficiencies of modern diets mean that exercise can leave us with a minus balance in our antioxidant account.

The assessment of antioxidant status in exercising individuals and athletes can be important to maximizing performance and good health. Different studies show that overexercise, heat, and environmental pollutants can all increase oxidative stress. The key to keeping fit in today's world lies in backing up your body's own defense and repair systems before strenuous exercise.

It has been shown that taking 1,200 IU of vitamin E for two weeks before strenuous exercise creates a significant reduction in oxidation during the exercise. In male college students who have done exhaustive exercise, those who ingested 300 IU per day of vitamin E for four weeks had lower levels of chemicals suggestive of free-radical damage immediately following exercise than those consuming a placebo.

The preventive role of antioxidants has also been demonstrated in marathon runners. Those who take 600 mg of vitamin C per day for twenty-one days prior to a 42 km run have a lower incidence of postexercise respiratory tract infection.

Interestingly, one antioxidant important to serious exercisers is at its highest levels in the organ crucial to any physical activity—the heart. This is the nutrient coenzyme Q10. Coenzyme Q10 works with vitamin C to prevent LDL cholesterol in the heart from oxidation and helps prevent damage to the arteries of the heart. This is typical of the cooperative interaction of antioxidants.

If you're serious about exercise, I recommend that you also get serious about taking your antioxidant supplements!

The "Big Three" Antioxidants

In addition to the super antioxidants, I'll be telling you about what I call the "big three" stars of the vitamin antioxidant world: beta-carotene, vitamin E, and vitamin C. They should be taken in addition to the super antioxidants, as they work hand in hand with each other. Every super antioxidant mentioned in this book works better with the "big three." Although I won't discuss selenium in detail, it is a mineral antioxidant that should be included in your daily multivitamin, as it also enhances many of the other antioxidants.

Even mainstream medical doctors tend to agree these days that taking the "big three" will help you stay healthier. The "big three" stop or slow the oxidation process by neutralizing free radicals. These antioxidants also help the body fight disease and the effects of aging in other ways. And yet Americans aren't getting enough of them. A study evaluating three national surveys of more than thirteen thousand Americans found that the majority of those surveyed were getting less than the RDA for these vitamins. (And the RDA is far less than I recommend!)

In a study at the University of Toronto, people with bladder cancer who took high daily doses of vitamins A (40,000 IU), B_6 (100 mg), C (2,000 mg), and E (400 IU) had 40 percent fewer tumors than a control group that took no vitamins, and they also lived almost twice as long. Researchers concluded that high doses of vitamins may provide protection against the high recurrence rates that tend to be present with bladder cancer.

Doctors have used a combination of the "big three" antioxidants plus vitamin A and manganese, along with radiation and chemotherapy, for small-cell lung cancer. Patients lived longer and tolerated chemotherapy and radiation better than the group not given antioxidant supplements.

The famous Harvard nurses' and doctors' studies, which looked at the health of thousands of men and women over a period of many years, found that heart disease deaths were 60 percent lower in those who took vitamin E.

Another large, long-term study, called the Basel Study, found that when blood levels of vitamins C, E, and A and beta-carotene were low, there were increased rates of death from cancer and heart disease. For example, people whose levels of vitamin C and beta-carotene were low were more likely to die of heart disease. What's more, vitamin E has been shown in several studies to be a definite help to those already suffering from heart disease.

It's easy to see that there is a wide range of diseases where supplements of the "big three" antioxi-dants have been shown to play a beneficial role. In some cases, the doses needed haven't been very high. For example, a study published in the *Journal of the American College of Nutrition* showed that a moderate dose of just 300 mg of vitamin C daily reduced the risk of developing cataracts by 33 percent. Vitamin E in 400 IU daily doses also dropped the risk. That sounds like pretty good health insurance to me!

The Bioflavonoids

Bioflavonoids are organic compounds found in plants that are turning out to be key to the power of super antioxidants. All of the super antioxidants contain bioflavonoids as a major part of their active principles. These powerful substances reduce inflammation and pain, strengthen blood vessels, improve circulation, fight bacteria and viruses, improve liver function, lower cholesterol levels, and improve vision. Vitamin C works much more effectively when combined with bioflavonoids.

Bioflavonoids are found in a wide variety of plants. Some of the best food sources are the white material underneath citrus fruit peels, peppers, and and berries. Although bioflavonoids are not considered essential to life and therefore not classified as vitamins, it is becoming clear that they *are* essential to good health.

BETA-CAROTENE: THE COLORFUL ANTIOXIDANT

Vitamin A occurs in two forms—preformed vitamin A, called retinol (found only in foods of animal origin), and provitamin A, better known as beta-carotene (provided by foods of both plant and animal origin). Beta-carotene is made up of two vitamin A molecules. When the body needs vitamin A, it uses an enzyme to break the beta-carotene molecule in half, creating two vitamin A molecules. This is why beta-carotene is considered a safer way to get vitamin A, which can accumulate in the body and become toxic if taken in high doses over a long period of time.

Beta-carotene is a member of the carotenoid family of plant pigments and is a powerful antioxidant. As well as helping to prevent heart disease and cancer, it prevents vitamin C from being oxidized or destroyed. Beta-carotene and vitamin C working in concert are especially important in protecting the eyes. Beta-carotene's protective effect is also seen in the mucous membranes of the mouth, nose, throat, and lungs.

The carotenoids are the pigments that give vegetables such as carrots, squash, and tomatoes their bright colors. They also give flowers such as nasturtiums, pansies, and sunflowers their yellow color. These compounds were first discovered in carrots, which is how they got their name. Scientists have found nearly six hundred carotenoids. Of these, the body can use about fifty to create vitamin A.

A Carrot a Day Keeps the Doctor Away: Bugs Bunny Was Right!

Although I recommend that you take a beta-carotene supplement daily, you can get 15,000 IU of beta-carotene by eating one carrot. By getting daily beta-carotene from foods, you also get a full complement of carotenoids, not just beta-carotene. Studies have shown that lightly steaming carrots is the best way to maximize your absorption of the beta-carotene. I also recommend that you eat a raw carrot every day. Make carrot sticks and have them for lunch, or grate the carrot into a salad. In the famous Harvard Nurses' Study, eating one carrot a day reduced the incidence of stroke by 68 percent and the rate of lung cancer by 50 percent. If a prescription medicine showed that kind of success, it would be the best-selling drug in the world! Carrots also contain fiber and lower cholesterol.

This is also a good reason to take a natural beta-carotene supplement, which comes packaged as part of the carotenoid family, rather than a synthetic one that just isolates the beta-carotene.

Beta-Carotene and Heart Disease

One source of evidence for the protective effect of beta-carotene comes from a study of doctors with heart disease. A subgroup of the Physicians' Health Study of male physicians between forty and eighty-four years of age comprised 333 doctors with angina pectoris and coronary revascularization. Those assigned to 50 mg of beta-carotene on alternate days had a 44 percent reduction in all major coronary events, including death from heart failure. Those taking beta-carotene also had a 49 percent reduction in events connected with blood vessels, such as strokes, heart attacks, revascularization, or cardiovascular death. The beneficial effect of beta-carotene appeared in the second year of follow-up in this study, showing how this antioxidant had prevented further fatty degeneration of the walls of arteries.

Data from a Netherlands study of 674 patients who had heart attacks supports the idea that beta-carotene plays a role in protecting polyunsaturated fatty acids from oxidation. In this way, beta-carotene protects the heart muscle from further deterioration caused by the restricted blood flow that can result from this kind of oxidation.

Beta-Carotene and Cancer

Dozens of published studies show that a high carotenoid intake is directly related to a decreased risk of cancer. A variety of population studies have shown that a low intake of carotenoids results in an increased risk of cancer. This may be due to beta-carotene's unique ability to squelch the free radicals that can spur the process of malignant tumor formation.

In one study of fifty cancer patients, recurrence of cancer was prevented in a significant number of those who took beta-carotene and vitamin E supplements. Beta-carotene and/or vitamin E have also stopped cancer in its tracks in a variety of studies. This was best demonstrated in clinical trials on oral cancer.

Over the past few decades, numerous studies have shown high levels of beta-carotene to be protective against many types of cancer, working not just to suppress cancerous cells but also to completely prevent the onset of cancer.

People who are deficient in vitamin A/beta-carotene often have skin diseases that resemble precancerous conditions.

Beta-Carotene and Infectious Diseases

Vitamin A deficiencies are clearly related to a higher rate of infection and slower healing. There is a worldwide campaign on the part of health care workers to make sure that children in Third World countries are given vitamin A to prevent a long list of infectious diseases and deficiency diseases. Some estimates are that a few pennies' worth of vitamin A could prevent 35 percent of the deaths attributable to measles in Third World countries.

Beta-Carotene and the Immune System

One of the best ways to combat viruses is to boost the immune system and increase the number of T cells present. T cells play a critical role in attacking and eliminating viruses. A number of studies have shown that high doses of beta-carotene can raise T cell levels. This makes it important in the treatment of those suffering from AIDS and cancer as well as less deadly viruses such as shingles, herpes, and the flu.

Beta-Carotene and the Skin

Although too much beta-carotene will turn your skin an orange hue, too little will cause premature wrinkling and signs of aging. Various derivatives of vitamin A have been used to improve skin quality, but keeping your beta-carotene intake high will work even better as a preventive.

Beta-Carotene and the Eyes

My mother told me to eat my carrots so that I would have good eyesight, and there's plenty of truth to that advice. Deficiencies of vitamin A are associated with night blindness. There is also some evidence that high dietary levels of beta-carotene prevent cataracts.

How to Make Beta-Carotene Part of Your Daily Life

I recommend that you take 10,000–25,000 IU of beta-carotene daily with meals. In fact, beta-carotene works best with fats, so if you take it at the same time you're eating fatty foods, you'll get more benefit from it. You may get enough beta-carotene from a combination of eating fresh fruits and vegetables and taking a multivitamin. However, if there's any question of getting enough beta-carotene and other antioxidants, then add an antioxidant supplement.

What Is the Best Form of Beta-Carotene to Take?

I recommend that you take a natural form of beta-carotene that most commonly comes from a sea alga called *Dunaliella salina*. It is usually referred to on vitamin bottles as *D. salina* or as a "marine source" of beta-carotene. This form of beta-carotene is patented by the Henkel company and may also be referred to by its commercial name, Betatene. Natural beta-carotene in supplements also comes from carrots and other food sources. When you take natural beta-carotene, you get the whole family of carotenoids rather than just the beta-carotene found in the synthetic versions.

Are There Any Side Effects from Taking Beta-Carotene?

If you take high doses of beta-carotene over a long period of time, your skin may turn yellow. This will not hurt you. However, I don't recommend taking it in a high enough dose to create yellow skin. As with everything, moderation is the key. Also, don't take beta-carotene if you're taking the prescription drug Accutane, a drug used to treat severe acne.

What Foods Is Beta-Carotene Found In?

You already know that carrots are a good source of beta-carotene, and you've probably guessed that any of the orange or yellow vegetables are good sources of this powerful antioxidant. Beta-carotene is plentiful, too, in yellow fruits such as apricots and oranges. Sweet potatoes, spinach, and most green leafy vegetables are also good sources. Green tea, too, contains beta-carotene.

How Beta-Carotene Can Help You

- Prevents and reverses heart disease
- Prevents and reverses cancer
- Improves vision
- Protects the mucous membranes of the upper respiratory tract
- Lowers cholesterol
- Prevents cataracts
- Improves immune system function
- Shortens the duration of disease
- Prevents and cures skin disease
- Prevents age spots
- Promotes growth
- Promotes strong bones
- Promotes healthy gums
- Helps treat acne

VITAMIN C: THE ULTIMATE PREVENTIVE ANTIOXIDANT

Vitamin C (ascorbic acid) is one of the most important vitamins our bodies require and one of the most powerful antioxidants we know of. It also enhances the benefits of almost every other antioxidant. As *Homo sapiens*, our bodies don't have the ability to manufacture vitamin C, so we must replace this precious vitamin every day of our lives in food or supplements or suffer the consequences. Most animal life is able to synthesize its own vitamin C and manufactures between 1,000 and 3,000 mg a day. While beta-carotene works with the fats, vitamin C works with the watery parts of the body, including intracellular fluids, blood plasma, lung fluid, and eye fluid.

Vitamin C makes vitamin E work better by recycling it. Scientists working with vitamin C in solution found that it delayed by a factor of ten the time taken to use up both vitamin E and beta-carotene from the start of oxidation.

One of the most extensively researched nutrients, vitamin C is also one of the most easily available. Naturally occurring vitamin C always exists in association with members of another set of power-

ful antioxidants, the flavonoids, and they work best together.

Vitamin C and Disease Prevention

How many people do you know who consume the recommended five to nine portions of vegetables and fruits per day? And if they don't, are they taking supplements? There is increasing support for the concept that higher amounts than the RDAs of vitamin C and other antioxidant vitamins are needed to fight infection and chronic disease.

An extensive review of the literature suggests that populations that consume higher than the RDA levels of vitamin C (which is 60 mg per day from foods and other supplements) have a reduced risk of cancer at several sites, as well as a reduced risk of cardiovascular disease and cataracts. Higher-than-RDA levels of vitamin C have been associated with normal cholesterol and blood pressure levels and reduced risk of cardiovascular death.

Research shows that increased consumption of fresh fruits and vegetables, excellent sources of vitamin C, even without supplements, leads to a dramatic reduction in the incidence of gastric cancer and hypertension leading to stroke. It is in this way, too, that vitamin C plays a major role in parts of Asia in lowering the risk of cancer of the esophagus. It is thought that this is partly because vitamin C can neutralize and scavenge free radicals in the upper gastrointestinal tract.

Many controlled studies prove the value of vitamin C as a disease preventive. In addition, it's known to contribute to resistance against pollution in air, water, and food and to support the manufacture of white blood cells and interferon. Even before it was isolated as a specific substance, the food sources of vitamin C received official recognition in the fight against disease.

You may know the story of "limeys." This was the nickname given to British sailors when, in 1753, the navy instructed all Admiralty ships to carry limes and fresh vegetables to prevent the debilitating disease called scurvy. Symptoms included livid spots on the skin, bleeding gums, and exhaustion. Until the new orders, sailors' fare consisted mainly of bread and salted meat. The fresh rations had spectacular results. From 1,754 cases in just one naval hospital in 1760, there was only one case in 1806.

Over two hundred years later, much more is known about the beneficial effects of vitamin C, and the research continues. One study, reported in the *British Medical Journal*, covered 730 men and women with no history of cardiovascular disease and evaluated seven-day dietary records. In these elderly subjects, the mortality from stroke was highest among those with lowest vitamin C intake. This study followed up its elderly subjects over a twenty-year period, revealing vitamin C status to be as strong a predictor of death from stroke as diastolic blood pressure. The study concluded that a high intake of vitamin C should be encouraged in the elderly. But don't wait. Starting young brings the full preventive benefits.

Vitamin C and other nutrients could benefit the national economy, too. Many Americans have vitamin C intakes at levels associated with increased risks of degenerative diseases such as cancer, cataracts, and cardiovascular disease. Today there is great concern worldwide, but particularly in the United States, about the high costs of diagnosis and treatment of such diseases, not to mention the common cold and other infectious illnesses. Just applying what we know about micronutrients like vitamin C would have a major impact in controlling and actually lowering the costs of medical care.

Vitamin C and Collagen

Vitamin C is essential for the formation of collagen in the body. Collagen is a protein substance that holds together the cells needed to make tissue. Collagen is necessary for structural soundness of bones, teeth, connective tissue, cartilage, and capillary walls. It also plays a role in wound and burn healing; it is necessary for the formation of healthy connective tissue used by the body to knit together a wound or burn. Moreover, collagen may play an important role in protecting the body from infection. A current theory holds that healthy collagen means stronger tissue, which enables the body to resist invasion by disease microorganisms.

Vitamin C and Your Skin

After your skin is exposed to sunlight, its vitamin C levels drop significantly. Cream or lotion containing vitamin C can help you guard against skin cancer and wrinkles. Yes, you read it right. Vitamin C on the skin will penetrate deeply, reducing the damage to your skin from ultraviolet light and thus reducing the wrinkles formed when skin is damaged. According to a study reported in the *British Journal of Dermatology*, vitamin C applied to the skin of pigs protected them from ultraviolet light damage. By applying the vitamin C to *your* skin, you get twenty times more into your skin than if you took it by mouth (but do keep taking it by mouth!). Vitamin C applied this way penetrates into the skin and can't be rubbed, sweated, or even washed off. The beneficial effects can last up to twenty days, but according to the pig study, the skin is most protected when the vitamin C is applied regularly.

Vitamin C and Allergies

If I could only recommend one thing to help with allergy symptoms, it would be vitamin C. Large doses of vitamin C can decrease allergic symptoms, especially a runny nose and cough.

It is the body's release of histamines that causes allergic symptoms such as red, itchy eyes and sinus congestion. Vitamin C performs an important antihistamine action in the body, making it a critical ally in fighting allergies. This essential vitamin, which many Americans are deficient in, works directly to lower histamine levels in the body and supports the immune system in many ways. If you suffer during allergy season, I recommend you take at least 1,000 mg of vitamin C three times daily, and if your symptoms continue or get worse, increase that to 1,000 mg every 3 or 4 hours.

Vitamin C and Asthma

Vitamin C, along with other antioxidants, has been shown to be beneficial for treating asthma and preventing attacks. Vitamin C is the major antioxidant present in the airway surface liquid of the lungs. It helps to open up the airways and liquefy the mucus buildup caused by the allergic reactions underlying asthma.

Many physicians have noted that vitamin C can diminish, if not prevent completely, the symptoms of byssinosis, a lung disease that strikes textile workers who breathe fiber dust. This was proven in an actual study in which textile workers were given 250 mg of vitamin C every few hours. Those who received vitamin C had significantly less incidence of the disease.

It is now known that low dietary intake of vitamin C puts people at risk for asthma. In fact, low levels of vitamin C are common in people with asthma. A report in the *American Journal of Clinical Nutrition* revealed that asthma sufferers unfortunately often show a decreased preference for foods containing vitamin C. The report also revealed that several studies have shown that vitamin C supplementation of 1–2 g daily improves respiratory measurements in asthmatics.

Vitamin C crystals have been used to stop an asthma attack, and in one study, athletes with asthma brought on by vigorous exercise had fewer asthma attacks when they took vitamin C just before and just after exercising.

There is evidence that exposure to oxidants produced both in the body and in external substances may be a causative factor for asthma, particularly in infancy.

Vitamin C and Heart Disease

Many studies have shown that vitamin C helps reduce cholesterol levels and helps prevent heart disease. Other studies have shown that those who have certain types of heart disease have lower levels of vitamin C in their blood. People who take vitamin C also show a much lower risk of life-threatening blood clots that can cause a stroke.

Myocardial infarction is a disease involving the death of heart muscle tissue due to an obstruction of the blood supply. In one study, five hundred patients with acute myocardial infarction were put on either a control or an intervention diet within 48 hours of the infarction. The intervention diet was designed to be antioxidant rich. Sure enough, vitamin C levels in the blood increased more in the intervention group than in the control group. The intervention group had safer levels of harmful enzymes and, not surprisingly, lower levels of free radicals. This put the intervention group at less risk of death or further injury from their illness. It's clear that a diet rich in vitamin C and other antioxidants is a sensible precaution against heart disease.

Vitamin C and Colds and Flu

Numerous studies have shown that vitamin C gives the immune system a big boost in its job of fighting off colds and flu. Other studies show that once a cold or flu is in progress, taking vitamin C can reduce the severity of the symptoms and shorten the duration of the illness. One study discovered that patients taking 1,000 mg (1 g) of vitamin C every day and increasing that dose to 4 g at the onset of a cold, had a 9 percent reduction in the frequency of colds and a 14 percent reduction in sick days.

Vitamin C and Cancer

The protective effect of vitamin C against cancer is well established. Over and over again, in population studies, those whose diet includes significant amounts of vitamin C show a lower risk of most kinds of cancer. Other studies show that vitamin C actually blocks the formation of certain substances in the body that cause cancer. Small studies done on the ability of vitamin C to block cervical cancer show great promise, and more research is needed. Vitamin C has also been shown to reduce the ability of cancerous cells to form in the stomach.

Most of the research on vitamin C and cancer shows that vitamin C is a *preventive* more than a cure, but vitamin C can also assist if you're fighting cancer. Some researchers believe, as did Dr. Linus Pauling, that the studies on vitamin C and cancer already in progress have been flawed and that better studies are needed.

Vitamin C and Diabetes

Diabetics who take vitamin C supplements can often reduce their insulin intake. One of the major complications of diabetes is the weakening of blood vessels, which can cause circulatory problems, infection, and eye problems. Vitamin C has been shown to reduce these complications. However, diabetics who are having kidney problems should not be taking megadoses of vitamin C. If you have diabetes, check with your doctor first before taking vitamins to reduce insulin intake.

How to Make Vitamin C Part of Your Daily Life

People are becoming more aware of the need to supplement their diets with extra vitamin C. Unfortunately, most people think that by taking an ordinary vitamin C tablet in the morning with their breakfast, they will be covered for the rest of the day. Actually, the vitamin C is metabolized, and any excess is excreted in about 2 hours, depending on the quantity of food in the stomach.

It is very important to maintain a high level of vitamin C in the bloodstream, since vitamin C can be destroyed by stress and any number of environmental pollutants, from cigarette smoke to carbon monoxide from exhaust fumes. You can do this by eating plenty of raw fresh fruits and vegetables (cooking destroys vitamin C) and by taking a vitamin C supplement with every meal. I actually recommend taking an antioxidant supplement that combines vitamins A, C, and E at every meal.

You should take as much vitamin C as your body can use without giving you diarrhea. When you are healthy, unstressed, and in a relatively clean environment, your need for a vitamin C supplement will probably range from 500 to 3,000 mg daily. If you are ill, stressed, or being exposed to pollutants and toxins, your need for vitamin C could increase by as much as one hundred times the normal amount.

What's the Best Form of Vitamin C to Take?

There are many forms of vitamin C on the market: buffered, esterified, with bioflavonoids, timed release, and ascorbates, to name the major ones. Vitamin C (ascorbate) as it is found in nature is combined with substances called bioflavonoids. Please take your vitamin C with ascorbate *and* bioflavonoids; they work best in combination.

Vitamin C is buffered, esterified, or made in timed-release form to prevent a common side effect of too much vitamin C: diarrhea. Timed-release vitamins often cause gas or tend to pass right through the system without ever dissolving. The esterified forms of vitamin C work best to prevent diarrhea, but you can also buy the cheaper forms of vitamin C if you're willing to test your tolerance for it. You do this by increasing your dose of vitamin C until you get diarrhea, and then back off until it goes away. This will be the amount of vitamin C your body can use effectively.

How Long Will Vitamin C Last on My Shelf?

Vitamin C is very stable in tablet form. Long-term and short-term tests indicate that under normal storage conditions, commercial vitamin C tablets are stable for periods in excess of five years (95 percent potency retention). But I hope that your vitamin C will never be around for this long!

What Foods Is Vitamin C Found In?

Most fresh, raw vegetables and fruits contain at least some vitamin C. Cooking destroys vitamin C. One of the best sources of vitamin C is citrus fruit such as oranges and grapefruit. Kiwi fruit contains high levels of vitamin C. Other good natural sources of vitamin C are broccoli and red bell peppers.

How Vitamin C Can Help You
- Prevents heart disease
- Prevents cancer
- Prevents stroke
- Prevents allergies
- Reduces inflammation
- May enable diabetics to reduce insulin intake
- Protects against pollutants and other toxins
- Shortens the duration of colds and flu
- Prevents asthma and reduces severity of attacks
- Protects the lungs from airborne pollutants
- Protects the skin from sun damage
- Reduces arthritis pain and inflammation

VITAMIN E: THE HEALTHY HEART ANTIOXIDANT

Vitamin E is one of our most important vitamins and a powerful antioxidant. If all Americans took vitamin E, it would save an estimated $8 billion a year in health care costs.

Vitamin E is another antioxidant, like beta-carotene, that works with the fats in our bodies. Vitamin E works most specifically to combat rancidity in our cells. Rancidity is caused when free radicals go after fat cells and oxidize them. Our cells contain membranes made of fatty substances called lipids, and vitamin E protects those membranes from free-radical damage. Vitamin E also works in our blood to neutralize free radicals by absorbing their free electron.

The unsaturated vegetable oils are extremely susceptible to rancidity or oxidation, and eating them greatly increases our need for vitamin E to combat this oxidation. These oils literally start turning rancid as soon as the bottle is opened, and some of them may already be rancid. (In fact, I recommend that you only buy vegetable oils that are preserved with vitamin E or that you add a capsule of vitamin E to your vegetable oil as soon as you open it.)

Vitamin E and Disease Prevention

For over twenty-five years, I have been urging you to take a supplement of vitamin E daily. Although scientists found vitamin E in the 1920s, and many nutritionists and scientists have also been recommending it for years, we are only recently proving beyond any doubt that vitamin E plays an important role in the maintenance of health—and particularly in a healthy heart.

Vitamin E and Your Lungs

Vitamin E can help protect the lungs and other air passageways against environmental pollutants such as air pollution, pesticides, and industrial pollutants. In a recent study of nonsmokers, taking vitamin E was associated with a 45 percent lower risk of lung cancer.

Vitamin E and Wound Healing

Vitamin E is a powerful wound healer, and when it is used, scarring tends to be greatly reduced. Vitamin E has also been used successfully in treating burns. It accelerates the healing rate of burns and lessens the formation of scar tissue. When applied to the skin, the antioxidizing effect of vitamin E prevents bacteria from growing. The British medical journal *The Lancet* reports that animal studies have shown that vitamin E also helps lessen tissue damage. It's known, too, for its anti-inflammatory action and for boosting the immune system's response to injury.

Vitamin E and Heart Disease

There are literally hundreds of good, solid, scientific studies showing that vitamin E can prevent and even reverse many kinds of heart disease. Let's review just a handful of these studies.

A review of European populations cosponsored by the World Health Organization (WHO) showed that those with higher levels of vitamin E had a lower rate of coronary artery disease. The same result was true in the majority of countries in studies of European and non-European nations, even where saturated fat intake was high.

Finland's Laplanders showed a 17 percent lower death rate from heart disease than their southern neighbors. A study of 350 people revealed a northern diet high in antioxidants, including vitamin E–rich reindeer meat!

The Nurses' Health Study of over 87,000 women showed that those who took vitamin E supplements greater than 100 IU per day had a 40 percent lower risk of coronary artery disease than those who took no vitamin E.

The Health Professionals' Follow-Up Study of over 39,000 males showed that those who took vitamin E supplements greater than or equal to 100 IU per day had a 37 percent reduced risk of coronary heart disease compared to those who took none.

A Harvard University study of 130,000 men and women found that daily doses of vitamin E of 100 IU or more taken for at least two years resulted in a whopping 46 percent lower heart disease risk for women and a 25 percent lower risk for men.

Just 100 IU of vitamin E helped produce less constriction of heart blood vessels over two years in one group, compared to those not taking the vitamin.

This was shown in a study at the University of Southern California School of Medicine. These results were supported by another study at the New Mexico School of Medicine of 440 patients who underwent successful angioplasty. During a three-year follow-up, patients who did not take vitamin E regularly saw almost double the recurrence of blood vessel constrictions compared to those who did take vitamin E.

The evidence grows for the beneficial effects of vitamin E to surgery patients. Another study from the University of Southern California School of Medicine evaluated 156 men between forty and fifty-nine years of age who had previous coronary bypass graft surgery. Results showed a reduction in coronary artery lesion for those taking vitamin E supplements.

A report in the *Medical Tribune* found that even at low doses, vitamin E came through as the heart's key protective nutrient. Even the medical establishment has jumped on the vitamin E bandwagon, with many MDs routinely prescribing it for themselves and their patients.

Here are a few of the effects that vitamin E has on the cardiovascular system:

- It combats oxidation of cholesterol, preventing and reducing accumulation on the arteries.
- It is a natural anticoagulant, dissolving blood clots safely.
- It permeates the tiny capillaries, assisting in bringing nourishment to all body cells and thereby supplying oxygen to the muscles (especially the heart muscles).
- It prevents undesirable excessive scarring of the heart after a heart attack, while it promotes a strong "patch" scar during the healing process.
- It is a natural vasodilator, meaning that it opens up the blood vessels.
- It allows a greater flexibility in cells and muscles, preventing hardening of the arteries.
- It is an anticlotting agent, helping to prevent blood clots in arteries and veins.
- It helps dissolve existing clots.
- It increases the blood's available oxygen (improves the transportation of oxygen by the red blood cells).
- It reduces the need of the heart for oxygen by making the heart become a more efficient pump.

Vitamin E and Diabetes

Diabetics have been found to be able to reduce their insulin levels when given vitamin E. Some people with type II diabetes have even been able to get off insulin completely by taking vitamin E supplements. (If you are diabetic, please check with your doctor first.) Because one of the main effects of vitamin E is its anticlotting effect, it can greatly aid in preventing the damage to blood vessels that frequently causes serious problems for diabetics.

Excessive levels of free radicals are a feature of diabetes and are possibly involved in triggering the disease. Three small trials reported by the American Diabetes Association all showed decreases in substances such as fatty acids in the blood vessels of diabetics given vitamin E supplements—confirmation, again, of the important effects of this antioxidant.

Vitamin E and Cataracts

It has been shown that a deficiency of vitamin E can contribute to the formation of cataracts and other vision problems. Supplementing your diet with vitamin E is good health insurance for the eyes. It works best when combined with vitamin C and selenium.

Vitamin E and Cancer

Vitamin E probably works best as a cancer preventive. The Chinese Linxian Study showed that 30 IU of vitamin E, taken along with beta-carotene at 15 mg and selenium at 50 mcg, lowers the risk of dying from cancer by 13 percent.

Vitamin E has been found to prevent the growth of breast tumors and can help protect against bowel cancer. In population studies, high levels of vitamin E in the diet have been linked to a decreased risk of lung cancer and stomach cancer. In one study, two groups of hamsters were exposed to a strong carcinogen. The group given vitamin E did not get cancer; those in the group that did not get vitamin E all got cancer.

Vitamin E and Neurological Disease

One of the roles of vitamin E has to do with proper neurological functioning of the body. Vitamin E has been found to be deficient in many people who have neurological diseases, including Parkinson's, cystic fibrosis, and epilepsy. There is some evidence that it may help alleviate or lessen the symptoms of these types of diseases in some people. Vitamin E is an oil- or fat-soluble vitamin, which means that it can be stored in the liver. Toxicity studies have shown that 3,200 IU of vitamin E given daily to patients with Parkinson's disease did not have any side effects. This therapy did show a significant slowing of the progression of the condition. Some health practitioners believe that high doses of vitamin E can even prevent and reverse some neurological diseases.

Vitamin E and Your Hormones

A vitamin E deficiency decreases the production of all pituitary hormones, including ACTH, essential to stimulate the adrenals, and the hormones that stimulate the thyroid and sex glands. With regard to fertility, vitamin E may help prevent free-radical damage to the sperm.

How to Make Vitamin E Part of Your Daily Life

Vitamin E is not found in large amounts in any food, so it's a good idea to take a vitamin E supplement regardless of your diet. A *Lancet* report found vitamin E to be very safe compared to other fat-soluble vitamins, with few side effects reported, even at doses as high as 3,200 mg daily. I recommend, though, that you take from 400 to 800 IU (dry form) daily, with meals and in combination with two other important antioxidants, vitamin C and beta-carotene.

What's the Best Form of Vitamin E to Take?

In nature, vitamin E is made of substances called tocopherols. Some vitamin E is made of just one type of tocopherol, such as *d*-alpha-tocopherol, whereas other kinds are made from mixed tocopherols. If you are over the age of fifty, I recommend the *d*-alpha-tocopherol in succinate (dry) form, because it is easier to absorb than the oil.

Vitamin E also comes as an oil, in its natural form. Whether the oil or dry form is best for you depends on how your body works. If you need vitamin E for problems such as dry skin or hormonal balance, the oil form may work best.

There is a synthetic form of vitamin E called *dl*-alpha-tocopherol, which I *do not* recommend. It is not absorbed as well in the body and is also not retained as well. In fact, I do not recommend any synthetic vitamins, as they put unnecessary stress on the liver, which has to work harder to eliminate them.

What Foods Is Vitamin E Found In?

Vitamin E is found in dark green leafy vegetables, such as broccoli and kale, as well as in soybeans, eggs, wheat germ, organ meats, many of the nuts, and unrefined vegetable oils. Most vitamin E is made from soybeans.

How Vitamin E Can Help You

- Prevents and reverses heart disease
- Reduces oxidation of cholesterol
- Increases fertility
- Prevents damage to sperm
- Supports the adrenal glands
- Enhances production of steroid/ sex hormones
- Supports the thyroid gland
- Speeds wound healing
- Decreases the risk of cancer
- Reduces need for insulin intake in diabetics
- Prevents capillary damage in diabetics
- Decreases scarring
- Lessens the symptoms of some neurological diseases
- Prevents cataracts
- Prevents macular degeneration
- Protects the lungs against airborne pollutants

PCOs: THE "DO-EVERYTHING" SUPER ANTIOXIDANTS

Now that you know something about how antioxidants work, I want to tell you about the "super" antioxidants—the most powerful free-radical fighters known. The star of the super antioxidants is a complex of substances called proanthocyanidins, known for short as PCOs. I've told you how important bioflavonoids are to your health, and PCOs rank as our most powerful flavonoids.

Pine Bark Tea Got Indians and Sailors Through the Winter

For centuries, sailors exploring the world feared one thing more than typhoons and sea monsters, and that was scurvy, a fatal disease caused by vitamin C deficiency. In those days, however, they had no idea that their diet of biscuits and salted meat was causing disease. Early scientists who suggested that a lack of fresh fruits and vegetables might be the problem were laughed at and called quacks.

When the French explorer Jacques Cartier became trapped in the ice on the St. Lawrence River in the winter of 1534, his 110-man crew began dying of scurvy. Some 25 of them had died of this horrible disease, and 40 were not far from death, covered with sores and suffering from weakness, rotting gums, and swollen legs. A passing Indian named Agaya gave Cartier a tea made from pine bark, claiming that it would cure the men of just about anything they were ailing from. Sure enough, the tea worked, and the men rapidly recovered.

A Modern Researcher Discovers Grapeseed Extract

Some four centuries after pine bark tea saved Cartier's men, Professor Jacques Masquelier of the University of Bordeaux, France, read Cartier's account of the expedition and decided to study the components of pine bark. His research led him to identify substances called pycnogenols, a generic term he used to describe a large group of what are now called proanthocyanidin complexes. He later found that the proanthocyanidins were in grapeseed, lemon tree bark, peanuts, cranberries, and citrus peels. Groups of these molecules, now called oligomeric proanthocyanidin complexes (OPCs) or procyanidolic oligomers (PCOs), were found to be even more potent. With all the wine making in France, Masquelier soon found that grapeseeds were a cheaper and more potent source of PCOs than pine bark. He and others carried out extensive research on PCOs using grapeseed extract.

The term *pycnogenol* is now a registered commercial trademark of a Swiss company that sells PCO supplements extracted from pine bark. I personally recommend grapeseed extract because it was the substance used for most PCO research, it is more potent than pine bark, and it is less expensive.

Extensive research done on the PCO extract from grapeseed between 1951 and the late 1970s has shown it to be one of the most potent antioxidant substances known. It is fifty times more powerful at scavenging free radicals than vitamin E and twenty times more powerful than vitamin C. Furthermore, it enhances the potency of both these vitamins.

In addition to its ability to neutralize free radicals, grapeseed extract strengthens capillaries, veins, and arteries, increases intracellular vitamin C levels, and strengthens collagen, the basic building block of our skin, tendons, ligaments, and cartilage.

PCOs and Disease Prevention

If you suffer from memory loss, varicose veins, diabetes, heart disease, arthritis, high cholesterol, allergies, or macular degeneration, I recommend that you take a PCO supplement. This product has received more rave reviews from people with these illnesses than anything else I've recommended in years.

PCOs Prevent Heart Disease

I predict that in the not-too-distant future, we will be measuring antioxidant levels rather than cholesterol levels to predict the risk of heart disease. Nearly every symptom related to heart disease, such as a high level of oxidized LDL cholesterol, has a deficiency of antioxidants as its root cause. PCOs work specifically to stop "bad" cholesterol from forming, oxidizing, and sticking to your artery walls. They also prevent the artery damage that attracts oxidized cholesterol and lower the overall level of LDL cholesterol.

A number of studies have shown red wine to be protective against heart disease. Researchers agree that it's most likely the proanthocyanidins found in red wine that carry the protective factor. Another long-term heart disease study published in the prestigious medical journal *The Lancet* showed that the higher the bioflavonoid intake, the lower the risk of heart disease, and conversely, the lower the bioflavonoid intake, the higher the risk of heart disease.

Only relatively recently have the benefits of PCOs for a healthy heart become known. Scientists exploring the antioxidant abilities of PCOs found that these substances work on many fronts to nip oxidation reactions in the bud. They have the basic antioxidant ability to neutralize free radicals by trapping them. But PCOs are unique in that they not only neutralize a wide variety of free radicals in different stages of activation but actually *prevent* free-radical formation before it begins. PCOs can neutralize the free radicals associated with the by-products of cellular energy production, with rancid fats and oils, with excess iron, and with tissue inflammation and degradation. All these types of oxidation reactions can contribute to heart disease.

Add this potent ability to wipe out all types of free radicals to PCOs' ability to strengthen blood vessels (and capillaries in particular), and you have a powerful weapon against heart disease.

PCOs Improve Circulation and Protect Against Stroke

The fact that PCOs strengthen blood vessels makes them very important in reducing your risk of ailments associated with weak blood vessels, such as certain types of stroke. All diabetics, who nearly always eventually suffer from diseases of poor circulation, should be taking some type of bioflavonoid daily. Since PCOs seem to have the best ability to strengthen blood vessels, they should be at the top of the list.

The rupture of small blood vessels in your legs, called varicose veins, can be unsightly and uncom-

fortable, but the rupture of veins in you debilitating or even deadly. If you are stroke or have had one, I highly recomm make PCOs a permanent part of your da ment routine. Most strokes occur when the blood gets "sticky" and clots, creating a logjam effect in an artery to the brain or in the brain. PCOs help prevent platelet aggregation, the process of clotting that can lead to a stroke.

If you have varicose veins, PCOs could be your key to preventing any further formation. Of course, you should also get some daily exercise, drink plenty of water, and eat plenty of fiber, since a major cause of varicose veins is straining to have a bowel movement.

PCOs Improve Vision

A primary reason that eyesight fails as we age is that the blood supply becomes reduced. This can happen because capillaries rupture or become weak and unable to supply the eye with oxygen and nutrients. Two of the most crippling of these types of eye disorders are diabetic retinopathy and macular degeneration. Both have responded to PCOs in studies with humans.

PCOs also improve other aspects of eye health. In one study, one hundred volunteers with healthy eyes received 200 mg per day of PCOs or a placebo for five to six weeks, and a control group received no treatment. The PCO group had significant improvement in their night vision and after-glare vision compared to the placebo group.

PCOs Maximize Athletic Performance

PCOs are very useful for athletes who want to maximize their performance and minimize tissue damage. While PCOs are enhancing the ability of your blood to deliver oxygen to your cells by improving capillary action, they are also keeping your tissues strong and elastic and promoting rapid healing to tissues that may have been damaged by overexertion.

PCOs Keep You Looking and Feeling Young

Scientists who study the process of aging tend to agree that oxidation reactions are one of the primary causes of aging and diseases related to aging. Thus, it makes sense to protect against the physical toll that the years take by taking antioxidants. Because they are so potent and their effects so wide-ranging, PCOs may be one of our best antiaging supplements. They will work to keep your skin looking young, increase energy, and improve flexibility. They are protective against heart disease, cancer, stroke, and arthritis, the major diseases of the elderly.

How to Make PCOs Part of Your Daily Life

If you're over the age of fifty, I recommend that you include 50 mg of PCOs in your daily supplement regimen as an antiaging and preventive measure. If you're using it therapeutically for a specific ailment, you can take 150–300 mg daily.

I recommend the grapeseed PCO extract that comes in a "phytosome" package, meaning that the molecules are combined with phosphatidylcholine, a natural component of lecithin. This new process allows the body to absorb and utilize much more of the PCOs than it would otherwise.

GREEN TEA: HAVE A CUP OF SUPER ANTIOXIDANTS

Super antioxidants can come from unexpected sources. Who would have guessed that a humble little cup of green tea could protect you from cancer, heart disease, viruses, and a long list of other ills? That's right, green tea, the most popular of Asian drinks, turns out to have a long list of health benefits. And by the way, being the most popular Asian drink also makes green tea the most widely consumed beverage on the planet after water—some 2.5 million tons a year!

A British study evaluating the antioxidant activity of green tea, pouchong tea, oolong tea, and black tea extracts found that all of the tea extracts showed antioxidant activity. The antioxidants specific to green tea are bioflavonoids known as polyphenols, and the specific type of polyphenol found in green tea is called a catechin. About half the polyphenols in green tea are epigallocatechin gallate (EGCG), the most biologically active polyphenol. Other ingredients in green tea include the amino acid theanine, carotenoids, chlorophyll, and the proanthocyanidins also found in grapeseed extract, pine bark, bilberry, and ginkgo.

How PCOs Can Help You

- Lower your risk of heart disease
- Strengthen capillaries and blood vessels
- Increase vitamin C levels
- Inhibit the destruction of collagen (the substance that holds the skin together)
- Strengthen tendons, ligaments, and cartilage
- Reduce inflammation caused by arthritis
- Improve athletic performance by minimizing tissue injury and inflammation
- Enhance immune response
- Promote faster healing
- Combat cancer
- Retard the aging process
- Promote greater flexibility
- Lower your risk of heart disease

- Promote healthy, beautiful skin
- Reduce water retention and bloating
- Increase resistance to bruising
- Reduce susceptibility to colds and flu
- Improve night vision
- Improve "after-glare" vision
- Improve overall vision
- Prevent cataracts and macular degeneration
- Reduce PMS symptoms
- Enhance energy
- Improve memory
- Improve resistance to radiation
- Improve resistance to environmental toxins
- Reduce or eliminate allergy symptoms

While there are three thousand varieties of tea in the world, it is the variety called *Camellia sinensis* that is consumed in such quantities and has such health benefits. In the West, we're familiar with *Camellia sinensis* as black teas such as Earl Grey, orange pekoe, and English breakfast, which are crushed before drying to allow some fermentation to take place. Green tea comes from the same plants but is simply picked and dried without fermentation, allowing more of the original catechin content to remain intact. Oolong is a semifermented tea that falls in between black and green tea. Green tea contains 30 to 42 percent catechins; oolong tea contains 8 to 20 percent catechins; and black tea contains 3 to 10 percent catechins.

A cup of green tea contains about 35–50 mg of caffeine. In contrast, a cup of coffee contains 75–95 mg of caffeine. Contrary to popular opinion, tea does not contain tannins. It is the polyphenols that give it the acrid taste that reminds us of tannins.

Green Tea and Disease Prevention

The polyphenols in green tea act as super antioxidants by neutralizing harmful fats and oils, lowering cholesterol and blood pressure, blocking cancer-triggering mechanisms, inhibiting bacteria and viruses, improving digestion, and protecting against ulcers and strokes.

Green Tea Inhibits Cancer

The studies showing that green tea inhibits cancer are impressive. In one study, the lung cancer rate in mice fed green tea was reduced by 45 percent. Other animal studies suggest that green tea can cut the rate of stomach and liver cancer and slow the progress of skin cancer.

In Shizuoka Province in Japan, where green tea is produced and heavily consumed by residents, cancer rates are sharply lower than in other parts of the country. Green tea's protective effect may also explain why lung cancer rates are lower among Japanese smokers than among American smokers.

Because the rate of breast cancer is so low in Japan, much research has been done to find out whether green tea plays a protective role. Animal studies, population studies, and anecdotal evidence all suggest that green tea contributes significantly to Japan's lower breast cancer rates. In the largest study comparing the power of a variety of antioxidants to block breast cancer in animals, green tea catechins were the most potent inhibitors of the cancer.

Green tea has also been tested for its ability to protect against skin cancer, and once again came out a winner.

You've probably heard that substances called HCAs (heterocyclic amines) formed during the cooking (and especially the charring) of meat can be carcinogenic. Well, have a cup of green tea with your charbroiled meat, because green tea neutralizes those substances in the stomach. In one study, EGCGs (making up, as noted earlier, about half the catechin content of green tea) were 85 percent effective in reducing the formation of HCAs. Now, that's potent stuff!

With the wide variety of testing that has been done on green tea's cancer-blocking effects, I think it's safe to assume that green tea can make a significant positive difference with just about every type of cancer. Researchers believe that green tea blocks the progression of cancer by blocking the formation of cancer-causing compounds, suppressing the activation of already-present carcinogens, and trapping and neutralizing toxins that could promote cancer. According to Japanese studies, very low doses of green tea added to the water of laboratory rats prevented colon cancer, and an extract of EGCG prevented liver tumors from forming. A Chinese study showed that green tea powerfully inhibited intestinal cancer in rats.

Green Tea Keeps Viruses at Bay

The Chinese have studied various green tea extracts against many viruses, among them a form of HIV, hepatitis, and herpesviruses. In every case, the extracts significantly inhibited the activity of the viruses. This indicates that green tea enhances the ability of the immune system to stop viral attacks. Adding plenty of green tea to your winter diet should help keep the flu at bay.

Green Tea Promotes a Healthy Heart

Like other polyphenols, green tea promotes a healthy heart by preventing the oxidation of LDL cholesterol and raising the level of "good" HDL cholesterol. As a bonus, it also lowers triglyceride levels. In fact, in a series of Japanese studies, green tea extracts prevented oxidation in fatty substances better than glutathione, vitamin C, synthetic vitamin E (*dl*-alpha-tocopherol), and BHT, a synthetic antioxidant often used as a food preservative.

Green Tea Protects the Brain and Liver

It's important to keep your liver in tip-top shape so that it can efficiently dispose of waste and toxins in the body, and green tea has been shown to be protective of the liver. The same mechanism that protects your liver also protects your brain from oxidized fatty acids. One study showed green tea to be two hundred times more protective against oxidation in the brain than vitamin E.

Green Tea Is an Antibacterial

Maybe we should add green tea to our municipal drinking water instead of chlorine, because it powerfully protects against nearly all types of bacteria, including cholera, salmonella, and typhoid. And unlike antibiotics, green tea is selective about what bacteria it kills, leaving the "good" intestinal bacteria such as acidophilus and going after those that cause digestive disturbances and damage.

Green Tea Cures Gum Disease

A dentistry school in Japan tested the effectiveness of green tea in reducing gum disease and found that in some people, it completely cured severe gum disease.

How to Make Green Tea Part of Your Daily Life

There are a variety of ways to integrate green tea into your daily diet. One is to have a cup or two of the hot brew in the morning. In fact, replacing coffee with green tea might be one of the healthiest moves you could make. And you can replace iced black tea with iced green tea.

If sipping beverages isn't your cup of tea (sorry!), you can find green tea extract in capsules at your health food store. You need to drink a lot of green tea—ten to twenty cups a day—to take complete advantage of green tea's protective properties. Since that's way too much for most people (and more caffeine than I would recommend), if you have a specific illness that you want to prevent or treat with green tea, I recommend using the extract.

Ten to twenty cups a day represents about 1–2 g of polyphenols, 0.5–1 g of EGCGs, and 0.5–1 g of caffeine. The extracts contain a higher concentration of polyphenols and a lower concentration of caffeine. I would recommend taking one to two tablets or capsules of 30 percent polyphenol green tea extract daily, with meals, for disease treatment and prevention.

How Green Tea Can Help You

- Protects against breast cancer
- Protects against lung cancer
- Protects against colon cancer
- Protects against liver cancer
- Protects against intestinal cancer
- Protects against skin cancer
- Protects against stomach cancer
- Prevents oxidation reactions in the brain
- Acts as an antibacterial against harmful digestive bacteria
- Cures gum disease
- Lowers oxidized LDL cholesterol
- Raises HDL cholesterol
- Lowers triglycerides
- Inhibits viruses, such as HIV, hepatitis, and herpes
- Provides antioxidant protection against damaged arteries

GINKGO BILOBA: THE BETTER MEMORY SUPER ANTIOXIDANT

Ginkgo biloba is an herb that comes from one of the most ancient species of trees on the planet. These magnificent trees, which can grow to be huge, have been around for at least three hundred million years! Some people refer to ginkgo as a "living fossil." It's so old that it has no known living relatives—ginkgo is an entity unto itself. The very properties that have helped ginkgo survive over the millennia may very well be the same properties that give it such potent medicinal value. Ginkgo is sacred to the Buddhists and features prominently in Chinese and Japanese medicinal folklore.

You've probably seen ginkgo trees on the sidewalks of American city streets, where they are used both for their decorative value and their ability to withstand the ravages of air pollution, periods of heavy drought or rain, and competition from concrete sidewalks. The leaves have a distinctive fan shape with parallel veins and are divided up the middle.

The Chinese prize ginkgo leaves for their ability to improve blood flow to the brain, open up congested lungs, and improve blood flow to the extremities. Ginkgo has been used in Chinese medicine for at least five thousand years.

In the past decade or so, this amazing plant has been as well studied and researched as most pharmaceutical drugs. Ginkgo has been the subject of over three hundred scientific studies. It is one of the best-selling medicines in Europe, sold to an estimated ten million people there every year. GBE, a standardized ginkgo biloba extract, is a government-approved medicine in Germany and is covered by health insurance there. Ginkgo was reviewed in the prestigious British medical journal *The Lancet*, and it was suggested that it may be a powerful antiaging aid, particularly in regard to improving brain function.

Ginkgo and Disease Prevention

In general, ginkgo's healing abilities have to do with improving circulation and improving the flow of oxygen to the brain and extremities. However, its spectrum of activities is wide, thanks to the wide variety of substances it contains, including flavonoids, terpenoids (ginkgolides, bilobalide), ginkgo heterosides, proanthocyanidins (PCOs), and organic acids.

GBE, the standardized extract most widely used in Europe, contains 24 percent flavonoid glycosides and 6 percent terpenes. The flavonoids scavenge free radicals, protect against cell membrane damage, and inactivate harmful enzyme reactions. Ginkgolides can protect against stroke by keeping certain parts of the blood from clumping or clotting, and bilobalide may inhibit swelling of the brain. You're familiar with the PCOs, which in combination with the other ingredients in ginkgo reduce blood pressure.

Ginkgo Improves Circulation, Especially in Diabetics

In addition to improving circulation to the extremities, ginkgo improves "microcirculation," which is the blood flow into the tiny capillaries feeding into larger blood vessels. This makes it useful for treating vision problems such as cataracts and macular degeneration, as well as varicose veins, cold or numb feet and hands, and ringing of the ears (tinnitus).

One of my favorite ginkgo stories is of an elderly diabetic man who had a sore on his big toe that was down to the bone and wouldn't heal. His doctors wanted to amputate his foot. Naturally, he had some resistance to that idea, so he decided to try some ginkgo as a last resort. Within ten days, his toe had healed and his foot was a rosy pink color instead of its usual gray.

Ginkgo improves the symptoms of peripheral vascular disease, such as pains in the legs at night, cramps, numbness, and impotence. Studies show that taking ginkgo for several weeks, up to six months, brings about a 48 to 68 percent increase in walking distance.

Ginkgo's ability to improve blood flow to the brain and strengthen blood vessels contributes to its ability to protect against strokes caused by weakened blood vessels.

Ginkgo Can Help Dizziness, Vertigo, and Tinnitus

These three symptoms tend to go together, and ginkgo has been found to be effective in treating all of them, as well as the symptoms that tend to accompany vertigo, such as nausea, vomiting, headaches, and hearing difficulty. Those who suffered from vertigo were able to travel, turn their heads, and bend down without symptoms. The patients in the studies were given 60–160 mg of ginkgo extract daily, and they consistently showed a 40 to 80 percent improvement after one to three months of treatment. Even cases caused by disease or injury tended to respond favorably to ginkgo. These symptoms can be caused by impaired blood flow to the inner ear, making ginkgo the perfect medicine.

Ginkgo Boosts Brainpower

Ginkgo's best-known and most noticeable effects are in improving blood flow to the brain, with the result of improving memory and cognitive (thinking) abilities. It is thought that a large part of this effect is created by the action of the terpenes present in ginkgo, particularly one called ginkgolide. Ginkgolide inhibits platelet-activating factor (PAF), which is known to weaken blood vessels with the result of impairing blood flow to the brain.

Ginkgo is clearly effective and safe for treating what is called in medical circles "cerebral insufficiency," or impaired blood flow to the brain, particularly in parts of the brain where blood flow has been interrupted by damage. These effects also fall under the category of improving brain disorders caused by atherosclerosis, or blockage of blood vessels.

In some cases, ginkgo helps relieve and control the symptoms of Alzheimer's disease. This may be due to its unusual ability to enhance the effects of norepinephrine, which tends to be depleted in some areas of the brain in Alzheimer's patients.

In a French double-blind study of 166 patients with aging-related memory and cognitive problems, the treated group showed significant improvement compared to the untreated group after three months. The authors of the study noted that those who had the severest problems seemed to be the ones who were helped the most. The many similar studies done in England and Germany produced similar results. Some of the aspects of brain function tested were orientation, communication, mental alertness, recent memory, and freedom from confusion.

Ginkgo can improve the ability to remember, the speed of memory, and mental performance, as well as

other symptoms of cerebral insufficiency, such as headaches, dizziness, ringing in the ears, clumsiness, and hearing impairment.

The benefits of ginkgo are not restricted to the elderly. Ginkgo extracts have become popular among college students writing papers and preparing for exams.

Ginkgo Protects Against Heart Disease

Many of the same substances that give the other super antioxidants their heart-protecting power are found in ginkgo. In that respect, it lowers LDL cholesterol, reduces the amount of oxidized LDL cholesterol circulating, raises HDL cholesterol, and lowers triglyceride levels.

Ginkgo also protects against heart disease by improving circulation to the heart and improving the delivery of oxygen to the heart muscle.

Ginkgo Can Cure Leg Cramps

Intermittent claudication, a condition caused by restricted blood flow in the arms and legs, causes painful muscle cramping and difficulty walking. If you have intermittent claudication, keep walking as much as you can, because that will steadily improve your circulation. But you can also use ginkgo. In numerous studies, ginkgo has been shown to increase pain-free walking distance in those with intermittent claudication or any other circulation problems.

Ginkgo Protects the Eyes

Because ginkgo improves blood flow, it can also improve vision and prevent a range of vision problems caused by impaired blood flow, including cataracts. In both animal and human studies, ginkgo extracts decreased damage to retinal blood vessels induced by oxidation, and protected them from damage. The flavonoids present in ginkgo also contribute to its ability to strengthen the small blood vessels in the eye, improving both circulation and the delivery of other nutrients, including oxygen. When ginkgo was given to patients suffering from macular degeneration, 90 percent of the ginkgo group showed improvement in their vision, while only 20 percent of the control group showed improvement.

How to Make Ginkgo Part of Your Daily Life

Ginkgo may be one of our most important antiaging medicines. I know many, many people who swear by ginkgo and take it every day, and I recommend you do the same if you're over the age of sixty.

Ginkgo biloba has a delayed onset of action, and it may be a few weeks before you notice results, especially for problems such as tinnitus, which can take months to clear up. The effects of ginkgo do not generally show up after a single dose. It is not used in massive doses but in repeated doses that can produce beneficial effects over a relatively long period of time.

The best way to take ginkgo is in a liquid extract called GBE (ginkgo biloba extract) that is standardized. GBE is a concentrated and semipurified extract designed to enhance ginkgo's health benefits and provide a consistent level of ginkgolides, the most active principles.

I recommend that you find a GBE extract containing at least 24 percent ginkgo flavoglycosides. You can take 60 mg tablets, two to three times daily with food, or use the liquid preparations in a dosage of one to three dropperfuls up to three or four times a day, but check the label for recommendations.

SOY: THE SUPER ANTIOXIDANT ANTICANCER FOOD

If I've already got you drinking green tea, perhaps you're ready to try something else from Asia. Many scientists believe that the frequent consumption of soy foods is a major factor in Japanese health and longevity. Soy contains a fascinating combination of beneficial chemicals, many of which have antioxidant properties that make this food one of nature's healthiest choices.

Soy is the name for food made from soybeans. Soybeans are related to clover, peas, and alfalfa and are sometimes called soya. The beans are processed in different ways, making, for example, sauce, drinks, and curds.

Soy is one of the few plant foods that contains the proper balance of the eight essential amino acids. This makes it a valuable protein source, especially since it is also low in fat and high in fiber.

The Isoflavone Called Genistein Is Soy's Antioxidant Star

Isoflavones are compounds found in soy that contribute to its antioxidant powers. Study after study has shown

---

How Ginkgo Biloba Can Help You

- Improves memory
- Improves balance
- Improves ability to communicate
- Improves dizziness
- Improves headaches
- Improves hearing
- Relieves symptoms of senility
- Prevents and cures leg cramps
- Improves circulation
- Strengthens blood vessels
- Lowers LDL cholesterol and oxidized LDL cholesterol
- Raises HDL cholesterol

- Lowers triglycerides
- Improves circulation to the heart
- Improves circulation to the extremities
- Prevents and improves effects of poor circulation in diabetics
- Improves or cures tinnitus (ringing in the ears)
- Warms up cold hands and feet
- Improves vision
- Prevents cataracts
- Prevents macular degeneration
- Protects against stroke
- Protects against damage from head injuries

just how effective isoflavones can be, and one isoflavone in particular turns out to be a real star. Genistein came to the attention of the research community in the 1960s. It has already been the subject of about four hundred scientific papers, with more than thirty laboratory studies confirming that genistein inhibits the growth of cancer cells. The only source of genistein is soy.

One fascinating study found that when the diet of mice was supplemented with genistein for thirty days, there was a significant increase in the activity of antioxidants in their skin and small intestine. In another study, Japanese researchers were looking for anticancer agents produced by bacteria. The most effective substance found was not made by the bacteria at all. It was genistein, and it was found in the soy medium used to grow the bacteria!

It's a fact that autopsies of Japanese men show that prostate cancer is as common in Japan as it is in the United States, but the cancer seems to grow much more slowly—so slowly, in fact, that many men die without ever developing clinical disease. Now researchers suspect that genistein blocks the growth of these tumors. A Finnish researcher and his colleagues compared the levels of isoflavones in Japanese and Finnish men. The levels of isoflavones were more than one hundred times higher among the Japanese men, with genistein occurring in the highest concentration of any other isoflavone. The researchers' conclusion, published in *The Lancet*, was that maintaining a lifelong concentration of isoflavones in the blood could be the reason Japanese prostate cancers remain latent.

A 1990 study by scientists at the University of Alabama showed that genistein reduced the number of mammary tumors in breast cancer experiments on animals. The researchers found that genistein doesn't block just estrogen but also cancer cell growth.

All these studies and their results show that genistein, unique to soy, its fellow isoflavones, and other important components of soy are very interesting characters in the unfolding story of cancer prevention and protection.

Soy and Disease Prevention

If you would like to keep your cholesterol levels low and your cancer risk to a minimum, soy should be a regular part of your diet. Soy also reduces unpleasant menopausal symptoms, can lower the need for insulin in diabetics, and has been shown to aid in osteoporosis prevention.

Soy Lowers Cholesterol and Helps Prevent Heart Disease

There have been hundreds of studies examining the effect of various forms of soy on blood fat levels in both animals and people. Most have shown that soy is a powerful cholesterol buster. Its antioxidants work to prevent LDL (or "bad") cholesterol oxidation and help reduce blood cholesterol levels.

In one groundbreaking study, laboratory rabbits were fed a cholesterol-free diet containing 38 percent milk protein. Despite the cholesterol-free regimen, the rabbits on milk protein eventually developed high cholesterol and severe thickening and hardening of the main heart artery. However, when the milk protein was replaced with soy flour, the cholesterol levels stayed low and the rabbits remained healthy.

A Japanese study published in the *Annals of the New York Academy of Sciences* found that the oxidation of LDL, or "bad," cholesterol was greatly reduced in rabbits fed on soy milk.

A study in Milan found a similar preventive effect in a group of volunteers who were all on low-fat diets and had high cholesterol levels. Those adding soy to their diets saw a drop in their cholesterol within just two weeks, while levels did not fall in those not eating soy. Even when cholesterol was deliberately added to their diet, soy eaters still experienced the same drop in cholesterol.

In rare cases, children are born with a genetic tendency to develop extremely high cholesterol. In a recent study involving eleven children with very high cholesterol, researchers found that isolated soy protein could reduce LDL cholesterol more effectively than the standard low-fat diet. When isolated soy protein replaced the animal protein in their diet, the cholesterol levels dropped even further.

Soy is even given official recognition in Italy where the National Health Service provides soy protein free of charge to doctors for the treatment of high cholesterol. The evidence is in. Let's hope that many more countries will choose to help soy play a similar role in heart disease prevention.

Soy Cuts Cancer Risk

There is significant evidence that diets containing large amounts of soy products are associated with an overall reduction in cancer deaths. There are good studies showing its preventive effect in cancers of the colon, breast, prostate, lung, esophagus, and pancreas.

The proven anticancer effects of substances in soy are causing a real stir in the scientific community. Many studies have been prompted by the fact that Asian populations have markedly lower cancer rates than those in the West. Dietary factors are very important and are seen, for example, in Asian immigrants to the United States who rapidly assume the risks of prostate cancer and breast cancer seen in Americans.

Possibly the most effective cancer blockers in soybeans are the isoflavones. They resemble the hormone estrogen, so they occupy estrogen receptors, but they don't behave like estrogens, which in excess are well-known carcinogens. Isoflavones are thousands of times weaker than the estrogens and actually act as anticancer compounds. This is similar to the way tamoxifen, the most widely used drug in breast cancer treatment, works. A study carried out in Cincinnati and England shows that isoflavones can be an effective treatment for premenopausal women with breast cancer and other cancers associated with estrogen.

A 1991 Singapore study, reported in *The Lancet*, found that the risk of breast cancer in those who rarely ate soy foods was twice as high as for those who ate soy frequently. This was after all other foods and lifestyle habits were accounted for.

A similar cancer comparison even shows up within the United States. A Harvard researcher found that Americans in South Dakota and Wyoming who regularly ate soybeans had less than half the risk of getting colon cancer as those who didn't eat soy.

The National Cancer Institute released a report showing that soy inhibits cancers of the mouth.

Some soy antioxidants are poorly absorbed in the intestines and go directly to the colon. Once there, these substances play an important role in reducing the development of colon tumors.

Japanese experiments with soy show that the antioxidants found in soy prevent cellular mutations that would lead to cancer. In the laboratory, soy antioxidants prevent cellular DNA from being attacked by carcinogens.

Soy Reduces Menopause Symptoms

Did you know that there is no word to describe "hot flash" in Japanese? In fact, many studies show that most Japanese women never experience hot flashes and complain of far fewer unpleasant symptoms of menopause than do Western women.

A recent Canadian study of Japanese women and menopause reported that hot flashes were mentioned by only 12 of the 105 women interviewed, and no one talked about night sweats. Another study compared menopausal Japanese, Canadian, and U.S. women. The Japanese women had far fewer physical and mental complaints than did the Western women. While over 30 percent of both the Americans and Canadians experienced hot flashes, lack of energy, and depression, the figures for the Japanese women did not go above 12.4 percent. In fact, researchers reported that few Japanese women were on hormone replacement, but they did use more herbs and herbal teas.

Many scientists now agree that diet, including the amount of soy products, is a major factor in accounting for results like these.

Soy Lowers Need for Insulin in Diabetics

Diabetics can reduce the amount of insulin they need by including a product made from soybean fiber. It can also be useful in weight control. This was a discovery made by Dr. Yoram Kanter, head of the Diabetes Service and Research Unit at a hospital in Haifa, Israel.

Soy and Cataracts

A Columbia University animal study suggests that genistein has the ability to inhibit the formation of cataracts. This probably reflects its ability to act as an antioxidant in the oxygen-rich parts of the eye.

Soy for Healthy Kidneys

People with kidney disease would do well to make soy their main source of protein. Soy is one of the few complete plant proteins and has been shown to be much easier on the kidneys than protein derived from a meat diet.

Soy Fights Osteoporosis

Osteoporosis is the thinning down of bones, leaving them weak and vulnerable to fracture. It is a disease of aging and is related to a variety of factors, including exercise, diet, protein intake, and the production of hormones. Theoretically, Caucasian and Asian women, especially those who are thin boned and petite, run a much greater risk of osteoporosis. However, even though Asian women are small boned, they have far fewer hip injuries than do Caucasian women. In fact, Japanese women have roughly half the hip injuries of U.S. women, and women in Hong Kong and Singapore fare even better. Excess protein causes calcium to be leached from the bones. Soy consumption results in far less calcium loss than does animal protein. This was demonstrated in a study by the University of Texas Health Sciences Center. Volunteers replacing animal products with soy foods in their diet saw a 50 percent drop in calcium in their urine.

Other studies suggest that the isoflavones in soy may help retain bone mass. Recently, two University of North Carolina animal studies showed that low-dose genistein was almost as effective as a synthetic estrogen in preventing bone loss in rats without a natural supply of estrogen.

How to Make Soy Part of Your Daily Life

Japanese men consume between 40 and 70 mg of genistein per day. U.S. men eat less than 1 mg. We need to change those numbers for both men and women. I recommend that you make soy part of your daily diet.

There are many, many ways to incorporate soy into your diet, from soy protein powders to soy milk, miso soup, and tofu. My book *Earl Mindell's Soy Miracle* (Simon and Schuster, 1995) will give you lots of recipes and helpful tips on making soy a part of your diet.

Soy comes in many different forms, including soy milk, tofu, tempeh, miso, soy sauce, and flour. These are all made in different ways, including fermenting, soaking, grinding, frying, steaming, and sprouting.

Studies on which forms of soy confer the most health benefits show that tempeh and tofu are among the best ways to eat soy. Soy sauce contains the least amount of beneficial nutrients and is high in sodium, so I don't recommend it in large quantities.

Remember, soy can't do the job on its own. Make it a part of a diet low in fat, high in fiber, and rich in other whole foods and vitamins.

How Soy Can Help You

- Prevents heart disease
- Lowers LDL cholesterol
- Reduces menopause symptoms
- Prevents many types of cancer
- Prevents cataracts
- Maintains healthy kidneys
- Reduces diabetics' need for insulin
- Helps prevent osteoporosis

GLUTATHIONE AND CYSTEINE: THE ANTIAGING ANTIOXIDANTS

Glutathione (known as GSH) defends the body against oxidation and toxins on three major fronts. This humble little protein is found in the cells of nearly all living organisms on earth, and its primary job is waste disposal.

GSH has three main detox jobs in the body:

1. When there are free radicals lurking about, threatening to start an oxidation reaction, GSH catches them, neutralizes them, passes them on (often to another antioxidant such as vitamin E), and begins the cycle anew.

2. In the liver, GSH latches on to toxic substances and binds to them, so that the liver can excrete them without being damaged.
3. GSH prevents red blood cells from being damaged by neutralizing unstable forms of oxygen.

We literally cannot survive without this miraculous antioxidant. GSH also plays a role in fighting cancer, stabilizing blood sugar, and repairing cells after a stroke.

As glutathione does its detox work, it transforms itself into a number of different substances, including an enzyme, while always retaining its basic structure. Each substance has a different name, such as glutathione peroxidase and glutathione disulfide, but for the purposes of this chapter, we'll use GSH or glutathione as a generic term for the whole spectrum of glutathione transformations.

How We Deplete—and Replace—Glutathione

GSH levels drop as we age and can also be depleted by:

- Chronic diseases such as cancer and arthritis
- An overload of rancid oils (such as polyunsaturated and partially hydrogenated vegetable oils)
- Overexposure to poisons such as pesticides
- Pharmaceutical drugs that stress the liver, such as acetaminophen (Tylenol) and aspirin
- Birth control pills and hormone replacement therapy

Moreover, because glutathione often passes off its neutralized waste products to antioxidants such as vitamins C and E and also needs the minerals selenium, copper, and zinc to do its cleanup work, a deficiency of these vitamins and minerals can impair its function.

Because glutathione is so unstable by nature, it is difficult to stabilize in a supplement. However, cysteine, when taken as a supplement, will raise glutathione levels. Cysteine is used routinely in hospital emergency rooms to prevent liver damage when people overdose on drugs or alcohol; to detoxify in cases of heavy-metal poisoning; and to protect against the harmful side effects of chemotherapy and radiation. Cysteine is currently being used successfully to raise T cell levels in AIDS patients.

The most commonly used form of cysteine is *N*-acetylcysteine, known as NAC. It has been used in Europe for thirty years to treat a variety of lung diseases involving excess mucus production.

It is important not to take too much cysteine, since the body works hard to keep it in just the right balance.

Supplementation with selenium and vitamin E can also raise glutathione levels in the body.

Glutathione and Cysteine and Disease Prevention

Glutathione's antioxidant work is the frontline defense for preventing oxidation of LDL cholesterol, which damages the arteries. It's also crucial in protecting the lymphatic system and the digestive system from an overload of unstable fatty molecules. It maintains the integrity of red blood cells and prevents damage to them. If glutathione levels drop anywhere in the body, the burden of toxic stress goes up.

Cells with decreased levels of glutathione are more susceptible to the harmful effects of radiation, free radicals, and many pharmaceutical drugs.

In addition to the many benefits of glutathione, supplementing it may be useful in modulating blood sugar in diabetics and in boosting performance in athletes. There is also evidence that raising glutathione levels in stroke victims can significantly reduce injury to the brain.

GSH is one of the most abundant substances in the body, and as long as we have a good supply of its building block cysteine (glycine and glutamic acid are rarely in short supply) and its cofactor selenium, it will be hard at work doing its detoxifying chores.

Glutathione Keeps the Elderly Healthy

Glutathione levels drop as we age, which no doubt contributes greatly to the aging process and diseases of aging. A study done in England in a community of elderly people showed that low glutathione levels were associated with a 24 percent higher rate of illness and death, higher cholesterol, and higher body weight. Those who had heart disease, cancer, arthritis, and diabetes had significantly lower levels of glutathione than those who were healthy.

Many elderly people suffer from malnutrition because they are unable to shop or cook healthy foods or because their digestive system is working inefficiently and they aren't absorbing nutrients. This leads to a depletion of antioxidants in the tissues, setting the stage for cancer to take hold.

Cysteine Breaks Up Mucus in the Lungs

NAC is used in Europe for coughs, asthma prevention, and chronic bronchitis because it is very effective at breaking up mucus in the lungs. A lung infection gets serious when the mucus gets so thick that you can't cough it up. Cysteine is currently undergoing clinical trials in Europe to find out how well it works at preventing lung disease.

Cysteine liquefies the mucus, making it easy to cough up. If you have a tendency to get a winter cough, put some NAC in the medicine cabinet and take it at the first sign of lung troubles.

Glutathione and Cysteine Boost the Immune System

An important study done in Germany showed that HIV-infected humans and SIV-infected monkeys had low levels of cysteine and glutathione. Raising the levels of these substances increased T cells, a key marker of good immune system function. In the published study, the authors hypothesized that part of the mechanism that causes those who are HIV positive to develop AIDS is very low cysteine and glutathione levels. A number of anecdotal reports suggest that cysteine supplements are helping dramatically in HIV-infected people.

Try cysteine supplements if you have any type of acute viral infection, such as the flu, or a chronic viral infection, such as herpes. While this is still experimental, there is enough evidence to warrant trying it.

If you're fighting a serious virus, don't make the mistake of thinking that megadoses of cysteine will work better than the recommended doses. You will only stress your body's systems further if you take too much cysteine.

Glutathione and Cysteine Keep Cancer at Bay

Some cancer researchers theorize that one way cancer gets a foothold in the body is by taking advantage of cell weakness caused by oxidation. When free radicals are running amok, cancer cells have an opportunity to get into a cell, damage its DNA, and get their own growth pattern going.

Here are some of the ways that glutathione and cysteine may prevent and reverse cancer:

- By neutralizing free radicals
- By blocking the action of toxins that are carcinogenic
- By preventing carcinogens from interfering with DNA
- By preventing carcinogens from altering chromosomes
- By suppressing the action of cancer promoters, such as excess estrogen
- By suppressing the growth of tumors

A study done in India with women suffering from cervical cancer found that the further the disease progressed, the lower the levels of cysteine and glutathione dropped and the higher the levels of lipid peroxides, harmful oxidized fatty substances.

A report from scientists in the Netherlands on using cysteine to treat lung cancer points out that tumor growth can only happen when detoxification pathways are saturated. They state that cysteine provides protection against mutagens and carcinogens at many different stages.

Glutathione and Cysteine Protect the Digestive System

Glutathione also works hard to keep the digestive system healthy, neutralizing free radicals, particularly those caused by unstable fats and oils. It indirectly keeps digestion healthy by being a key part of the liver's ability to detoxify the body. In a small Italian study of people with Crohn's disease (a serious chronic bowel disorder), it was found that levels of glutathione were much lower in those with Crohn's disease than in controls. Some preliminary data suggest that cysteine supplements may be useful in treating Crohn's disease and other bowel disorders.

Glutathione and Cysteine Are Crucial for Eye Health

The health of the eye, and in particular the macula, is dependent on a long list of antioxidants and their cofactors. This includes vitamins C and E and beta-carotene; the minerals zinc, selenium, and copper; superoxide dismutase; and glutathione and riboflavin.

We've known since the early 1900s that *all* people with cataracts have low levels of glutathione in the lens of the eye. In a study from the National Cataract Study Group, it was reported that there was approximately a 35 percent reduction in cataract formation in the study group with the higher antioxidant levels. Another group reports a reduction in vision loss among those taking zinc supplements.

Low glutathione levels are also directly related to macular degeneration. The macula of the eye is an oxygen-rich environment where there's a large turnover of oxygen, generating a large amount of free radicals. Several studies have indicated that higher blood concentrations of antioxidants such as glutathione, beta-carotene, and vitamins C and E are associated with lower levels of macular degeneration.

Glutathione and Cysteine Promote Heart Health

Underlying many of the risk factors for heart disease is a deficiency of antioxidants, which allows arteries to be damaged and oxidized cholesterol to float around in the bloodstream, where it will attach itself to the damaged arteries. Glutathione is the body's first line of defense against oxidation of cholesterol. An Italian animal study even suggests that giving cysteine supplements after a heart attack could greatly reduce damage done to the heart.

How to Make Glutathione and Cysteine Part of Your Daily Life

Measuring glutathione levels is expensive at this time, but if you have heart disease, are at a high risk for it, or have high LDL cholesterol levels, I recommend that you try raising your glutathione levels. The best way to raise glutathione levels is by taking a cysteine supplement, preferably in the more stable form of NAC (*N*-acetylcysteine).

To convert the cysteine to glutathione, you also need vitamins C and E, beta-carotene, and selenium. One of the best food sources of cysteine is eggs, which I encourage you to eat a few times a week, since they are full of nutrition and in most people won't raise LDL cholesterol, in spite of rumors to the contrary.

Other foods that contain high levels of cysteine include watermelon, onions, garlic, yogurt, wheat germ, and red meat. The cruciferous vegetables, such as broccoli, cauliflower, and cabbage, stimulate the body's production of glutathione.

The recommended dosage of NAC is 500 mg one to four times daily. Over that amount can upset the balance of your body's chemistry just as much as a deficiency can.

How Glutathione and Cysteine Can Help You

- Prevent cataracts
- Prevent macular degeneration
- Prevent cancer
- Suppress tumor growth
- Detoxify the liver, cells, and lymphatic system
- Break up mucus in the lungs
- Prevent heart disease
- Prevent arthritis
- Prevent diabetes
- Stabilize blood sugar
- Protect the digestive system
- Boost the immune system
- Slow the aging process
- Boost athletic performance
- Reduce injury to the brain caused by stroke
- Reduce damage to the heart from a heart attack
- Reduce cholesterol
- Protect red blood cells from damage
- Prevent LDL cholesterol from being oxidized
- Protect cells from oxidation damage

3 TRACE MINERALS ~

THE ROLE OF TRACE MINERALS

The story of minerals is as old as the earth, with billions of years of participation in the very formation of life on this planet. Before animal and vegetable, there was mineral in the form of chemical elements such as iron and silicon. Primeval rains created the first oceans and washed minerals into the seas, quickening the pace of evolution in the first chapter of life.

The sciences of biochemistry, physics, and geology continue to unravel the mysteries of the minerals needed for life. According to a *New York Times* story about sulphur, some researchers believe that the asteroid collision thought to have led to the extinction of the dinosaurs resulted in wide distribution of the trace element sulfur. The asteroid was especially rich in sulphur and is thought to have vaporized, creating more than 100 billion tons of mainly sulphur dioxide in the atmosphere, increasing the availability of sulphur for the life-forms that evolved after the dinosaurs.

What Are Minerals?

To be technical, minerals are inorganic chemical elements. Inorganic means not bound to carbon. Sometimes minerals are described as inorganic when they have not been dissolved in water or transformed by plants. "Inorganic" minerals are harder for the body to absorb than those in organic form. While the chemical structure of the minerals themselves doesn't change, they may be attached to other molecules that give them different properties.

Since the origin of multicellular life, minerals have been important for their ability to bond to themselves and other substances in animals and plants. In this way, they help create important chemical compounds. The trace mineral cobalt is a component of vitamin B_{12}, and iron is a part of hemoglobin. A total of about twenty-two dietary minerals are needed for optimum human health.

Rocks remain the original source of minerals, since living matter cannot synthesize them as it can most vitamins. Fortunately, we don't have to serve up pebbles and stones with our meals! Nature has instead provided pathways for minerals, taking them from soil and water to plants and animals. Wise eating, drinking, and use of supplements ensures that we take in just enough dietary minerals to keep our bodies fully functional.

What Are Trace Minerals?

Everyone has heard of the essential minerals calcium and magnesium, but relatively few know of the importance of the trace minerals, such as chromium, vanadium, and selenium. Although the trace minerals comprise less than 4 percent of our total body weight, their presence, absence, or imbalance can mean the difference between health and illness—and even between life and death.

In a 150-pound body, some 2 to 3 pounds is the mineral calcium, which we need to get from the food we eat. Vanadium, in contrast, would be difficult even to measure, and yet it is a trace mineral that in the form of the compound vanadyl sulfate can help reverse adult-onset diabetes.

The definition of what exactly a trace mineral is varies, but in general it is a mineral that makes up less than 0.01 percent of body weight. The major minerals, or macrominerals, each make up more than 0.01 percent of body weight. Although a few trace minerals, such as zinc, are needed in milligram amounts daily, most are needed in only microgram amounts. Trace minerals are sometimes called trace elements, and those needed to maintain health are called *essential* trace minerals or elements.

The macrominerals essential to human health are calcium, phosphorus, magnesium, potassium, sodium, and chloride. The trace minerals we will cover in some detail in this chapter, either because they are essential to optimal health or because they can play a key role in healing, are boron, chromium, cobalt, copper, fluorine, iodine, iron, lithium, manganese, molybdenum, selenium, vanadium, and zinc. Trace minerals that are found in the body but which are poisonous in very small amounts when inhaled, absorbed, or ingested include arsenic, aluminum, cadmium, lead, mercury, nickel, and tin. Toxicity caused by these metals is largely a result of by-products of manufacturing and pollution.

What Do Trace Minerals Do?

The tiniest amounts of trace minerals are all that is needed to keep body functions running smoothly, but a deficiency has quite obvious effects. For example, in the absence of only a little over a millionth of an ounce of iodine, the thyroid gland enlarges.

The nutritional role of copper and iron may have been unknown in ancient times, but along with other minerals, they were believed to possess spiritual powers. Although the story of essential trace minerals and humans began hundreds of thousands of years ago, it remained mostly untold until the twentieth century. In 1928, just three trace elements were recognized: iron, which was found in the seventeenth century to be needed for healthy blood; iodine, shown in 1859 to prevent goiter (thyroid deficiency); and copper, found in 1928 to be needed for the absorption and utilization of iron. In the ensuing decades, other trace minerals were found to play a role in maintaining health. It wasn't until the 1980s that boron and vanadium were added to the list of important trace minerals.

Vitamins cannot function without trace minerals. Trace minerals also play a role in regulating hormones, enzymes, amino acids, and the immune system. They are required to build and maintain the structure of the body, to maintain proper brain function and blood sugar balance, and to keep the intestines healthy and fully functioning. In other words, trace minerals are involved in every aspect of health and balance in the human body. Whereas the body can synthesize certain vitamins, it cannot manufacture a single trace mineral and can withstand a deficiency of vitamins longer than a deficiency of minerals. In turn, vitamins play a role in the uptake and utilization of trace minerals.

Although trace mineral consumption is tiny compared to that of energy-providing foods, they perform fundamental chemical tasks in an extremely wide range of vital animal and plant functions. While many "major" minerals, such as calcium and magnesium, are needed in milligram amounts, most trace minerals are needed in only microgram amounts. But the small quantities of minerals required are no measure of their importance in the human body. True, the minute amounts of trace minerals needed meant that their importance was largely undiscovered until the twentieth century. But once uncovered, the activity of trace minerals opened a giant chest of subtle but very powerful tools for fine-tuning the body for optimal health, increasing the benefits of exercise, and even preventing cancer, heart disease, and diabetes.

Where Are Trace Minerals Found?

Trace minerals are washed from rocks into streams and lakes, and they are naturally found in food. Tiny mineral particles also form layers of subsoil and are absorbed by water passing by or through. Plants need minerals to function and have evolved methods for absorbing them efficiently from soil and water. In turn, animals meet most of their mineral needs by eating plants. Humans meet their mineral needs by eating both plants and animals and by drinking water. The cycle continues as humans, animals, and plants die, eventually returning their mineral content to the environment.

It is impossible to specify the quantities of any trace mineral likely to be found in foods. Soil conditions, time of year, weather, and environmental pollution all influence mineral levels. The way a trace mineral is chemically packaged within a food is as important as its quantity. Different mineral compounds are absorbed differently during digestion. Spinach, for example, has traditionally been considered a rich source of iron. In fact, it contains iron oxalate, which makes the iron only partially available to the human body. Parsley offers a form of iron that is much easier for the body to assimilate.

Knowing which foods are typically high in a particular trace mineral is useful when it comes to planning a healthy diet. Just one Brazil nut (find an unshelled, organically grown one if possible) a day, for example, can provide a daily dose of selenium. However, it remains important to eat a variety of foods to increase the number of sources and varieties of trace minerals in the diet.

THE POWER OF TRACE MINERALS

Copper, iron, manganese, and zinc are trace minerals needed by all bacteria, algae, fungi, and higher plants for survival. Boron is required by green plants and algae; some also need cobalt and molybdenum. This has been true for billions of years, since the first primitive organisms in the world's oceans began to develop. As life evolved, relatively advanced chemical structures were created, with minerals as major components. One such structure was chlorophyll, the substance in plants that uses the energy of light to convert carbon dioxide and water to carbohydrates. At the center of chlorophyll is the major mineral magnesium. In this way, the same silver-white flaring metal used in flashbulbs and fireworks is crucial to any vegetable or part of a grazing animal you might eat.

The trace mineral molybdenum is used by blue-green algae and other plant life to turn nitrogen into a usable compound essential to all life. Wherever we turn, minerals are in action contributing to processes that are key to life on earth.

In humans, trace minerals are involved in protein, hormone, and vitamin formation, as well as in immunity, muscle function, and nerve transmission. Zinc, for example, is used in practically every cell process. The strong, consistent structure of minerals makes them essential in the body's structures, from the cal-

cium, phosphorus, and boron in the bones to silicon, which is an important component of collagen, the principal structural component found in skin. Silicon forms long, complex molecules, suitable for parts of the body, like skin, that need to be strong and flexible. Vitamin C is another major component of collagen.

Minerals are well known for their role as catalysts, speeding up chemical reactions in the body. Catalysts help the formation or breakdown of substances to occur with less energy than the original chemicals involved would need on their own. Needing less energy, life processes such as digestion and healing can occur more quickly and efficiently. Without catalysts, many essential biological reactions would take place too slowly to sustain life. Throughout any reaction, in a very neat arrangement, catalysts themselves remain unchanged, ready for reuse. The trace mineral molybdenum, for example, activates an enzyme (another type of catalyst) that detoxifies harmful preservative compounds called sulfites.

You could say that minerals act as wheelbarrows, forklifts, gears, conveyor belts, and electronic switches in the factory of the body, assisting at every step from unloading the fuel trucks and stoking and damping the boilers to switching the wiring and oiling the machinery.

The importance of all this work? Tachycardia—rapid heartbeat—can be caused by a lack of potassium; diabetes can be brought on by a shortage of chromium and zinc; anemia can be caused by a lack of iron through a deficiency of cobalt, which is also required in vitamin B_{12} and is needed for the absorption of iron.

Prevention of disease through adequate mineral uptake should be a natural result of our nutritional intake. The increasing pollution, intensive farming, deforestation, food refining, and use of medical drugs during the twentieth century, however, have depleted dietary minerals and increased our exposure to minerals that are toxic in small amounts. The need is greater than ever to ensure an adequate mineral supply for anyone interested in maintaining good health.

The Electrolyte Power of Minerals

The best minerals come shaken, not stirred. Minerals are at their most powerful in forms that conduct electricity. Electrically charged minerals are known as ionized salts, or electrolytes. Electrolytes are produced naturally as minerals are swept up and tumbled by water rushing past rocks. Homeopathic medicines, often diluted forms of minerals, are produced by deliberately simulating this natural process through vigorous shaking. The electrical charge of electrolytes makes them valuable triggers of processes in cells. Ionized mineral particles are small enough to pass directly through cell walls, bypassing the digestive process, to be absorbed within minutes of being taken. In this way, minerals can act like a charge to cells, which in turn are like batteries supplying energy to the body.

Solutions of ionized minerals are described as "crystalloid." Crystalloid solutions increase the availability of minerals to the body. Minerals also exist in more inert forms as parts of "colloid" suspensions. *Colloid* is the term used for fairly large particles unable to dissolve but able to remain partially suspended in water. Minerals in colloidal form do not pass through animal and plant membranes as easily as electrolytes in crystalloid solutions. The best of both worlds would be to combine ionized and colloidal minerals in one supplement. If they are packaged in soy phosphatide microspheres, they can be absorbed through the membranes in the mouth. With this type of delivery system, the minerals can be absorbed directly into the bloodstream rather than having to pass through the harsh digestive system.

Soil and plants in good condition contain all the ingredients necessary to ionize colloidal minerals, preparing them for absorption. Similarly, a healthy diet ensures a nutritionally balanced body that is adapted to absorb minerals. Hydrochloric acid softens minerals, making sure, with the help of vitamins, that they travel from the gut and into the bloodstream. Once in the bloodstream, vitamins and other substances help to ionize minerals as necessary, which enables them to move into the tissues of the body, where they are required.

Mineral supplements become necessary because modern farming, irrigation, pollution, and water cleansing have produced food and water supplies robbed of electrolytes. Food produced using modern methods may be cheaper, but it is a nutritional rip-off. Buy organic as much as you can, and rest assured that the extra dollars are harnessing valuable electrolyte power.

HOW MINERALS ARE DEPLETED FROM THE SOIL

Evolution has led to a system in which minerals move from soil and water to plants, animals, and humans. Sustainability marks the beauty of the system, as minerals return intact to soil and water through the rot and decay of organic matter. Until the industrial revolution of the nineteenth century, the cycle of minerals was mainly undisturbed, and vegetables, meat, fish, and dairy foods were reliable sources of most minerals.

Ironically, as science continues to reveal more and more about the value of minerals, they have become less and less available from food. The story behind this unhappy scenario is largely one of refined foods, medical drugs, chemical fertilizers, pollution, and deforestation. The mineral depletion so evident in today's crop-growing soils and fast foods is reflected in the depleted state of health of people all over the world, with escalating rates of killer illnesses like cancer and heart disease.

Bringing our individual mineral intakes up to par is an important dietary action. It's also worth remembering that our own actions as consumers, workers, drivers, and gardeners are influencing the minerals of the world we live in.

Soil Loss Is Mineral Loss

The mineral-rich result of one hundred to one thousand years of natural processes is 1 inch of topsoil rich in minerals and other nutrients. An unprotected layer of soil ten times this thick can disappear in the trail of a bulldozer or the puff of a violent storm. Environmentally unsound farming practices and the paving of civilization have led to a steady depletion of a precious natural resource the world over.

According to Bernard Jensen and Mark Anderson in the important book *Empty Harvest* (Avery Publishing, 1993), when pioneers first crossed North America, they settled on land with topsoil 18 to 25 inches deep. Today, the figure in most states is around 6 inches, often less. Out of the total measurement of soil erosion in the United States, 90 percent occurs on farmland. Midwestern states like Wyoming and Nebraska have seen their soils literally blown away, creating huge "dust bowls" where farmers once led prosperous lives. The days of the farming disasters of the Great Plains are still with us. North Dakota lost 3.5 million acres of topsoil to wind in 1988 alone. In the drought years of 1988–89, soil loss through wind and water was estimated at 6 billion tons per year.

The U.S. Department of Agriculture estimates that a 6-inch loss of topsoil can reduce crop yields by 40 percent a year. Until topsoil is seen as a complex store of minerals and organic matter of great value, it will be easy to abuse. Often soil has been seen only as a useful medium because it holds plants upright and can receive the water they need. The loss of essential dietary minerals has gone unnoticed. The remaining land has been forced to produce more food artificially and unsustainably. Salty, overirrigated soils and creeping desert conditions are two of the results— hardly conducive to good human nutrition.

Keeping Our Soil Mineral Rich

In its natural state, quality soil is 45 percent minerals and is full of "good" bacteria. A teaspoon of good soil contains billions of living creatures. Soil is the major source of nutrients for most plants. Mineral-rich soil supports soil microbes that break down anything falling onto the soil, from dead leaves to picnic leftovers. In this way, matter is rotted down into its basic elements, including minerals, which then form part of the soil. This cycle keeps soil mineral rich in a self-perpetuating cycle.

People often forget that bacteria are not usually disease agents but actually perform very useful functions. Only when there are not enough bacteria to do the work required or the bacteria start to function where they are not needed does trouble begin. What prevents bacteria from devouring living plants? Plants are protected by a natural balance of fungi and bacteria. The fungi, called mycorrhizae, live along plant rootlets and secrete toxins that act against bacteria. The toxins, in a word, are antibiotics, just like the famous example produced from the *Penicillium* mold. By fending off bacteria, the mycorrhizae play an essential part in plant immunity and help create healthy crops.

When the uptake of minerals is out of balance, the result is deformity or deficiency. Mycorrhiza fungi help plants keep their mineral intake in balance. If mycorrhizae did not act as a buffer, plants would simply absorb minerals in proportion to the amounts found in soil, which would not necessarily match the plants' need for each mineral. The mycorrhizae perform this balancing action by binding needed minerals to protein, a process known as chelating. Chelation ensures that plants take in the minerals they need rather than the minerals in greatest quantity around them.

Healthy soil, then, is rich in bacteria that recycle matter into its basic elements, which in turn help keep soil bacteria rich. Plants benefit from the products of soil bacteria and don't get rotted down themselves because they are protected by fungi. Mycorrhiza fungi also protect plants from over- and underconsumption of the minerals they need. Such natural checks and balances in soil and plant life pay wonderful dividends to human beings in strong, healthy crops that can never be bettered by artificial, unnatural tinkering. And of course, when we eat plants with the right balance of trace minerals, we're consuming the trace minerals essential for our own good health.

Artificial Fertilizers and Pesticides Lead to Mineral Loss

Topsoil loss is bad enough. The quality of the soil remaining is in many ways producing a slow starvation— not of calories, but of minerals. Since the industrial revolution and the technological advances of the nineteenth and twentieth centuries, farming itself has become an industry. Early scientific discoveries focused on boosting plant growth and killing agents of crop disease. Human-made fertilizers and pesticides did in fact produce initial dramatic increases in crop yields and led to a large-scale shift from traditional farming practices.

The invention of the tractor in the early twentieth century distanced farmers even more from soil as the most vital resource of their work. Land began to be overworked and underfed at an unprecedented rate. It no longer seemed necessary to let fields lie fallow for a time or to dig crop remains back into the soil. Soil-rejuvenating crops known to host beneficial bacteria were no longer grown in years between crops reared for greater profit. Deficient soils unable to support livestock profitably were forced to grow crops for humans.

Soils in many areas have now become so deficient in enzymes, microbes, worms, and insect life that crop remnants sit unrotted and do not become compost.

Science produced powerful chemicals in the form of pesticides that could kill disease-producing organisms in plants. Pesticides changed the focus of farming from raising strong crops to treating sick ones or eliminating sources of sickness.

Chemical fertilizers are also part of the trend, substituting crop boosting for crop nurturing. Today, we pay the price of foods kept artificially free of disease and blemishes in mineral depletion and the risks that it brings.

Naturally caused inequalities will always exist in crops. Mineral variations are to be expected according to time of harvesting, climate, and geology. However, the use of artificial fertilizers, whose formulas are influenced by cost and profit rather than the actual needs of the soil in any given location, has created unbalanced soil that is too high in some minerals and too low in others.

Chemical fertilizers contain relatively few minerals. This in itself leads to deficiencies in the "fertilized" plants. The chemical contents of artificial fertilizers are concentrated and acidic, typically mixtures of ammonia and nitrogen, and often strong enough to cause skin burns. Chemical fertilizers blaze a path through soil, destroying soil matter that would normally rot into a rich source of nutrients and killing the microbes and other life that would achieve this. While chemical fertilizers cause the release of minerals from rocks in the soil, the microbes and mycorrhiza fungi disappear, making the released minerals unavailable to the plants. The same destructive process occurs with acid rain.

The combination of chemical fertilizer and pesticide use produces apparently healthy crops. The illusory appearance of large, good-looking fruits and vegetables masks the reality of severely compromised plant immunity brought about by inadequate nutrition. Nature would normally see to it that inferior plant life would not survive, but modern chemical treatments remove the fungi, insects, and other life-forms designed to carry out nature's work. Eventually, however, extreme natural conditions such as drought or frost reveal the serious inherent weaknesses of plants and soils treated with artificial fertilizers and we have farming disasters.

Good Trace Minerals Down, Toxic Elements Up

Feed soil superphosphate fertilizer, and crops grown on it will develop high levels of the toxic trace element cadmium. This has been known since work in the 1920s by soil scientist Dr. G. H. Earp-Thomas. Studies of trace elements show that under certain conditions, toxic minerals can displace their beneficial cousins. This applies in the human body and soil alike. Cadmium and essential zinc are good examples. A plant growing in unbalanced soil containing high levels of cadmium will take up the toxic mineral in preference to zinc, actually blocking the plant's ability to absorb that essential element. The probable result for humans is an increase in uptake of cadmium, with its unfortunate ability to interfere with processes in the body that normally use zinc. The fact that Americans tend to be deficient in zinc owes much to this scenario.

The cadmium-zinc problem is only one of several examples. Where lead is present in high levels and calcium and magnesium are low, the body will take up lead instead of calcium and magnesium. This is a double whammy! The body is deprived of an essential mineral *and* poisoned with a toxic mineral.

Earp-Thomas also found that in the presence of too little sulfur, a plant may take up toxic levels of selenium, and that chemical fertilizers high in phosphate will block the uptake of boron, a trace mineral increasingly accepted as essential. Studies have shown that boron decreases the loss of calcium and magnesium. Boron is also thought to be involved in the production of vitamin D and the synthesis of hormones, including estrogen.

It's important to remember that handy nutrition tables listing the amounts of vitamins and minerals in foods can only serve as rough guides. They cannot tell you, for example, if produce was grown in a mineral-balanced soil or a polluted soil. Nor can they give any indication of naturally occurring variations, such as selenium deficiency in high-rainfall areas of the United States. Chromium, iodine, and selenium are three trace elements in particular that vary widely in soils from different geographical areas. What's more, many nutrition tables have not been updated in twenty years or more! In almost a century of practices that have continued to rob the soil of vital mineral content, even one year can make a difference to food values.

Studies show that natural farming produces foods of greater nutritional value than those grown with artificial fertilizers. Organic foods are also far less contaminated by chemicals. A study from the Universities of Maine and Vermont, published in 1987 in the *Journal of Food Quality*, found much lower levels of calcium, magnesium, beta-carotene, and vitamin C in produce grown using chemicals than in naturally grown vegetables. Several studies have shown that the protein content of grains is increased when natural farming methods that maintain the mineral content of soil are used. Minerals play a key role in the formation of proteins. Molybdenum, for instance, is believed to be required by bacteria that convert nitrogen into a usable plant form. The resulting nitrates are used by plants as the basis of proteins.

FOOD AND WATER AS MINERAL SOURCES

Your best source of minerals is the food you eat every day. Taking supplements is important, too. It's a form of health insurance that acknowledges that nobody's diet is perfect and that a certain percentage of the food we eat will not be supplying us with the vitamins and minerals our bodies need for optimal health.

Cooking for Minerals

How you cook your food can make all the difference between getting the minerals you need and becoming deficient in minerals. You could buy a fresh, crisp head of organic broccoli, wash and chop it carefully together with tender, organic carrots and new potatoes, then drop them lovingly into a pan full of boiling water for 10 minutes. You could do all this and watch the trace elements and other nutrients go up in steam and down the pan. Alternatively, you could steam your veggies for just enough time to create succulent rather than soggy servings and preserve the nutrients. Stir-frying can seal in nutrients when done fast, hot, started with water, and finished off with a small amount of olive oil. If you use frozen vegetables, steam them without thawing. Of course, frozen meat and fish should always be thawed thoroughly before cooking.

For meat and vegetable cooking, stewing can be healthful as long as meats are browned first and drained of fat. Mineral and vitamin contents do leach out into broth but will be consumed along with the finished stew.

Baking and roasting are both methods that cook using hot air. Bake or roast and you lose the fatty disadvantages of frying and the watery nutrient losses of boiling and steaming. Deep-frying only adds calories and potentially harmful chemicals. Cooking over charcoal and broiling bring the danger of contamination with chemicals in smoke from ignited fats. Broiling from above can help prevent this problem.

Microwave ovens should be reserved for rapid heating and defrosting. Long cooking with microwaves can change the chemistry of foods containing protein. Always use ceramic or glass containers for microwave preparation, as the heat causes chemicals to leach out from plastic and plastic wrap.

Foods lowest in fat content are foods richest in mineral nutrients. Selecting healthy foods and preparing them well prevent avoidable depletion of trace minerals, vitamins, and other valuable nutrients.

Water Is Not the Mineral Source It Used to Be

Running water is nature's primary delivery source of minerals. Its rushing, turbulent energy transports minerals from oceans and rocks to soil. It also leads to their existence in the highly available forms of electrolytes. Research findings are now confirming that mineral absorption is highest when they are taken in dissolved form. Medical studies have shown this to be true of toxic minerals as well as dietary elements. One advantage that unpolluted, mineral-rich water has over foods is the absence of factors that can block mineral absorption. Such factors can be natural substances or chemical residues.

Ideally, drinking water should be an important source of trace elements. Unpolluted water from mountain and spring sources used to provide us with a range of beneficial minerals in a readily available form. Unfortunately, technology has created treatable water for mass distribution that protects us from diseases such as cholera but adds aluminum, chlorine, and fluoride. Tap water is often also polluted with lead and copper from old plumbing. In high doses, these substances compete with other important trace minerals for absorption.

In much of the industrialized world, municipal water treatment systems add aluminum to the water. Aluminum blocks other minerals in the body, accumulates in the brain, liver, lungs, and thyroid, and is a nerve poison in high amounts.

Chlorine, used to kill bacteria in water, is another toxic pollutant of tap water. In the gut, chlorine continues its sterilizing work, disturbing the balance of bacteria and potentially opening the door to an unfriendly overgrowth of organisms such as *Candida albicans*. Chlorine is also easily absorbed through the skin, especially in a hot shower, when pores are open, adding to the body's overload.

Unless your water comes from a well that you check regularly for groundwater contaminants, I highly recommend that you purchase a water filter. A good one is expensive but well worth the price for the health benefits, as you avoid chlorine, aluminum, benzene from petrochemical pollution, and many other potential hazards from treatment systems, industrial wastes, and groundwater pollutants.

The Fluoridation Controversy

Many "health myths" have been sold to the American public in the name of profits. These myths creep in on the back of advertising, marketing, lobbying, and political favors and kickbacks, and pretty soon they're taken as the gospel truth, even though they're far from it. There's the margarine-is-heart-healthy myth (the truth is that it has caused much more heart disease than it has prevented); there's the estrogen myth (it's more like the Grim Reaper than the Fountain of Youth); and there's the fluoride myth. I know, the common and seemingly irrefutable wisdom is that the number of cavities has been greatly decreased by the addition of fluoride to our drinking water and toothpaste. I'm very sorry to say that it's not true and that fluoride is probably doing a great deal of harm.

Here's the story behind the story. During World War II, we learned how to manufacture things from aluminum: airplanes, buildings, and pots and pans, to name a few. We also greatly increased our production of chemical fertilizers. The downside of both these manufacturing processes was a by-product called fluoride. Although fluoride is a trace mineral naturally occurring in our food, in anything but those trace amounts it's a more potent poison than arsenic. Disposing of the thousands of pounds of fluoride by-product became a major problem in American manufacturing. The manufacturers tried blowing it out their smokestacks, dumping it into rivers, and burying it in the ground, but the immediate result was dead and deformed cows and other animals within miles of the smokestacks, rivers full of dead fish, and poisoned water aquifers. In fact, its primary use was as a rat poison.

Finally, no doubt pushed by manufacturers' political pressure, the U.S. Public Health Service did a study claiming to show that one part per million of fluoride in water reduced tooth decay by 60 percent. Thus began the trickling of fluoride into our water supply.

The price of fluoride went up 1,000 percent almost overnight, and the problem of how to dispose of a potent toxin was solved. The practice of water fluoridation was further justified by more glowing studies claiming to show that communities using fluoridated drinking water had a much lower rate of tooth decay than those using unfluoridated water. The fluoride and cavity myth has been perpetuated by the fact that the rate of dental cavities has dropped steadily in the past thirty years, approximately the amount of time that our water has been fluoridated. So it must be good for us, right? Wrong.

The studies that were supposed to show how well fluoridated communities did are highly suspect. The original U.S. Public Health study on fluoridation was supposed to compare hundreds of communities, but the final study only included a few dozen, presumably those that fit the desired prefluoridation profile. And even those were flawed. For example, in the most widely cited study, two towns in Michigan were compared for dental cavities, but those children studied in the fluoridated community had higher incomes, received regular dental checkups, and agreed to brush their teeth twice a day. It wouldn't seem strange that they would have a lower rate of cavities, with or without fluoride!

"But," I hear you saying, "I had lots of cavities when I was a kid, and my kids hardly have any. It must be due to fluoride." Not so. In both fluoridated and unfluoridated areas in North America and Europe, the decline in tooth decay has been the same for thirty years. This even holds true for entire countries in Europe that have not had fluoridated water or toothpaste. What has changed is that dental hygiene has improved, nutrition has improved, and access to dental care has improved. Studies do show a strong correlation between higher rates of tooth decay and lower economic status.

Japan and all of continental Europe either rejected the fluoride concept from the beginning or have stopped the practice. Most of Great Britain has also discontinued fluoridation, and Australia and New Zealand are in the process of reversing the trend. A 1994 study of virtually all New Zealand schoolchildren showed no benefit in dental health in fluoridated communities.

What's so bad about fluoride? There is good, solid evidence in eight reputable studies that fluoridated drinking water increases your risk of hip fractures by 20 to 40 percent. For a while it was thought that fluoride might actually help prevent osteoporosis. But long-term studies with hundreds of thousands of people proved the wisdom of checking things out thoroughly. There is a clear correlation between bone fractures and fluoridation. It turns out that while fluoride does create denser bone, it is poor-quality, structurally unsound bone that is actually more prone to fracture over time.

So much fluoride has been put into our water and toothpaste over the past thirty years that levels in our food chain are very high. Just by following a normal diet, the average person exceeds the recommended dose. A potent enzyme inhibitor, fluoride interferes with enzymes in the body, particularly in the lining of the intestines, causing stomach pain, gas, and bloating. This enzyme-inhibiting effect also interferes with thyroid gland function. Some studies indicate that fluoride damages the immune system, leading to autoimmune disorders and arthritis. There is also evidence that communities with fluoridated water have a higher incidence of heart disease and higher rates of bone cancer in young men. Some 30 percent of children in fluoridated communities have fluorosis, a malformation of tooth enamel that causes discoloration (usually chalky white patches) and brittleness. This is a permanent change in the teeth that has also been associated with abnormal bone structure.

Advocates of putting fluoride in toothpaste and mouthwash argue that it is not swallowed and therefore not ingested. However, fluoride is absorbed through the mucous membranes of the mouth, and young children do not have control over their swallowing reflex. There have been numerous reports of children poisoned by ingesting high levels of fluoride through school fluoride mouthwash programs or fluoridated toothpastes full of sweeteners that kids want to swallow. (Please avoid both!) Who knows how many stomachaches in kids and adults alike have been caused by unknowingly ingesting too much fluoride?

While it is clear that fluoride can be helpful in the year or two when a child's adult teeth are growing in, there is absolutely no evidence that it is helpful before or after that time, and there are reams of evidence that it is harmful. A child's fluoride needs can be handled perfectly well by brushing with fluoride toothpaste for a few years. Other than that, I recommend that you and your loved ones avoid fluoride in all forms, including toothpastes. This substance has crept into every link in our food chain, and the evidence is that even without fluoridated water and toothpaste, we're getting a higher dose than is safe or recommended in our daily diets.

You can be thankful if you live in an unfluoridated community because it's not easy to get rid of fluoride in your tap water. Distillation and reverse osmosis are the only two reliable methods for removing fluoride. Other water filters may work at eliminating fluoride for a short period of time, but fluoride binds so strongly and quickly to filter materials such as charcoal that the binding sites become fully occupied after a short time. If you are at high risk for osteoporosis or heart disease or if you have chronic digestive problems, I recommend that you spend the money on a reverse osmosis water purification system.

Refining Foods—Mineral Robbery

A better phrase than "refined foods" might be "nutrient-free foods." The obsession with convenience that has filled American lives since the 1940s has brought increasingly dubious versions of food to TV trays across the land. When a food is refined, important parts of it are literally removed. White flour is produced by removing the outer husk of grains, which consists of the fibrous bran and germ, the part containing 95 percent of the nutrient value. The fiber is also removed from brown rice and whole sugar cane to give white variations of those foods. Advertising might lead us to believe that white sugar, rice, and flour are "pure" foods. What they are is pure starch. Although we do need starch, we also need essential minerals to aid in the digestion and processing of starch. The outer fiber of sugar and grains contains exactly the nutrients required to deal with the starch they surround.

Chromium found in the husk of grains is particularly needed in the processing of starch. Bran is itself fiber and contains other trace minerals like silicon and zinc as well as vitamin E and useful oils. Chromium is also found in unrefined sugar, where it is packaged with fiber and B-complex vitamins. Fiber in products like unrefined flour and sugar provides bulk, acting as a check on excess consumption. Fiber also slows digestion and aids excretion of unwanted substances.

Pure starch taxes the body, as it stresses the pancreas and draws on stores of elements, especially chromium, needed for its digestion and absorption. What's more, as refined foods are processed, the body's acid/alkaline balance shifts toward acid. As the body works to restore its chemical balance, it has to call even more on its mineral reserves. In this way, refining foods not only undersupplies but also depletes trace minerals. Depletion is bad enough, but an additional result of eating only the inner core of rice and wheat grains is increased uptake of the element cadmium, which can accumulate to toxic levels. Cadmium is found largely in the central, starchy part of wheat and rice grains.

Unrefined wheat and rice are packaged with zinc, mainly as part of their germ and bran. Zinc is absorbed by the body in preference to the toxic element cadmium. Take away enough zinc, and the cadmium is absorbed instead. White rice, white bread, white flour—all such refined products leave the door open to excess consumption of cadmium, which can inhibit the uptake of iron and block production of vitamin D.

Eating fresh, whole foods is like fitting the right keys into the locks of the body. Foods precooked, processed, or refined in any other way may pick the locks of digestion and energy production, but they can damage them at the same time. Leave the convenience, fast, and snack foods on the shelves and stick to whole, unrefined foods to keep your systems topped up with trace minerals and functioning smoothly.

"Enriched" Foods Are Mineral Poor

U.S. law requires the addition of iron sulfate wherever iron and other minerals are removed during the processing of foods. Iron is an essential trace mineral with several valuable roles, particularly in the transportation of oxygen by the blood. I suppose the intention of this law is positive, but in practice it's almost useless, because iron sulfate is a form of iron that is not particularly well absorbed. In addition, absorption of the added iron in enriched food made with white flour or rice is likely to be blocked by other food additives or cadmium. Cadmium as an iron blocker is made available by the incidental removal of zinc during refining.

Does this make any sense to you? Iron is removed from foods, then replaced in questionable form, facing obstacles to its absorption. It is the same story or worse for other nutrients. More than thirty nutrients are removed from white, bleached flour. Four are added back, creating an "enriched" product. Ironically, the extracted nutrients are sold as animal feed! To add insult to injury, manufacturers charge more for refined products sprayed with added nutrients. The only difference between one refined cereal and another can be sprayed-on vitamins and a higher price.

"Enriching" foods is nutritional nonsense. It plays havoc with the natural balance of trace elements established in foodstuffs. As seen with soil, mineral imbalances are perpetuated and worsened as nutrients are absorbed. The body has to scramble to provide the minerals needed simply to digest foods robbed of their natural content, and those minerals are not replenished. The selective replacement of a few nutrients ignores the fact that many work best when packaged with others that have not been restored.

Tinkering with the content of foods might pay the manufacturers, but it does not pay consumers in nutritional terms. Stay naturally enriched with trace minerals and other essential nutrients by steering clear of technologically "improved" food.

Fiber Is Good—In Moderation

Fiber is a perfect example of why moderation will keep you healthy in almost every aspect of your life. Fiber has been shown to be extremely important in the prevention of certain degenerative diseases, including colitis, diverticulosis, ulcers, and some cancers. Important minerals are packaged in the fiber around the energy-supplying starch in foods like rice and wheat. The body is adapted to absorb nutrients parceled in this way when they are consumed as part of a balanced diet.

The vast majority of Americans eat too many refined foods and don't get enough fiber. But too much fiber isn't healthy, either. Take in too much, and it will strip out trace elements and other nutrients. Fiber is largely indigestible and passes quickly out of the gut. Its ability to bind with toxins and other waste products is beneficial—in moderation. This ability simply extends too far when fiber levels are too high. It is

highly unlikely that anyone will get too much fiber from the food they eat; most often the culprit is a fiber laxative or stimulant, such as Metamucil (which is just psyllium with added colorings and sweeteners—the real thing is much cheaper and healthier).

If you're taking a fiber supplement such as psyllium, I recommend that you take it first thing in the morning, at least half an hour before breakfast. This way it can stimulate and clean your digestive tract without taking nutrients with it. For the same reason, it's smart to take supplements at least an hour or two after taking a fiber supplement.

HOW DRUGS DEPLETE YOUR BODY'S MINERALS

I'll bet that when you take an antacid or an antibiotic, it never occurs to you that you could be creating a mineral deficiency or imbalance, but many over-the-counter (OTC) and prescription drugs interfere with mineral balance.

Some medications reduce mineral absorption, while others cause minerals to be excreted in the urine in higher than normal quantities. Total intake of nutrients can change, too, as some drugs cause changes in appetite. In addition, the way a nutrient is used in the body can be altered by medications.

It is ironic that by disrupting nutrient uptake, medications meant to heal the body can weaken it. One of the systems most impacted is the immune system, which requires vitamins and minerals for full protection against illness. A lack of nutrients may well lie behind a gap in the body's defenses that allows infection to take hold in the first place. Poor diet puts patients, particularly children and the elderly, at great risk from nutritional interference by drugs, especially if usage is long-term.

Research on drug and trace mineral interactions is sparse, but remember—wherever major minerals such as calcium, potassium, and magnesium are lost, it's very likely that trace minerals are also being depleted.

Antacids

Antacids are not a good source of calcium, even though they may contain a great deal of it. In spite of advertising meant to convince you that stomach acid is your enemy, the truth is that heartburn and indigestion are most often caused by a *lack* of hydrochloric acid (HCl). Insufficient HCl leads to stomach churning and the fermentation of undigested food, which causes the food to be "burped" back up, burning the esophagus as it goes.

Taking antacids weakens or neutralizes acids for about an hour, relieving the symptoms but often causing rebound heartburn or indigestion as the stomach tries to make up for the stomach acid it doesn't have by working overtime. In fact, in the long run, antacids will make heartburn and indigestion worse.

Antacids are advertised as being a good source of calcium, but this is misleading. The aluminum and magnesium in most antacids tend to bind with phosphate, which can result in calcium *depletion*! Weakened stomach acids cannot soften minerals, including calcium, arriving in the stomach. Minerals taken in are unlikely to be absorbed and will almost certainly be excreted. The fact is that antacids can actually block calcium absorption and also tend to block iron absorption.

Some antacids deliver large amounts of compounds of aluminum, a trace element that can block mineral absorption and in large amounts can cause harm to the nervous system. Avoid taking antacids with citrus foods or drinks, as these increase the amount of aluminum absorbed. Aluminum hydroxides are the worst antacid culprits for blocking mineral absorption.

Used in too great amounts or for too long, antacids can produce vitamin and mineral deficiencies. If they do become necessary for extreme conditions, such as a true excess of HCl, their nutrient-blocking effects are lessened by taking them between meals or at night.

Most often I recommend that people with chronic heartburn and indigestion try taking betaine hydrochloride tablets before meals to aid digestion. Even simpler, just a warm glass of water with a tablespoon of apple cider vinegar can stimulate digestive juices and provide an acidic environment.

As an aside, please don't turn to the H2 blockers such as Tagamet, Pepcid, and Zantac for heartburn and indigestion. They have a long list of side effects and block the absorption of vitamin B_{12}, potentially causing symptoms of senility. Making these powerful drugs available over the counter is one of the most irresponsible actions that the FDA has ever taken.

Antibiotics

Antibiotics can be a powerful weapon against infection. Unfortunately they cannot distinguish between friend and foe. Antibiotics wipe out beneficial bacteria along with those causing harm. Take antibiotics and you will, for example, also destroy the bacteria in the gut that produce the B-complex vitamin biotin. Mineral disruption can occur with the antibiotic neomycin, which interferes with the absorption of calcium, iron, and potassium as well as vitamin B_{12}.

In some cases, the antibiotics interfere with the absorption of the minerals, and the minerals interfere with the absorption of the antibiotic. Tetracycline blocks the absorption of dietary minerals by interacting with calcium, iron, magnesium, and zinc, and taking these supplements will also block the action of the antibiotic. Antibiotics known as quinolones will block the absorption of calcium, iron, and zinc, and these minerals can also block the action of the antibiotic. Don't take tetracycline or the quinolones within two hours of taking a mineral supplement. Do not take antacids at the same time as these antibiotics, either, because the calcium and magnesium may block their action.

As a general rule, problems with nutrient absorption end when the course of antibiotics ends. It is not advisable to take antibiotics for longer than about two weeks.

Anticonvulsants

Anticonvulsants, such as carbamazepine, phenobarbital, phenytoin, and primidone, block adequate production of vitamin D in the body. A lack of vitamin D leads the body to draw on calcium from bones instead of from dietary uptake. This is why long-term use of anticonvulsants can result in bone disorders. Another possible contributory factor in bone deformities caused by anticonvulsants is a lowering of blood and tissue levels of the trace mineral copper. Levels of zinc are also seen to drop over the long term when these drugs are used, compromising, among other functions, tissue formation and the immune system.

Antidepressants

Antidepressants, such as fluoxetine, amoxapine, doxepin, imipramine, and lithium carbonate, may dampen the appetite and therefore indirectly cause nutrient deficiencies. Side effects such as abdominal cramps, diarrhea, dry mouth, nausea, and vomiting can occur with these types of drugs and with antianxiety medications like Librium and Valium. These symptoms can impair the absorption of nutrients. Long-term use of diazepam, for example, can disturb the balance of magnesium and calcium and increase the risk of bone disorders such as osteoporosis. Lithium disrupts copper absorption and may lead to a deficiency with long-term use.

Arthritis Medications

D-penicillamine and similar arthritis medications can cause serious nutrient deficiencies, including mineral loss. Some of its side effects include an altered sense of taste, diarrhea, intestinal and digestive fluid problems, nausea, sores of the mouth and tongue, and vomiting, all of which can cause a loss of minerals. D-penicillamine reduces absorption of the trace element zinc, producing signs of clinical deficiency, such as hair loss and skin changes. The drug binds to zinc and iron as well as other dietary minerals.

Aspirin

Aspirin can cause small amounts of blood to be lost in the stomach, and taking it regularly over a long period of time can result in enough blood loss to cause iron deficiency. I don't recommend that you take iron supplements; I recommend you avoid taking aspirin long-term. The painkiller indomethacin has the same problem.

Cholesterol-Lowering Drugs

Such drugs, including cholestyramine and colestipol, lower the body's stores of iron as well as the fat-soluble vitamins A, E, and K, which are all protective against heart disease.

Corticosteroids

Corticosteroids such as cortisone and prednisone are used to treat many illnesses, including arthritis and autoimmune diseases. They are also prescribed for skin problems, blood and eye disorders, and asthma. Researchers conducted a study of twenty-four asthmatics using cortisone-type drugs and found that their zinc levels were 42 percent lower than in patients not treated with corticosteroids.

Diuretics

Frequently used in the treatment of high blood pressure and heart failure, diuretics can cause minerals to be lost in urine. Their effect is strongest with the beneficial minerals calcium, potassium, and magnesium, but they also deplete the trace minerals iodine and zinc. Long-term diuretic use is definitely not encouraged. High blood pressure should always be vigorously treated first with lifestyle changes, such as weight loss, exercise, and a diet of nutrient-rich whole foods.

Laxatives

These drugs turn nutrients into whistle-stop tourists of the intestine. Before they've even had a chance to inspect stomach or intestinal tract linings, nutrients are whisked away by laxatives. Even when nutrients do get to pause, laxatives like senna, bisocodyl (Dulcolax), and phenolphthalein can interfere with the intestinal lining, possibly reducing nutrient uptake.

Mineral oil used as a laxative prevents absorption of vitamins A and D. Any laxative taken to excess can flush out large amounts of potassium, which can cause heart problems and muscle weakness.

Oral Contraceptives

These drugs tend to increase the levels of some vitamins and minerals, including copper, which in excess can cause a decrease in blood levels of iron and zinc.

Studies have shown that this type of medication can also lead to an increase in iron levels, possibly due to decreased menstrual flow.

Alcohol and Tobacco

Alcohol is one of our worst vitamin and mineral robbers. It depletes iron, selenium, zinc, and magnesium, in addition to many other important nutrients. It also reduces the intake of minerals and nutrients in general by causing loss of appetite. Alcoholic drinks like wine and whiskey are also relatively high in the toxic element cadmium, which is taken up in greater quantities when zinc levels are low.

While a glass of wine with dinner may be beneficial, tobacco is not suitable in any quantity. And remember that the harmful effects of tobacco extend to people breathing secondhand smoke. This is true especially because nonsmokers breathe in the unfiltered smoke, which contains more poisons than the smoke breathed through a filtered cigarette. The trace element zinc and many other nutrients drop to low levels in smokers, impairing the immune system as well as the ability to detoxify the poisons being absorbed. Low zinc levels lead to a greater uptake and absorption of the trace element cadmium, which happens to be one of the toxins in tobacco smoke. Pregnant women who smoke are more likely to give birth to zinc-deficient babies.

KEEPING THE TRACE MINERALS IN BALANCE

Wouldn't life be a lot simpler if nutrition were only a matter of opening our mouths and pouring down a liquid superfood? Well, yes, but *we'd* be simpler, too, possibly drifting as a single cell in the ocean. As complex organisms, we have complex nutritional needs that are automatically supplied by foods in their natural forms. For example, whole-wheat bread brings the elements needed to digest it, and fruit delivers fast energy supported by the nutrients required to process it. Yet the production of our foods has to be rooted in properly balanced soils to ensure that nutrients blend as nature intended and health requires. Trace mineral interactions are examples of the way partnerships of

nutrients abound. Research is increasingly showing the importance of nutrients in combination, which is powerfully demonstrated by the effects of trace minerals in and out of balance.

The Body Works to Create Optimum Trace Mineral Levels

The body is actually designed to maintain healthy levels of many trace minerals and hundreds of other biologically active chemicals. It performs constant, subtle adjustments in a wonderful, automatic effort to maintain balance, also known as homeostasis. (This word is somewhat misleading, because *stasis* means "standing" or "stopping," and maintaining balance in the body is one of the most active processes I can think of.)

Excess trace elements are removed by preventing their absorption or triggering their excretion. Excretion occurs through feces, urine, and sweat. Hair can also be a minor route of excretion for metallic trace minerals. Essential trace elements are nontoxic except in large amounts, and the body can temporarily tolerate a wide range between the highest and lowest levels associated with health. At low levels, the body can survive with an amount of a trace element sufficient for growth and maintenance but insufficient for optimum function.

Mineral balance can be interfered with and overwhelmed, leading to inadequate or excess absorption. Normally, the maintenance of optimum levels of trace minerals is affected by dietary consumption.

The intestines can reject excess amounts of trace minerals just as the kidneys can excrete them. However, both organs can only handle so much of any trace mineral. If that amount is exceeded, the body accumulates the mineral to poisonous levels.

Toxic Elements Can Take the Place of Trace Elements

All elements, even oxygen, can become toxic at high enough levels. Extremely poisonous chemicals, such as mercury, are simply those that have toxic effects in very small amounts. Fortunately for the human race, nature has locked away many of the substances that are harmful in low amounts. Humans, however, have been uncovering them at increasing rates, mining uranium and other heavy metals and minerals. We are also exposed to unprecedented levels of lead through car exhaust and to cadmium through poor agricultural processes. This has increased the need for trace elements required to help protect the body and process noxious chemicals. It has also led to a greater chance that toxic chemicals may be absorbed instead of essential trace elements.

Essential trace minerals belong to different families of elements that include toxic cousins. Just as with plants, if not enough of a particular trace element is present, the body will take up its nearest available cousin. Illness can be caused, for example, when cadmium displaces zinc, changing or inactivating enzymes. And disease can occur when insufficient iodine causes the thyroid gland to take up sodium fluoride instead. Iodine pills were issued by the Polish government after the nuclear disaster of Chernobyl in 1986. This was to try to prevent an uptake of radioactive iodine in place of essential iodine.

The best prevention of toxic element uptake is to avoid exposure by buying organic foods and living in an unpolluted environment. A healthy diet also protects you from harmful elements by maintaining trace element levels, filling any gaps a toxic cousin might fit. Optimum levels of trace elements also aid the body's detoxifying mechanisms.

How Essential Trace Elements Interact

The interaction of several trace minerals and other nutrients requires a cautious and intelligent approach to supplementation. The human body is geared to receive nature's own balanced recipes of nutrients that exist in individual foods. Ideally, trace elements and other nutrients should be readily available from whole-food sources without major concerns about their correct proportions or partners. Sadly, a compromised and polluted environment leads to an unbalanced uptake of nutrients and unnatural toxins. This generates a need for wisely chosen supplements and diet. Awareness of the types of stress that use up trace minerals helps to promote the use of supplements at the right time. Supplies of zinc, for example, are run

down with infection, and iron will be lost with extensive bleeding.

A good general rule is to avoid taking higher-than-recommended doses of any one mineral without taking into account the effect it will have on other minerals, especially when taking them long-term. Trace mineral interactions include the following:

Cobalt and molybdenum. Molybdenum antagonizes cobalt.

Cobalt and iodine. Cobalt antagonizes iodine.

Copper and molybdenum. Molybdenum may alter copper absorption, but copper is also believed to work against molybdenum.

Copper and selenium. Copper is believed by some investigators to be a selenium antagonist, probably competing for absorption.

Iron and magnesium carbonate. Excessive magnesium carbonate can reduce the absorption of iron. (*Note:* Magnesium carbonate is not a good magnesium supplement, since it is not easily absorbed.)

Iron, copper, manganese, and zinc. Take too much of one and you may cause a deficiency in another of these trace minerals, creating an increased risk of infection and other diseases. These elements compete for absorption in the small intestine. When in balance, copper enhances the absorption and utilization of iron. Zinc, in particular, competes against copper for absorption.

FOOD SOURCES OF ESSENTIAL TRACE MINERALS

The food values found in tables do not account for variations caused by climate, geology, time of harvesting, and chemical farming. However, they do provide basic information about which foods are usually comparatively high in certain trace minerals and other nutrients. It's a good idea to hedge against a depletion of nutrients in any one food by eating a range that in theory supplies the content you are looking for.

Boron. Good sources are fruits and vegetables.

Chromium. Good sources are black pepper, thyme, cheese, lean meat, and whole-grain cereals.

Cobalt. Good sources are meats and other foods of animal origin.

Copper. Good sources are shellfish, especially oysters, avocados, fish, poultry, dark green leafy vegetables, cooked soybeans, dried peas and other legumes, nuts, bananas and other fruits, whole-grain bread and cereals, and cooked carrots.

Iodine. Good sources include iodized salt, seafood, and seaweed.

Iron. Good sources (all better than spinach) include red meat, brewer's yeast, kelp, lima beans, chickpeas, duck, shellfish, molasses, wheat bran, parsley, and apricots.

Manganese. Good sources are whole grains, nuts, shellfish, and milk. Given soil that is not too alkaline, fruit and green vegetables can be moderate sources of manganese.

Molybdenum. Good sources are whole grains, dark green leafy vegetables, peas, beans, and milk. Crops grown on depleted soil can have molybdenum levels up to five hundred times lower than plants grown on soil rich in this mineral.

Selenium. Good sources are brewer's yeast, broccoli, cabbage, celery, cucumbers, fish, garlic, whole grains, mushrooms, and poultry. However, selenium levels vary greatly in soils. As a general rule, soils in the western states are lower in selenium than soils in the eastern ones.

Zinc. Good sources are fish, meat, oysters, and whole grains.

Kelp

Kelp, a seaweed, is an excellent source of minerals. It contains twenty-three minerals, the most important of which are present in the percentages shown here:

Iodine	0.15–0.20%
Calcium	1.20%
Phosphorus	0.30%
Iron	0.10%
Sodium	3.14%
Potassium	0.63%
Magnesium	0.76%

Sulfur	0.93%
Copper	0.0008%
Zinc	0.0003%
Manganese	0.0008%

Vitamins present in kelp are vitamin B_2, niacin, choline, and carotene. Algenic acid is also present. This remarkable food contains more vitamins and minerals than any other substance known. All these nutrients have been assimilated by the growing plant.

Kelp, because of its natural iodine content, acts to normalize the thyroid gland. Therefore, thin people with thyroid trouble may gain weight by using kelp, and obese people with thyroid trouble may lose weight.

If you need a good supply of highly absorbable minerals, try taking kelp supplements.

THE *GOOD* TRACE MINERALS FROM A TO ZINC

Minerals that are currently considered essential for human nutrition are calcium, phosphorus, iron, potassium, selenium, and magnesium. Chromium, cobalt, copper, zinc, and manganese are important in their own right, even though we only require them in very small amounts.

Unless you are trying to correct a specific nutritional deficiency under the supervision of a health care professional, minerals should only be taken in the recommended doses, as an excess can cause just as many problems as a deficiency.

Let's take a closer look at the trace minerals you should be getting in your daily vitamin and mineral program.

Boron

Boron is a trace mineral that helps retard bone loss, and it works with calcium, magnesium, and vitamin D to help prevent osteoporosis (brittle bones). Some studies suggest that a boron deficiency may aggravate arthritis and other degenerative joint conditions. Boric acids and borates have been used medicinally for centuries as disinfectants and to treat burns. As mentioned earlier in the chapter, we tend to be deficient in boron because the use of superphosphate fertilizers blocks its uptake by plants.

According to boron researcher Forrest H. Nielsen, of the Department of Agriculture's Grand Forks Human Nutrition Center, calcium cannot be properly metabolized without boron. Nielsen fed a low-boron diet (less than 0.32 mg per day) to five men, five postmenopausal women on bone-preserving estrogen therapy, and four postmenopausal women not on estrogen for sixty-three days. Then, for the next forty-nine days, they continued on the low-boron diet but added a daily 3 mg supplement of boron. On the low-boron diet blood levels of calcium decreased, along with other nutrients that affect bone health. When boron was added back in, all these measures improved, and copper levels improved as well.

You can take 1–3 mg of boron daily—not more than that—if you are at risk for osteoporosis. Otherwise, you can get boron in a healthy diet. Boron is abundant in pears, apples, and grapes and is also found in nuts, green leafy vegetables, and legumes such as soybeans.

Chromium

Chromium is one of our most important trace minerals and one of the most depleted. It works with insulin in the metabolism of sugar, helps the body utilize protein and fats, and lowers high blood pressure. It is best to take chromium in the form of chromium picolinate.

Recent studies suggest that chromium may help athletes by regulating the body's use of glycogen during exercise. In one study, weight lifters using chromium supplements had greater muscle and weight gains than a group given a placebo. In another study, chromium supplements lowered blood cholesterol levels.

Chromium is also very important to those with blood sugar and insulin imbalances, such as diabetics. Chromium is necessary for glucose to enter the cells, so it is essential in the efficient burning of carbohydrates. In fact, a chromium deficiency may cause adult-onset diabetes, especially in older people.

I know that the people who make those bottled "natural" fruit drinks and teas aren't going to like me for saying this, but I suspect that the steep rise in our consumption of high-fructose corn syrup has contributed to the rise in diabetes by depleting chromium. (Our consumption of high-fructose corn syrup has risen 250 percent in the past fifteen years, and our rate of diabetes has increased approximately 45 percent in about the same time period.) According to studies done at the Agriculture Department's Human Nutrition Resource Center, fructose consumption causes a drop in chromium as well as raising "bad" LDL cholesterol and triglycerides and impairing immune system function.

According to researchers, giving people with elevated blood sugar a chromium supplement will result in a significant drop in blood sugar in 80 to 90 percent of those people.

Chromium may also be important for skin health. In a study reported in *Medical Hypotheses*, when nine patients with acne were given 2 teaspoons daily of high-chromium yeast containing 400 mcg of chromium, their acne rapidly cleared up.

Please don't be scared away from chromium by recent media reports about it. Taking chromium picolinate supplements of 100–600 mcg daily is not the same as exposing hamster cells in a test tube to five thousand to six thousand times that dose every day, nor is it the same as factory workers breathing in chromium dust.

Most Americans are actually deficient in chromium, and at the recommended doses, it is very safe and very effective in helping stabilize blood sugar as well as helping burn fat during exercise and producing lean muscle tissue.

You can take 200 mcg of chromium daily, depending on your needs. Food sources of chromium include brewer's yeast, whole grains, nuts, molasses, and cheese.

Cobalt

Cobalt is a component of vitamin B_{12}, and as such is a stimulant to the production of red blood cells. It is also necessary for normal cell growth and healthy nerve tissue. A deficiency of cobalt/B_{12} can cause anemia. Although a deficiency of cobalt is rare, it can occur in vegetarians, since cobalt is mainly found in meat and shellfish in the form of vitamin B_{12}. Cobalt can also replace other trace minerals in enzyme reactions and is part of the enzyme action involved in forming some antioxidants.

Copper

A deficiency of copper can cause an excess of zinc and vice versa.

Copper works as a catalyst in the formation of red blood cells and is present in the hemoglobin molecule. It also plays a role in maintaining the skeletal system. Copper is essential before iron can be utilized and is necessary to prevent anemia. It is an important partner to vitamin C in the synthesis of collagen. You don't usually need to add copper to your diet. An excess can cause hair loss, insomnia, irregular menses, and depression.

Fluoride

Fluoride helps protect teeth from decay and may help protect against osteoporosis. Too much causes discolored teeth, and continued overuse of it may lead to bone fractures, abnormal bony growths, heart disease, and digestive disorders. Most Americans get excessive fluoride in their normal diet, just by drinking tap water, sodas, and other commercial products made with fluoridated water. I don't recommend that you supplement fluoride in your diet. (See our earlier discussion about the fluoridation controversy.)

Iodine

As far back as Hippocrates, physicians have known that something in seaweed and seafood prevents goiter, an enlargement of the thyroid gland. Iodine is the key component in a thyroid hormone called thyroxine, and a lack of it causes the thyroid gland to enlarge. Because the thyroid regulates our metabolism—how fast we use energy—iodine is an essential trace mineral. And yet, it is a trace mineral found in the sea and rarely inland. Many inland areas of the world are still deficient in iodine and suffer from diseases related to improper thyroid function.

Iodine is necessary for proper growth, and it promotes healthy hair, nails, skin, and teeth. A deficiency of iodine in pregnant women can cause retardation in their children, and children deficient in iodine may become retarded. A deficiency of vitamin A can make iodine deficiency even worse.

Iodine deficiency can be caused by eating too many vegetables in the cabbage family (kale, cauliflower, turnips) without a sufficient intake of iodine. A substance in these vegetables blocks the uptake of iodine. Disease conditions can occur when insufficient iodine causes the thyroid gland to take up sodium fluoride instead.

Sufficient iodine levels also confer some protection against radiation damage, as a lack of it will cause the thyroid to take up the radioactive trace elements instead. As mentioned earlier, it was for this reason that the Polish government distributed iodine pills after the Chernobyl nuclear disaster.

An oversupply of iodine can cause or aggravate acne in adolescents. Some researchers speculate that this is caused when the excess iodine is excreted through the pores, irritating the skin.

Seafoods are very high in iodine, and it is added to most table salt. Kelp is a good source of natural iodine. You should be getting 150 mcg (0.15 mg) of iodine daily as part of your food or in your multivitamin. Pregnant and nursing women should be getting 175–200 mcg daily.

Iron

Iron is required in the manufacture of hemoglobin, a component of blood that transports oxygen through the circulatory system. It works with many enzymes in biochemical reactions in the body, and to be used efficiently, it must also have copper, cobalt, manganese, and vitamin C present. B-complex vitamins, such as B_1, B_6, biotin, folic acid, and B_{12}, all work with iron to produce rich red blood.

In excess, iron is not efficiently excreted from the body. It can accumulate in tissues and become toxic. Although iron is an essential mineral, it is important not to take too much iron in supplement form. Recent research has shown that excessive amounts of iron in the tissues raise the risk of heart disease.

Iron deficiency can cause a specific disease called iron deficiency anemia. Women need more iron than men because of the loss of blood during the menstrual cycle, and their need for iron is increased during pregnancy and breast-feeding.

The most noticeable warning sign of anemia, a sign of iron deficiency, is fatigue. If you are getting plenty of rest but still feel tired and lacking in energy, your body could be telling you that you are becoming anemic. The hair, skin, and nails also show the effects of anemia. The skin tends to wrinkle more. Fingernails and toenails become brittle, break easily, and become tender. Hair becomes dry and lacks luster. Skin color becomes paler, even pasty and gray. The mouth and tongue begin to feel sore and tender.

Because the most available sources of absorbable iron are meat, vegetarians are at a greater risk of becoming iron deficient.

Sufficient iron levels are essential for top athletic performance. Since iron plays a role in delivering oxygen to the muscles, iron-poor blood can cause less efficient use of muscles and fatigue. Studies have shown that female athletes in particular may benefit from iron supplements, even when iron levels test as normal. A study of high school cross-country runners found that 45 percent of the female runners and 17 percent of the male runners had low iron levels during the competitive season. Another study of one hundred female college students showed that 31 percent had iron deficiency. The population most susceptible to iron deficiency is young women who are dieting to keep their weight down and also exercising strenuously. For young athletes, keeping the body well stocked with iron can improve endurance and keep red blood cells optimally healthy.

Iron supplements can cause constipation, diarrhea, nausea, and poor absorption of zinc. Your best bet is to eat plenty of iron-rich foods and keep iron supplements low. In fact, I don't recommend iron supplements except for young women and possibly pregnant women as needed, unless blood tests show low iron levels. Most iron deficiency anemia can be cured by proper diet. If you need iron supplementation, 10 mg daily is a reasonable amount to take. If you want to take more, do so under the guidance of a health care professional who can measure your iron levels.

Lithium

Lithium, a trace mineral only recently studied, is not needed in significant enough amounts in the body to be supplemented. However, lithium has been used successfully for years to treat manic depression, now known as bipolar mood disorder. It is a treatment that must be used with care, because lithium interacts with other substances and can cause kidney damage and death if it accumulates to a toxic level.

Some researchers have used lithium to successfully treat those attempting to withdraw from alcohol, cocaine, and other drugs.

The two most common side effects of lithium are weight gain and fatigue, which may be caused by reduced thyroid function, even though thyroid tests are normal. Lithium may also cause a deficiency of folic acid, which can increase the risk of heart disease and some cancers and cause a deficiency of vitamin B_{12}. A report from the National Institutes of Health suggests that taking the B vitamin inositol with lithium may reduce the side effects.

Lithium also replaces sodium where there is a sodium deficiency, which can upset the delicate balance of fluid in the cells, causing edema, nausea, and vomiting.

Many arthritis and pain medications interfere with lithium excretion and can cause a toxic buildup. These include aspirin, ibuprofen (Advil, Motrin), naproxen (Aleve), and indomethacin (Indocin). Both the thiazide diuretics (furosemide, bumetanide) and the potassium-sparing diuretics (spironolactone, triamterene) used to treat high blood pressure can also raise lithium levels dangerously. The same is true of the heart drugs known as ACE inhibitors, such as captopril, enalapril, and quinapril. The anticonvulsant caramazepine (Tegretol) can make lithium more effective in some people, but in others can cause toxicity.

I recommend that you use lithium only under the guidance of a health care professional. If you are taking it and experience nausea, diarrhea, or muscle weakness, call your doctor immediately.

Manganese

Manganese is another trace mineral that we're learning more about every day. It is an important trace mineral that activates numerous enzymes and is related to proper utilization of vitamins B_1 and E and iron. Manganese is also involved with thyroid function, the central nervous system, and digestion of proteins. It increases levels of the antioxidant SOD (superoxide dismutase).

Very little manganese is stored in the body, making it an important mineral to include in a supplement program. Too much manganese interferes with iron absorption, and conversely, too much iron can reduce manganese levels.

Although manganese deficiency is not well studied, some of the symptoms are middle ear problems, reduced fertility, retarded growth, and low blood sugar.

A study of trace metals conducted during autopsies of thirty-two people, of whom sixteen had blocked arteries, showed that those with the heart disease had low copper and manganese levels in the damaged arteries.

Manganese plays a role in the breakdown of collagen, and a deficiency can cause dermatitis, reduce levels of "good" HDL cholesterol, and cause bone loss and bone instability. A study of women with osteoporosis showed that they had low manganese levels, and rodent studies indicate that it is a crucial mineral in the formation of strong, normal bones.

Researchers all over the world have reported success in treating schizophrenia with manganese, and some theorize that it plays an important role in stabilizing nerve transmissions. It has also been used to treat seizures, and this may be connected to its important role in the middle ear.

Manganese is one of the important trace minerals removed when grains are refined. The prevalence of nutrition-free refined foods in America has made manganese deficiency common. Since manganese competes with calcium, it should be taken separately as a supplement.

I recommend that women at risk for osteoporosis add 5–10 mg of manganese to their daily supplements and that other adults include 2–5 mg daily.

Molybdenum

This trace mineral was once considered toxic because miners inhaling it became ill. However, we now know that it is important to human health in very small quantities. It is used by blue-green algae and other plant life to turn nitrogen into a usable compound essential to all life, so its presence is foundational to life as we know it.

A deficiency of molybdenum has been linked to age-related cataracts and cancer of the stomach and esophagus. It is one of the trace elements necessary for the metabolism of iron, and it plays important roles in at least three enzyme systems having to do with the metabolism of fats, carbohydrates, and proteins.

There is evidence that sufficient molybdenum is important to the formation of strong teeth, which makes sense, since it is a component of tooth enamel. It is also vital to the normal development of the fetus.

Since molybdenum and copper compete with each other, an excess of one can cause a deficiency of the other. Excess sulphur can also cause a deficiency of molybdenum.

Molybdenum is one of the trace minerals stripped out of refined grains and depleted from many soils. I recommend that you include 100–250 mcg of molybdenum in your daily supplement intake.

Selenium

Selenium is a trace mineral found in very small amounts in the body. However, its role in maintaining your health is anything but small. I have been telling my readers about this mineral for twenty years. In 1957, Dr. Klaus Schwarz and Dr. C. M. Katz established that selenium is essential to life, even though it is needed in very small quantities. But it was not until 1990 that it was designated as a recommended dietary allowance (RDA) mineral. This means that your body must have this mineral daily. If we need selenium in such small amounts, why do we need to add it to our diets? White bread is one answer. Processing grain to produce white flour robs it of 75 percent of its selenium content.

Selenium could be called the "anticancer" mineral. Over and over again, population studies have shown that people living in areas containing plenty of selenium in the soil have lower rates of cancer, and those living in areas with selenium-depleted soil have higher rates, especially of colon cancer.

Selenium is an antioxidant that also stimulates the immune system. A deficiency can lead to impaired immune function and reduced T cell counts.

Selenium works synergistically with vitamin E, each enhancing the actions of the other. Selenium is found in high concentrations in semen, and men seem to need more of this mineral than women. A selenium deficiency can cause dandruff, dry skin, and fatigue and may be associated with the development of cataracts.

Selenium is important in male hormone regulation and is found in large amounts in the prostate. Blood levels of both zinc and selenium are low in men who have prostate cancer. Men who live in areas where the soil is rich in selenium tend to have lower rates of prostate cancer.

Selenium is protective against heavy-metal exposure, specifically to mercury. It is also important in the formation of the antioxidant glutathione and has been associated with reductions in heart disease.

Selenium also aids in keeping youthful elasticity to your tissues, can help alleviate hot flashes and other menopausal symptoms, and helps in the treatment and prevention of dandruff.

If you're over the age of fifty, I suggest that you supplement your diet with up to 200 mcg of selenium daily.

Vanadium

Vanadium is a mineral mainly stored in our bones and fat. Although no human deficiency of vanadium has ever been identified, in test animals a deficiency caused impaired growth of teeth, bones, and cartilage; thyroid changes; decreased overall growth; and fluid retention. This mineral can also be used to build up teeth, bones, cartilage, and even muscle. It stimulates cell division but also has anticarcinogenic properties.

A substance called vanadyl sulfate, which is derived from vanadium, is used to increase muscle growth and development and appears to make muscles larger and denser more rapidly than would normally be the case.

Vanadyl sulfate is also very important in the treatment of diabetes. It helps insulin work more efficiently, and that may be why it also lowers cholesterol and triglyceride levels. If you have diabetes, I don't recommend long-term high doses of vanadium, but you can use it to help stabilize your blood sugar, and then cut back. Try starting with 6 mg daily and work your way up to 100 mg daily until you get results. Once you begin having results, stay at that dose for up to three weeks and then taper back gradually to 6–10 mg daily.

Normally, it is not necessary to include vanadium as a dietary supplement.

Zinc

Think of zinc as a traffic officer, directing and overseeing the efficient flow of body processes, the maintenance of enzyme systems, and the integrity of our cells. It is a tiny but powerful catalyst that is absolutely essential for most body functions.

Zinc is a trace mineral found in the thyroid gland, hair, fingernails and toenails, nervous system, liver, bones, pancreas, kidneys, pituitary glands, blood, and in the male reproductive fluid, or semen. It is the prime element in male hormone production. Zinc is a constituent of insulin, which is necessary for the utilization of sugar. It also assists food absorption through the intestinal wall.

Zinc governs the contractility of our muscles, stabilizes blood, and maintains the relationship of acidity and alkalinity in the blood and other fluids. Zinc is essential for the synthesis of protein and in the action of many enzymes. A lack of zinc can cause increased fatigue, susceptibility to infection and injury, and a slowdown in alertness and scholastic achievement.

Zinc exerts a normalizing effect on the prostate, and a lack of the mineral can produce testicular atrophy and prostate trouble. Zinc is necessary for the proper functioning of the prostate gland. In men, higher concentrations of this mineral are found in the prostate than anywhere else in the body. A recent study looked at zinc supplementation in young men and found that when plasma zinc levels were low, there was a corresponding drop in testosterone. There have been many clinical studies showing that zinc supplementation can reduce the size of the prostate gland, along with troublesome symptoms.

Zinc supplements during pregnancy appear to promote an increase in birth weight. It's important for athletes to take a zinc supplement, because vigorous exercise leads to significant loss of this mineral.

Most zinc available in foods is lost in processing. For example, 80 percent of the zinc in white bread is destroyed by processing. White spots or bands on the fingernails may indicate zinc deficiency.

Zinc supplements can be taken as lozenges, and in that form can cut down the length and severity of colds and flu, especially when combined with vitamin C.

Zinc is important in maintaining clear skin. Zinc stimulates antibody production to help fend off invading organisms on the skin surface. Some adolescent acne may be caused by a zinc deficiency.

As with all minerals, don't take zinc in excess, as it will cause other imbalances in your body. Zinc works best in combination with vitamin A, calcium, and phosphorus.

I recommend that all men take up to 15–30 mg of zinc daily and include zinc-rich foods in the diet such as oysters (well cooked, please!), lamb chops, and wheat germ. Pumpkin seeds are also a good source of zinc. Pregnant women and athletes can take 15–30 mg daily. Everyone else should include 5–15 mg of zinc in their daily supplements.

THE *BAD* TRACE MINERALS AND HOW TO AVOID THEM

The following trace minerals I have labeled as "bad" because, although they exist in the body in extremely small amounts, they can cause toxicity in minute doses, some as small as a few parts per million. Even the "good" trace minerals are only beneficial in very small amounts, becoming toxic in large amounts. The toxic metals tend to accumulate in the body, increasing their potential for toxicity. Some can enter the brain, causing serious biochemical imbalances. Industrial wastes, car exhaust, farming with artificial fertilizers, pesticides and fungicides, copper and lead in pipes, polluted groundwater, and cooking and eating utensils made of these dangerous substances have created an environment where metal poisoning is common in the industrialized world.

It's easy to become frightened after reading about the pervasiveness of these metals in the environment and the extent of the damage they can do to the body, and there is certainly cause for concern and watchfulness. Your best ally is education: finding out what the sources of these metals are and then avoiding them as best you can. A single exposure to toxic trace minerals is unlikely to cause serious illness unless it is a very large dose. Most poisoning occurs through small doses over time.

Exposure to toxic trace minerals can be insidious because the symptoms may be generalized and not severe enough to warrant a visit to the doctor or proper blood testing by a doctor, yet be severe enough to cause chronic fatigue, headaches, dizziness, and mental and emotional symptoms such as irritability, confusion, memory loss, hyperactivity, and even violent behavior.

According to research reported by the American Society for Reproductive Medicine, air pollution with heavy metals may be an unsuspected cause of infertility. Exposure to cadmium, nickel, manganese, and zinc at concentrations not high enough to be directly toxic can produce changes in sperm that cause infertility. Some estimates put it at 1 percent per year. (Exposure to hormone-altering pesticides is also playing a role in male infertility.)

Eating a balanced, nutritious diet, drinking plenty of clean water, doing moderate exercise, and taking a daily multivitamin will make a big different in your body's ability to detox and clear out any overload of toxic minerals. Getting the "good" minerals in your daily supplement regimen is particularly important, because many of the toxic trace minerals replace good minerals such as calcium, iron, and zinc.

Aluminum

Thanks to industrial pollution and the widespread use of aluminum in foods, medicines, municipal water treatment, and cosmetics, people living in industrialized nations are exposed to much higher levels of this metal than is safe.

Although it is the third most abundant element in the earth's crust, aluminum is only found in very small amounts in plants and animals. Up to a point, our bodies are well equipped to safely excrete most of the aluminum we ingest. But in larger doses, it becomes toxic, causing bone abnormalities, muscle weakness, loss of balance and coordination, memory loss, and depression. Because aluminum interferes with the absorption of important minerals such as selenium, magnesium, and calcium, its toxic effects can include the deficiency diseases caused by a lack of these minerals.

The fact that aluminum's toxicity remains controversial has more to do with greed and politics than a lack of scientific research. Aluminum in excess is clearly a poison, but it is also the third most used metal product in the United States. This means that the aluminum lobbyists are well endowed and powerful enough to discourage government action that might decrease our exposure to aluminum.

Because aluminum is so pervasive in the environment, it pays to avoid it whenever possible, because even then you're likely to be getting regular overdoses of it.

Aluminum and Alzheimer's Disease

Although research into the connection between Alzheimer's disease and aluminum remains controversial, it is clear from half a dozen good population studies that those with higher levels of aluminum in their water supply have higher levels of Alzheimer's. In fact, rats whose brains are injected with aluminum have symptoms similar to those of Alzheimer's. A Johns Hopkins University study found that those patients undergoing hemodialysis who had increased levels of aluminum also had decreased levels of cognitive brain function. The authors of that study theorized that aluminum may interfere with the brain's ability to use glucose and thus its ability to produce important brain chemicals, such as acetylcholine.

It may also be that some people have a genetic susceptibility to brain damage caused by a combination of factors, including aluminum. Whatever the cause or combination of causes, aluminum is clearly implicated in Alzheimer's disease, and for that reason alone I would recommend that you avoid it.

Sources of Aluminum

One of the most pervasive sources of aluminum is simply industrial by-products, blown out smoke-stacks, dumped into rivers and waste sites, and trickling into our water aquifers. The secondary effect of industrial air pollution is acid rain, which contains high levels of aluminum that leaches through the soil into groundwater over time.

Aluminum also enters water through municipal treatment plants because aluminum sulfate (alum) is used to clarify the water. To add insult to injury, there is some evidence that adding fluoride to the water makes the aluminum even more toxic by making it more difficult to excrete. Aluminum fluoride also crosses the blood-brain barrier more easily, exposing the brain to increased levels of both aluminum and fluoride. Ironically, the sodium fluoride pumped into America's water supplies is a waste product of aluminum manufacturing.

Aluminum is commonly used in processed foods as an emulsifier, to prevent clumping, and to whiten ingredients. It is found in processed flours of all kinds, baking powder, processed fruits and vegetables, and table salt. There are literally dozens of variations on aluminum additives, but some of the most common ones you'll find on food labels are alum, aluminum potassium sulfate, sodium aluminum phosphate, sodium silicon aluminate, aluminum calcium silicate, potassium alum, aluminum stearate, and aluminum hydroxide. Suffice it to say that anything with the word *aluminum* in it counts.

Probably the next most common source of aluminum is antacids. Antacid users can easily consume 5 g (5,000 mg) of aluminum per day. Since 150 mg a day is considered a safe level of aluminum consumption, antacids represent a major source of aluminum overdose. Indigestion and heartburn become more common as we age, and antacid use and abuse rise steeply in people over the age of fifty. (See chapter 5 for specifics on preventing and treating indigestion and heartburn naturally.) As we age, we accumulate heavy metals in our tissues, so throwing any additional burden on top of an already overloaded system may be pushing some senior citizens into symptoms of senility by blocking essential trace minerals such as selenium and causing brain chemistry changes. Antacids also interfere with the absorption of nutrients, so I recommend that you avoid them except for occasional use, and then use antacids that don't contain aluminum. The most common type of aluminum in antacids is aluminum hydroxide, which is transformed by hydrochloric acid in the stomach to aluminum chloride, which is easily absorbed in the intestines. Drinking citrus juice such as orange or grapefruit juice or taking vitamin C within an hour or two of taking an antacid can greatly increase the absorption of aluminum.

Aluminum is also put into deodorants designed to be absorbed through the skin, creating a daily source of aluminum consumption. Toothpaste is another source of aluminum compounds that can be avoided. Your local health food store will have aluminum-free deodorants and toothpastes.

Although aluminum pots and pans are not as large a source of aluminum as food additives, they remain a daily source of aluminum consumption for those who use them. Acidic foods such as tomatoes and coffee leach more aluminum from pots and pans, and there is evidence that as they age, these implements corrode, increasing the levels of aluminum ingested. It's safer for your health in the long run to use stainless steel pots and pans with copper or aluminum outer bottoms to conduct heat evenly, or you can use glass cookware.

Arsenic

When I think of arsenic, I think of Victorian-era detectives on the trail of an arsenic poisoning, and indeed, for centuries it was one of the most popular ways to kill someone. Arsenic accumulates in the body, so taking very small amounts over a long period of time will eventually cause poisoning. It's interesting that among the "bad" trace minerals, arsenic is not the most potently toxic. In fact, the "good" trace mineral fluoride is a much more potent toxin than arsenic and was used as a rat poison before it started being dumped into our municipal water supplies. (See our earlier discussion of water fluoridation.)

It may also surprise you to know that your body needs arsenic. It is a necessary nutrient—although in extremely small amounts, which you easily get just by eating and drinking. In industrialized countries, it's much more likely that you're getting an overdose of arsenic via industrial smokestacks, fungicides, pesticides, herbicides, and cigarette smoke.

Excess arsenic can cause high blood pressure; skin abnormalities such as odd pigmentation, lesions, and psoriasis; diarrhea; symptoms of heartburn and indigestion; cancer; and poor circulation. There is also some evidence that chronic overexposure to arsenic can be a causative factor in diabetes.

Cadmium

Our major source of overexposure to the trace mineral cadmium is agricultural dependence on superphosphate fertilizers. Crops grown with them will absorb higher than normal levels of cadmium from the soil. Cadmium is not only toxic in and of itself in small amounts; it also displaces zinc, one of our most essential trace minerals. Cadmium replaces zinc in plants and animals and is absorbed in greater amounts when zinc is deficient. Thus, like many of the toxic trace minerals, there is a double jeopardy, with overexposure to cadmium causing a deficiency of zinc and the potential for all the resulting illnesses. This is one of the best reasons I can think of to eat organic fruits and vegetables, aside from not being exposed to pesticides.

Cadmium is also an industrial waste product and can be poisonous in doses as small as three parts per million. Alcoholic drinks like wine and whiskey are relatively high in cadmium, and cigarette smoke is a significant source. In fact, cadmium is probably one of the main sources of illness in those exposed to secondhand smoke. Pregnant women who smoke are more likely to give birth to zinc-deficient babies.

Cadmium blocks the absorption of iron. And in studies on the effects of cadmium done with rodents, the immune system was compromised. Overexposure to cadmium also causes lung, kidney, and liver disease. Moreover, it can cause high blood pressure and may play a role in Alzheimer's disease.

Lead

According to the medical journal *The Lancet*, some historians believe that lead contamination in wine decanters and other cookware in ancient Rome led to its downfall owing to widespread lead poisoning among the upper classes. As far-fetched as this theory might sound, it's not implausible, because the effects of lead poisoning are subtle and insidious and lead to deterioration of the brain.

More recently, prior to the 1970s, lead was widely used in the United States in interior house paint. For this reason, lead is still an incredibly common source of poisoning, especially among children. If you live in one of the estimated forty million houses in the United States that still has lead-based paint inside, you, your family, and your pets may be breathing lead-laden dust. It's more than worth it, if you live in a house built prior to 1976, to have your house dust or paint tested for lead.

If you do find that you have high levels of lead in your house paint or dust, it's important to cover it or remove it. If you remove it, be sure to take precautions not to breathe the dust created or allow your family and pets to breathe it. Small children and pregnant women should not be allowed in a house where leaded paint is being removed. If you have lead paint on the outside of your house, it can wash off the side of the house and into the soil, polluting areas where children play or where pets spend time.

Those children most susceptible to lead poisoning live in urban slums where paint is peeling. And prior to the early 1990s, when leaded gasoline was finally phased out, there was excessive lead in the air from car exhaust.

And here's the typical toxic trace mineral double jeopardy: Zinc deficiency can exacerbate lead poisoning, and zinc supplementation may prevent it. While those in poverty in the United States aren't typically starving, their nutrition tends to be very poor, with an emphasis on refined white flours, chips, soda, sugary foods, and other processed foods devoid of essential trace minerals such as zinc. Children from low-income families have been shown to be deficient in dietary zinc, so not only are they overexposed to lead, but they are deficient in the very mineral that could help them avoid lead poisoning.

But lead doesn't just take up where zinc left off. Where lead is present in high levels, and calcium and magnesium are low, the body will take up lead instead of calcium and magnesium. Sufficient dietary calcium and magnesium can also help prevent lead poisoning.

Premature infants also tend to be deficient in zinc. Lead poisoning in children can cause mental retardation, stunted growth, hearing loss, anemia, high blood pressure, hyperactivity, aggressiveness, kidney disease, poor coordination, learning disabilities, and lower IQ. According to a report published in the *Journal of the American Medical Association*, a study that evaluated 503 first-grade children for lead exposure found that higher levels of lead were associated with antisocial and delinquent behavior. When nutrition is very poor and lead exposure very high, even death may result.

Another source of lead is tap water polluted by old plumbing soldered with lead. The EPA (Environmental Protection Agency) estimates that one out of every six households in America has toxic levels of lead in their water. Tin cans soldered with lead used to be a source of lead poisoning in the United States, and in many countries still are. Children may chew on toys with lead-based paints. Cigarette smoke is also a source of lead. Lead crystal decanters, if used to store wine or other alcoholic or acidic beverages, can be a significant source of lead. Even a lead crystal glass filled with wine will leach tiny amounts of lead.

One of the most common sources of lead poisoning among adults in North America is ceramic pots, plates, cups, pitchers, casserole dishes, and other cookware and food storage containers bought in foreign countries that don't regulate lead content, such as Mexico, South America, and Asia. If you buy these items outside of North America, I recommend that you test them for lead before eating off them or using them to store food.

Symptoms of lead poisoning in adults can include confusion, headaches, constipation, fatigue, weight loss, high blood pressure, kidney disease, degenerative brain diseases, reproductive abnormalities, and digestive problems. According to a study done at Harvard Medical School, even low levels of lead poisoning can cause kidney dysfunction in older men. Overexposure to lead is also associated with cancer, probably because lead interferes with the production of glutathione, your body's first level of antioxidant defense.

Mercury

The single biggest source of exposure to the toxic trace mineral mercury is dental fillings called amalgams, which contain a mix of metals, including mercury. Because mercury is a liquid metal at room temperature and changes easily with changes in temperature and pressure, it readily gives off fumes that are inhaled by those with amalgam fillings.

Unfortunately, the toxicity of mercury fillings is not acknowledged by the American Dental Association, presumably due to fear of billions of dollars in class action lawsuits if they admit to the dangers of this extremely toxic and volatile heavy metal. In other countries, mercury amalgams have been well studied, and it is clear that the more mercury amalgam fillings a person has, the higher the mercury concentrations in the blood and urine. Both dentists and dental assistants frequently show symptoms of mercury poisoning. Germany and Sweden have banned the use of mercury in dental fillings.

I strongly recommend that you not have any new mercury amalgams put in, and if you are suffering from symptoms of mercury poisoning, have your old amalgams taken out and replaced with porcelain fillings. (Gold fillings can contain high levels of cadmium.) There is no perfect substance to use for filling cavities in teeth, but porcelain seems to be the most benign right now.

Mercury is yet another heavy metal that is a common by-product of industrial wastes, and it is also a common waste product in hospitals. It is often dumped into waterways or the ocean, where it is ingested by shellfish and fish. Large fish that live near coastlines often have very high levels of mercury in their flesh. Swordfish and large tuna have the highest levels of mercury.

Mercury is one of the most toxic of the heavy metals, as it inhibits the body's use of the important B vitamin folic acid and alters protein structures, which are involved in every aspect of bodily function.

Symptoms of mercury poisoning can include birth defects in the children of mothers exposed to it in utero and central nervous system damage, such as is seen in multiple sclerosis and Alzheimer's disease. Other symptoms include insomnia, anorexia, chronic fatigue, depression, headaches, diarrhea, irregular heartbeat, hair loss, irritability, kidney damage, loss of sex drive, and muscle weakness. Mercury suppresses the immune system and creates a high susceptibility to infection.

If you break a thermometer in your home and spill mercury, cleaning it up can cause significant amounts of mercury to escape into the air, carpets, and dust of the house. Pregnant women and small children should be removed from the room for at least 24 hours, and the mercury should be carefully scooped up and placed in a closed glass container. The container should be disposed of at a hazardous waste facility. Then the area where the mercury spilled should be carefully vacuumed up and the bag immediately disposed of.

Nickel

Nickel is a trace mineral that is needed for the maintenance of health in very small amounts, but can quickly become toxic. Nickel is found in human RNA and is thought to play a role in enzyme function. Overexposure to nickel can cause heart disease, cancer, skin disorders, and thyroid malfunction. Because nickel is not a commonly used metal, overexposure is rare.

Tin

Poisoning from tin used to be a major health problem due to canning and storage of food in tin containers with no inner coating, but today it is rare. Caution should be used, however, when eating canned food outside North America. Some processed foods may contain tin-based preservatives and stabilizers.

Overexposure to tin may interfere with the body's production of glutathione, an important antioxidant, and block the absorption of copper, zinc, and iron.

Chelation Therapy and Other Detoxifiers

Mainstream medicine is largely at a loss to effectively handle heavy-metal poisoning, but for years, alternative doctors and other health care professionals have successfully used chelation therapy to rid the body of these toxins and also to treat heart disease. Chelation therapy is controversial largely because it competes with prescription drugs and is a safe and effective alternative to them. Opponents claim that EDTA (ethylenediaminetetraacetic acid), the synthetic amino acid used in chelation, can produce kidney damage. This has been caused by rapid administration of the EDTA solution. Today, the solution is infused very slowly, and there hasn't been an instance of kidney damage with EDTA use since the early 1960s.

Chelation therapy uses EDTA or other chelating agents, given intravenously over a period of many weeks or months in twenty to thirty treatments. At the same time, essential vitamins and minerals are given. EDTA essentially latches onto heavy metals that have accumulated in the tissues, combining with them to form compounds that can be excreted from the body. Chelation therapy is well studied and has

been used in at least half a million people. Remarkable results have been achieved with it for children with lead poisoning and for adults with heart disease, Alzheimer's disease, and arthritis.

Substances found in seaweed called alginates have been found to bind with some heavy metals, including strontium, cadmium, barium, radium, and lead. Regularly adding dried seaweed products to meals can be a kind of health insurance against heavy-metal poisoning.

Saunas and sweat baths are said to sweat out heavy metals, but this is hard on the body if you are already weakened by toxins.

One of the best allies against the accumulation of heavy metals in the body is proper nutrition. Getting plenty of the "good" trace minerals and enough of the body's other needed nutrients for optimal health will give your body the armament it needs to fight heavy metals.

4 HERBS FOR YOUR HEALTH~

HERBS, THE ORIGINAL MEDICINES

Can you imagine a world without bottles of aspirin and antibiotics? How would you feel if your doctor had no drugs to prescribe for serious illnesses? This was the world of our not-so-distant ancestors, and what's more, it still exists today in Third World countries. Yet it is precisely this primitive world that we owe for all the benefits of modern medicine we enjoy.

The pharmaceutical industry has learned to harness the power of many natural substances, producing synthetic versions that have become our prescription and over-the-counter drugs. These have brought undoubted advances, but often at the cost of debilitating side effects and complications.

Meanwhile, more and more scientific research is serving to remind us of nature's own safer, gentler packages of healing power that lie behind so many of today's drugs. The truth is that remedies like Grandma's elderberry wine and the Chickasaw Indians' infusion of willow root are scientifically proven. As more and more natural remedies are tested and refined, the apparent need for expensive drugs with dangerous side effects declines. Real medical advances are in store as we learn to combine the old wisdom with the new.

What Is an Herb?

Any plant with medicinal properties is called an herb. Of course, herbs can also be plants used as food, or in cosmetics, or for seasoning or flavoring. Herbs used to treat physical conditions are plants that in some way demonstrate a healing effect.

Herbs are the main source of medicine for the primary care needs of possibly 80 percent of the world's population. This was the World Health Organization's estimate in 1985. In the United States, herbs have been overtaken by manufactured drugs only in the past sixty years. Until World War II, the *U.S. Pharmacopoeia*, the listing of officially accepted medicines, included herbal preparations. Even today, nearly 40 percent of prescribed drugs dispensed in the United States either are based on or are synthesized versions of natural substances. In a way, herbs are the forgotten or hidden healing elements of modern medicine.

THE ANCIENT TRADITION OF HERBAL MEDICINE

Chrysanthemum as an antibiotic? It's true, and, believe it or not, used by chimpanzees! Zoologists in Africa have seen one species regularly dosing themselves with this potent plant. All of us have seen sick cats and dogs eating grass. Imagine human intelligence and curiosity combined with instinct, and it's easy to see how prehistoric cultures must have developed considerable knowledge of the medicinal properties of the plants around them.

We no longer have to chew on buckthorn and discover its purgative effects by accident. Someone long ago ate lobelia flowers and ended up with their head over an ancient toilet. It is modern science that labels these things as laxatives and emetics, but it was wise, observant people of the past who discovered them and realized that their actions could relieve illness. Indeed, the remains of herbal remedies such as bramble, crab apple, orache (a spinachlike weed), and wild service tree have been found in the pots and waste pits of Neolithic villages in England and Switzerland. The recording of such remedies began as civilization advanced, allowing us to trace fascinating herbal treatments from every culture far back into history.

Traditional herbal medicine in India, called Ayurveda, goes back more than five thousand years. As far back as 3000 B.C., official schools of herbalism existed in Egypt, teaching about plants like garlic, mint, and coriander. Cleopatra is said to have used cucumber to preserve her skin, and the *Ebers Papyrus*, written about 1500 B.C., recommends applying a moldy piece of bread to open wounds, thousands of years before Alexander Fleming developed penicillin from the very same mold.

The Chinese were using oil from hydnocarpus trees to treat leprosy as early as 2500 B.C. Centuries later came the *Shen Nong Ben Cao Jing*, China's first true herbal, describing more than 350 plants used for medicinal purposes. The Chinese were also using ephedrine, our over-the-counter cold medication, in the form of the shrub ma huang, over two thousand years ago.

Although a religious work, the Bible is another rich source of herbal references, from cinnamon to myrrh, with mandrakes even serving as aphrodisiacs in the Genesis story of Jacob's wives, Leah and Rachel.

Early European settlers in America were amazed at and often thankful for the range of medicinal applications of herbs used by the Indians, treating everything from headaches to heart conditions. Tribes such as the Iroquois and Mohegans treated colds and fevers with tea made from the boneset plant. Wormwood was a bronchitis and cold remedy used by Indians as far apart as New Mexico and British Columbia. Thompson Indians would stuff their nostrils with wormwood leaves to relieve nasal congestion and when burying decaying corpses. As America was settled, remedies were exchanged. Europeans, for example, learned of soothing witch hazel ointment from the North Americans, and Indians learned to use dandelion remedies for conditions like heartburn as the plant was introduced to their country.

Some American Indian, European, and Eastern remedies were often selected in a similar manner, referred to as the Doctrine of Signatures. A plant would be used to treat a condition of a body part that it resembled. Liverleaf, with liver-shaped leaves, for example, was used to treat liver disorders. Science has even proven links for plants such as red bloodroot as a "blood purifier" and the yellowish goldenseal root for the treatment of jaundice.

European herbal remedies, passed down through village wise women, sold by wandering herbalists, and often copied by monks from ancient Greek and Roman writings, were used by royalty and peasants alike. Queen Elizabeth I is said to have favored meadowsweet, used to treat flu, fever, and arthritis. From Roman times, lavender was known to promote relaxation, while chervil was recommended as a stimulant—one that also reportedly cured hiccups if you ate the whole plant! Arabs, too, used Greek and Roman texts, elaborating on remedies with often highly sweetened preparations and exotic spices. Herbs such as ginger and cardamom were believed to prevent illness.

The herbals of sixteenth- and seventeenth-century Europe make colorful reading today. Would you swallow sumac powder if you were advised that it had "great efficacy in strengthening the stomach and bowels"? Would you wash "pestiferous sores" with wild succory? How about calamint to kill "all manner of worms in the body"? We might smile and raise our eyebrows at some of these ancient herbal treatments, but science today is telling us loud and clear that many a plant prescription makes as much (if not more) sense as a modern drug equivalent.

FROM FOLKLORE TO PHARMACEUTICAL

Observation, trial and error, and faith seem to have been key to the practice of early Western herbalism. It came with no real system or rules until the second century A.D. and a Greek called Galen, physician to a Roman emperor. Galen's herbal marked the beginning of a trend separating the professional physician from the traditional healer. Influenced by Galen and his rigid rules, medicine began to be taught in

Europe as a superior art, favoring exotic medicines with aggressive treatments such as bloodletting and purging.

Following the failure of this style of doctoring to help in the Black Plague of 1348 and again with outbreaks of syphilis, Galenic practice began to be challenged in Europe in the sixteenth and seventeenth centuries. Herbalists such as the famous Englishman Nicholas Culpeper helped expose the false mystery and monopoly of "official" medicine and brought simple, garden-grown remedies back to popularity. Brutal attempts at dramatic cures with practices like medical bleeding eventually died out, but not before George Washington was bled to death in 1797 during treatment for a sore throat.

The Swiss physician and alchemist Paracelsus, who developed laudanum, also influenced the return to the idea that medicines were found by searching for cures held by plants. He even predicted that pharmacologically "active principles" would be found in herbs. Ironically, it may have been the observation of just such active compounds in the plant digitalis that set orthodox medicine on the path of the synthetic drugs that came to replace herbs. In 1785, the English doctor William Withering detailed the biological effects and recommended doses of the plant digitalis. His work eventually led to the discovery of the modern heart stimulants digoxin and digitoxin.

Digitalis probably helped standard physicians continue to focus on the "quick fix"—in demand, too, of course, by the public. Although prominent figures like Thomas Jefferson still cultivated herbs in kitchen gardens, eighteenth-century chemists worked hard in laboratories to isolate and synthesize active ingredients and bypass the plants themselves. In this way, the modern pharmaceutical industry was born.

In a move to help companies recover the costs of research and development of synthetic substances, the U.S. government passed a patent medicine law in the late 1800s. This gave companies the exclusive seventeen-year rights to sell patented drugs. Unfortunately, it also gave them an incentive to discredit the use of natural remedies in order to maximize profits from synthetic ones. Formation of the Federal Drug Administration (FDA) made this situation even worse for natural remedies. There is no incentive at all to gain FDA approval for an herbal medicine when it takes ten to eighteen years and costs millions of dollars with no patent protection at the end of it all!

In countries like France and Germany, however, the system for approval of medicines is different, and many natural medications are sold over-the-counter and prescribed. No health claims can be made in the United States for herbal remedies, which must be sold as foods or supplements. Thanks also to the American Medical Association's (AMA) support and huge marketing campaigns, it's not surprising that synthetic drugs have dominated American medical teaching and treatment since the 1950s. However, surveys show that the majority of Americans take supplements of some sort, and increasing numbers of physicians are beginning to integrate modern and traditional practices. The Program in Integrative Medicine at the University of Arizona, for example, is part of a new teaching trend that integrates alternative medicine with mainstream medicine. The future of medicine will be all about combining ancient knowledge with modern technology.

NATURAL OR SYNTHETIC? A QUESTION OF BALANCE

Heart attack? Broken leg? Life-threatening infection? Western emergency medicine is the proven choice. But it's estimated that emergencies make up only about 20 percent of conditions treated by doctors. Viral infections, degenerative diseases, cancers, autoimmune diseases, and other illnesses make up the other 80 percent. With the majority of illnesses, the focus of modern medicine has been the relief of symptoms. The aim with herbal remedies, on the other hand, is the restoration of health by treating the underlying cause.

Early herbalists regarded themselves as "nature's servants" and respected the body's natural efforts to return to wellness. Western pharmaceutical companies act more like nature's masters, attempting to manipulate biochemical functions in isolation from each other. The drugs they produce are concentrated versions of compounds recognized by the cells of our bodies. This is why they achieve their often fast and dramatic effects. However, to make an effective substance patentable, drug companies must add molecules that make the drug synthetic, or not found in nature. These extra molecules create additional biological reactions as they are processed—reactions we call side effects.

In contrast, herbal remedies package their active chemicals with beneficial substances that ameliorate side effects. This packaging can make the active compound more easily absorbed, as with the uptake of iron aided by the vitamin C in plants like watercress and rose hips. Other chemical combinations in herbs seem to be built-in safety measures. Ephedrine, isolated from the ma huang plant, was once prescribed for asthma but produced the side effect of dangerously high blood pressure. The whole plant has been used for thousands of years with no harmful results. The difference? There are six related chemicals in the herb itself, one of which actually lowers blood pressure and reduces heart rate. Aspirin can relieve pain and fever but may cause stomach bleeding. Its natural derivative, white willow bark, is without this unwanted effect.

Scientific analysis bears out the observation that the effects of chemicals in plants often have parallel effects in humans. Plants such as cranberries contain substances that help to preserve them by killing bacteria. The same substances have similar effects in our bodies. This sort of phenomenon is not surprising, since every living thing is made of the same basic constituents, such as proteins and sugars, and since they have all evolved from the same origins.

Medicinal plants also echo the body's own life-maintaining system of checks and balances. Ginseng, for instance, contains hormonelike substances called saponins. Some have a sedative effect; others are stimulating. The body, then, will naturally utilize the different saponins according to its needs. Ginseng, as a result, is a body stabilizer, increasing the ability of the body to withstand stress. Hawthorn berries work on blood pressure in the same way with a mixture of compounds that either raise or lower blood pressure. Expert herbalists are able to extend this process by creating remedies that are a combination of plants with a selected balance of effects.

Western medicine's pill-popping habits have led to passive, often fearful, and unquestioning patients who do not expect to take much part in their own recovery. Herbal medicine differs in that it demands a review of the body's overall condition as well as specific symptoms. Herbs themselves, and the way they are used, are more likely than synthetic drugs to address underlying conditions. The care, cultivation, and mixing of herbs also bring respect for and conservation of natural resources.

While the advances brought about by modern medicine are obvious, Western levels of conditions like heart disease, hypertension, and cancers are appallingly high. Complications from prescription drugs result in 40 percent of hospitalizations and cause twenty thousand to thirty thousand deaths every year in the United States. Yet this is an age where a balance can be struck. Powerful, short-term treatment with synthetic drugs is a proven option. Gentle, safe longer-term herbal medications deserve a role alongside them as nature's complete pharmacy, evolved in natural harmony with the human body.

Science Proves the Value of Herbs

Slaves building the Egyptian pyramids once went on strike over their rations of garlic! Today they would have scientific proof of its benefits—so much of it that even the U.S. medical establishment cannot falsely claim that none exists. Recent years have produced two thousand studies on garlic by researchers all over the world. Garlic has been shown to be antimicrobial, antibiotic, antiviral, antiparasitic, and anticancer as well as being an immune booster. Substances found in garlic include antioxidants, smooth muscle relaxants, and four powerful anticlogging agents. Studies have shown how these substances help garlic prevent and relieve heart disease. Garlic also inhibits an enzyme that generates an inflammatory chemical, explaining claims for its use with asthma.

Another ancient remedy proven effective by science is chamomile, used for centuries in Europe against infections and aches. Modern analysis shows that it is an antispasmodic in the bowel and stomach, with a sedative effect on the central nervous system. It also contains anti-inflammatories, which contribute to its usefulness in ointments and lotions.

A North American remedy now validated scientifically is the purple coneflower, echinacea. Native Americans used this plant medicinally more than any other plant. Echinacea treatments existed for wounds, burns, abscesses, insect bites, snake bites, toothaches, joint pains, and infections. Chemical analysis of echinacea reveals a fascinating combination of substances, including some with antiviral and anticancer properties and others that regenerate tissue. Interestingly, the antibiotic properties of echinacea are mild. Instead, scientists have found that it is the strong immune-enhancing activity of echinacea compounds that lies behind its power against internal and external bacterial infections.

A popular folk remedy for colds and flu, elderberry has high concentrations of bioflavonoids. These could account for the recently proven ability of elderberry extract to kill flu viruses. A recent double-blind study using the commercial elderberry extract Sambucol more than halved the recovery time for sufferers of flu compared to subjects given placebos. As a winter tonic, elderberry is now official.

Chemicals called PCOs are the main effective agents in the bilberry, or European blueberry. Bilberry jam was eaten to improve the night vision of World War II pilots. Bilberry extract has indeed been shown to improve the ability of the eyes to adapt from dark to light. It also prevents and retards cataracts and ulcers and lowers blood sugar, proving its folk use in the treatment of diabetes. What's more, its relaxing effects on smooth muscle have been demonstrated in experiments, showing exactly why it became a treatment for vascular disorders.

Another herb that shines under the spotlight of modern science is ginger. Used for thousands of years in China, ginger is shown to be high in antioxidants, to inhibit inflammation triggers and blood-clotting agents, to kill bacteria, and to reduce cholesterol levels. Animal studies confirm ginger's traditional use in warming the body and treating ulcers.

Experiments also show important differences in the composition of dry and raw ginger. They serve, too, to show why the effects of herbs like garlic and licorice change, depending on their form. The standards of modern analysis and testing producing these kinds of observations give added reassurance to users of herbal remedies. They form a technological supplement to the huge volume of historical evidence for the efficacy of herbs. And they often stem, ironically, from the research used to produce synthetic drugs. Perhaps the pendulum is due now to rest between traditional herbal and modern medicines.

The Race for Modern Herbal Discoveries Is On

Did you know that a major ingredient of birth control pills comes from wild yam or that quinine, the malaria drug, is derived from the Peruvian "fever tree," the cinchona? A surprising amount of the world's harvest goes to help produce the drugs of our time. Unhappily, the potential harvest has been dwindling at an amazing rate as land is cleared or developed. Experts like Tom Eisner, Schurman Professor of Biology at Cornell, point out that only about 2 percent of known plant species have been analyzed thoroughly for their pharmacological effects. Even worse, botanists estimate that millions of plants have still to be named, and many have already been lost forever to environmental destruction. Only recently, logging operations in Pacific Northwest forests burned Pacific yew as slash. Then came the discovery of the anticancer drug taxol in, yes, the bark of the Pacific yew tree. There is no doubt that many effective compounds must have already been lost as unknown species have been wiped out.

Naturalists and scientists have been spurred to work together to fully investigate the wealth of species already collected and to campaign for environmental preservation measures. The profit motive actually brings the cooperation of drug companies, too, which continually search for new plant drugs to synthesize. The payoff can be big, in medical and money terms, with finds like the rosy periwinkle, which has produced two anticancer drugs used successfully to treat childhood leukemias and Hodgkin's disease. This was an accidental spin-off of a drug company's search for antidiabetic agents. Drugs like the fungus-derived cyclosporin, an immune suppressant used in organ transplants, and ivermectin, a parasitic worm killer, have also been uncovered relatively recently.

Only a small percentage of known plants have already yielded tremendous medical benefit. It's simply common sense to continue the research and investigation of the depleted stocks of the laboratory we call earth while ensuring, too, that we don't burn down the laboratory itself.

Medicinal Herbs in Other Cultures

Because herbs are the main form of medicine for most cultures of the world, and because pharmaceutical drugs are, relatively speaking, much more expensive and cause thousands of deaths every year, the World Health Organization is studying and promoting herbal medicines. Natural medicines have come into their own as inexpensive, safe, and effective treatments easily accessible to their native users. There is a real opportunity for developing cultures to integrate natural remedies with the benefits of modern medicine and none of the penalties.

China, with its established and ancient herbal tradition, has been integrating positive aspects of Western medicine faster than natural remedies have been revived in the West. A revival is happening, however, and on an international scale. Many physicians from India also train in the United States and Europe, blending Ayurvedic and Western medicines in their practices. Scientific research has spurred fresh interest, seeing sales of herbal products pass $4 billion in Germany alone and higher figures in Japan.

Use of herbal remedies as standard medicines in different countries probably never dipped as low as they did in the United States with its restrictive FDA regulations. Herbal medicines and modern drugs face the same legal tests in Germany, and insurance reimburses the costs of herbal remedies sold in pharmacies when they are prescribed by a doctor. One of the three most widely prescribed drugs in both Germany and France is ginkgo biloba, used to treat certain vascular disorders. In the United States, ginkgo biloba can only be sold as a food supplement. German physicians might also prescribe the herb valerian to treat mild anxiety. Homeopathic remedies are very widely prescribed in France. In Great Britain, natural remedies have always sat side by side with synthetic remedies on drugstore shelves.

Around the world, cultural gravity seems to be working to pull Western medicine back down to its herbal roots. The weight of scientific evidence only adds to the pull, with the message that stronger links with nature are good medicine everywhere on earth.

A WORD OF CAUTION ABOUT HERBS

As modern technology becomes increasingly sophisticated, we are discovering more and more about just how complex plant ingredients are. We used to believe that beta-carotene was the only useful vitamin in a carrot. Now we know that in a raw carrot there are hundreds of carotenoids, of which beta-carotene is only one. In addition, a raw carrot is packed with vitamins, minerals, sugars, enzymes, fibers, and dozens of other substances we don't fully understand yet.

Think of celery and lettuce. For years we were told they had no nutritional value. Now we know that if you eat six stalks of celery a day, your blood pressure will almost certainly drop. And lettuce contains ingredients that can make you sleepy. It's not that these vegetables had no nutritional value; it's just that until recently, our technology and science weren't advanced enough to understand them.

Any healing herb or medicinal plant is a veritable chemistry lab of ingredients with specific biochemical actions and reactions in the human body. These include volatile oils, which give plants their aroma; sterols, which are similar to our own steroid hormones; saponins, which have "soapy" qualities; and alkaloids, which are often poisonous to the liver but which sometimes have profound healing properties.

Each healing herb has specific effects on the body, based on its chemical makeup. The chemicals that have the strongest effects on the tissues and organs of the body are called *active principles*. Plants rich in active principles are the most valuable as medicines. It is the active principles in plants that the pharmaceutical companies attempt to isolate, patent, and turn into pharmaceutical drugs. But what we have found, over and over again, is that once an active principle is isolated from the other ingredients in a plant, it has side effects. Somehow in the miraculous wisdom of nature, a whole herb prepared and taken properly has very few, if any, side effects. The synergy or combination of ingredients working together in a plant brings a balance to it as a medicine that makes herbal medicine gentle and yet still effective.

While herbal medicines are more gentle than pharmaceutical drugs, don't be fooled into thinking that herbs can be used carelessly. A wide range of potency and toxicity exists among the healing herbs. Women who are pregnant or nursing, as well as anyone with a serious chronic illness such as diabetes or heart disease, should carefully research an herb or consult with a health care professional familiar with herbs before using it.

For example, angelica can be a wonderful herb for indigestion and for inducing sweat in a cold. But because it increases circulation, it can also promote menstruation, so it shouldn't be used by pregnant women. Another active principle in angelica can increase the amount of sugar in the blood, so angelica should not be used by diabetics without supervision.

Your doctor is unlikely to encourage you to use herbal medicine. He or she was told in medical school that herbs were unscientific, superstitious folklore. Doctors are trained to believe that their job is to diagnose a disease and then find a drug to prescribe for the symptoms of the disease. While I know that you're going to get a negative response ranging from condescension to dire warnings if you tell your doctor that you're taking herbs, I encourage you not to self-treat yourself with herbs if you have a serious or chronic condition. Seek out a doctor who uses natural medicines, or find a naturopathic doctor. Many chiropractors are also skilled in the use of natural medicines. And before taking any herb, do your homework. That could be as simple as referring to this book, or it could mean buying a more detailed herb book and doing some in-depth research. Don't use an herb long-term without thoroughly checking it out. Powerful herbs, such as ephedra, should never be used for more than a week or two at a time.

If You're Taking Other Medications

Be aware that mixing herbs with pharmaceutical drugs can cause the drug to overreact or underreact. For example, ephedra may help dry up your sinuses, but it also can raise blood pressure and increase heart rate, which can be dangerous for someone taking a heart drug. And echinacea won't interfere with an antibiotic, but because it stimulates the immune system, it could interfere with an immunosuppressive drug, such as a cortisone.

On the other side of the coin, taking herbs that support your body can help alleviate the side effects of a prescription drug. For example, if you're taking acetaminophen (Tylenol), which is very hard on the liver, taking milk thistle (silymarin) will help support your liver.

I realize that you can't possibly figure out all the possible interactions of drugs, foods, and herbs. But you need to be aware that herbs do have specific biochemical actions in the body, so you should use caution. My best advice is to use common sense and moderation and follow the proper dosage instructions.

As a pharmacist, I am well aware that no two people respond to a medicine in the same way. Each person's biochemistry is unique. Your weight, age, sex, and diet, as well as how much you exercise and whether you use drugs such as alcohol and caffeine will all affect how you respond to an herbal medicine.

If you try an herb and feel worse, stop taking it. If you try an herb and nothing happens, try half again to twice as much. If there is still no result, this probably isn't the herb for you. (Some herbs take two to four weeks to affect the system in a noticeable way. Again, do your research.)

If You're Pregnant

When you're pregnant, you want to avoid putting anything into your body that would disrupt or interfere with the growth of the fetus. Do not take herbs of any kind if you're pregnant without checking first with an experienced health care professional familiar with herbs. There are a few herbs, such as raspberry leaf, which can be beneficial when you're pregnant, and there are specific herbs to help with labor and to start breast milk flowing. However, these should only be used as directed by an experienced professional.

MY TOP THIRTY HEALING HERBS

Here's a comprehensive list of my favorite healing and health-promoting herbs.

Aloe Vera *(Aloe barbadensis)*

It's common to see a spiky houseplant with thick, rubbery, tapering green leaves edged with spiny teeth in a pot sitting around a home. Those wise to the ways of herbal healing keep it in the kitchen. The plant is aloe vera, or lily of the desert, and for most people it is there waiting to exude a mucilaginous sap when broken as first aid to quickly spread over a burn to relieve pain and prevent blisters. However, the skin-healing properties of aloe are not limited to burns.

In Africa, prior to hunting, natives rub the gel of the aloe over their bodies to remove the human scent. Women all over the world apply aloe gel on their skin to keep it supple and to clear blemishes. Greek history records the use of aloe as a healing herb for wounds two thousand years ago. Legend has it that Cleopatra massaged the gel into her skin every day. Napoleon's wife, Josephine, is said to have used a lotion of aloe and milk for her complexion.

In Ayurvedic medicine, aloe gel is a tonic for the female reproductive system. At one time, people rubbed it into their scalps, believing that it prevented hair loss. The gel is used to treat ulcers, ringworm, and shingles and to repel insects.

Aloe reportedly helps to clear pimples and acne. Dermatologists have also had success treating oily skin, dandruff, and psoriasis with aloe. By applying aloe to their nipples, nursing mothers can begin to reduce the supply of milk, thereby serving as an aid to weaning. And aloe has been found to aid in the treatment of frostbite.

The medicinal properties of aloe have now been scientifically substantiated. Research documents its healing effect in all kinds of burns and the itch caused by poison ivy and poison oak. Additional studies have confirmed the anesthetic, antibacterial, and tissue-restorative properties of this remarkable herb. The gel does indeed heal burns from the sun or a hot pan, and when not severe, regenerates tissue without scarring.

Aloe is believed to improve wound healing by increasing the availability of oxygen and by increasing the synthesis and strength of collagen and tissue.

Arnica *(Arnica montana)*

Also commonly called leopard's bane, arnica is a perennial herb found singly or in small clusters in mountainous regions. Its bright yellow, daisylike flower heads bloom around July.

The volatile oils from the dried flower heads of European arnica have been used since the eleventh century largely as a topical pain reliever and as an application to treat bruises and sprains. The Catawba Indians used a tea of arnica root resins for treating back pains. In old Russia, the herb was used internally to reduce cholesterol, promote production of bile, stimulate the nervous system, stop bleeding, and strengthen the heart.

Externally, the classic use of arnica is for muscle, joint, or cartilage pain that is generally aggravated by movement and alleviated by rest. Typically, arnica is rubbed on the skin to soothe and heal bruises, sprains, hyperextensions, wounds, and irritations and to provide relief from muscle spasm, arthritis, and bursitis. Placed on the stomach, a compress containing arnica can relieve abdominal pains. Applied as a salve, arnica is also good for chapped lips, irritated nostrils, and acne. Only a highly diluted form of arnica should be used when the surface of the skin is broken. Too strong a concentration can cause blistering. There are a wide variety of arnica creams and salves available at your health food store.

Internally, tinctures of arnica are used for mental and physical shock, pain and swelling, concussion, fractured bones, sprains, dental extractions, and headache. Some doctors have used the herb for internal bleeding, obstinate sore throat, and inflammation of the mouth. Arnica should never be used internally without medical direction because an overdose can be fatal.

Arnica works by stimulating activity of white blood cells (macrophages) that perform much of the digestion of congested blood and by dispersing trapped, disorganized fluids from banged, bumped, and bruised tissues, muscles, and joints.

Bilberry *(Vaccinium myrtillus)*

The bilberry, or European blueberry, is a perennial shrub that grows in meadows and woods in Europe. Only the blue-black berries of the plant are used. These differ from the American blueberry in that the meat of the bilberry fruit is blue-black throughout.

Bilberry has long been a folk remedy for poor vision and night blindness. During World War II, British Royal Air Force pilots reported improved vision on night bombing raids after eating bilberry jam.

Clinical tests confirm that bilberry given orally to humans not only improves visual accuracy in healthy people but also helps those with eye diseases such as retinitis pigmentosa, glaucoma, and myopia. Components in the herb work specifically to improve vision by improving microcirculation and speeding the regeneration of retinal purple, a substance required for good eyesight.

Bilberry extract has been widely used in connection with vascular, or blood vessel, disorders. Specific studies reveal a positive effect in the treatment of varicose veins, thrombosis, and angina. The active components of bilberries are its flavonoids, which prevent capillary fragility, inhibit platelet aggregation, and stimulate the release of vasodilators, substances that open up blood vessels and improve the flow of blood, thus increasing the level of oxygen in tissues.

Recent research has also indicated that bilberry extract possesses significant preventive and curative antiulcer properties, attributed to the strengthening of the defensive barriers of the digestive system.

Calendula (*Calendula officinalis*)

A featured plant in many ornamental gardens, calendula, or pot marigold, is a hardy, many-branched annual, almost entirely covered with fine hairs. The yellow-to-deep-orange flowers ray out from a central head and close up at night.

Ancient Romans named this plant, noting that the flowers were in bloom on the first day, or calends, of every month. They also grew calendula to treat scorpion bites. In early use, the herb was also used to treat headaches, fevers, and toothaches. A sixteenth-century concoction that called for the use of calendula was thought to enable one to see fairies. Calendula came to America with settlers from Europe and was used during the Civil War to stop bleeding and promote the healing of wounds.

Medically, calendula flower tinctures have been recommended in the treatment of a wide variety of ailments, including fever, cramps, flu, and stomachaches. Others apply calendula-based remedies to external sores, cuts, bruises, burns, and rashes. Calendula flowers are said to relieve the pain of bee stings. And when applied directly to the ear, calendula oil can reduce earache pain. Mothers find it works well as a solution for diaper rash. Calendula and arnica are often combined in commercial skin ointments for burns and bruises.

Calendula tea can be used as an eyewash for sore, reddened eyes. As a cosmetic, calendula brings out highlights in blond and brunette hair and is found in herbal bath mixtures to stimulate the body.

The flavor and color of calendula account for its widespread use in cooking, particularly soups, cheeses, and salads.

The volatile oils in calendula stimulate blood circulation and induce sweating, thus aiding fevers to break, and accelerate eruptions like measles or rashes. Calendula also increases urination, aids digestion, and acts as a general tonic. The herb's antiseptic value is likely related to its content of natural iodine.

Cat's Claw (*Uncaria tomentosa*)

We keep hearing about the medicinal potential of plants growing undiscovered in the Amazon jungle of South America. One that is showing great potential as a healing herb has been brought to this country. It is called cat's claw, or una de gato, its Spanish name.

Scientific studies on cat's claw are in progress, but Indians native to the Amazon rain forest have long relied on this herb to heal a range of ills. Although many, many claims have been made for the various healing powers of cat's claw, studies on it are limited. The herb does, however, seem to hold promise for enhancing the immune system and as an anti-inflammatory, meaning that it may well deliver relief from joint pain like arthritis.

At this time, scientists have not isolated the active constituents of cat's claw in their quest to manufacture a patentable drug. In other words, the whole plant works very effectively, but there doesn't seem to be one single ingredient that's responsible for its healing powers.

If you have arthritis, you may want to try cat's claw, particularly if other things you have tried for inflammatory conditions have proved unsuccessful.

One caution: Natives of Peru reportedly use cat's claw for birth control, so don't take it if you are trying to become pregnant.

Dong Quai *(Angelica sinensis)*

This fragrant perennial herb grows in China, Korea, and Japan. The root of the plant is described as having a head, body, and tail to correspond with the herb's various applications.

The reputation of dong quai in Asia is second only to ginseng. Regarded as the ultimate, all-purpose woman's tonic herb, it is used for almost every gynecological complaint, from regulating the menstrual cycle and treating menopausal symptoms, such as hot flashes caused by hormonal changes, to assuring a healthy pregnancy and easy delivery. Chinese women have used dong quai for centuries to stop painful menstrual cramps caused by uterine contractions.

Herbalists today use dong quai for menopausal symptoms such as hot flashes, for PMS, and to stimulate regular menstruation when women go off birth control pills.

Scientific investigation has shown that dong quai produces a balancing effect on estrogen activity. The herb, rich in vitamins and minerals, has also been used to promote blood circulation and correct anemia in both sexes, as well as to treat insomnia, lower high blood pressure, and alleviate constipation.

Most recently, studies involving dong quai have indicated that the herb regulates irregular heartbeat, may help prevent heart disease, and acts as an immunostimulant to suppress tumors.

Echinacea *(Echinacea angustifolia)*

Resembling a black-eyed Susan, echinacea, or purple coneflower, is a North American herbaceous perennial that is also called snakeroot because it grows from a thick black root that American Indians used to treat snake bites, indicative of the blood-cleansing quality attributed to this herb.

Native American tribes of the Great Plains are known to have used echinacea for medicinal purposes, notably as an antispasmodic or analgesic (painkiller). They also used the juice of the plant to bathe burns, and the root to treat toothaches and sore throats as well as colds and flu. They would sprinkle the herb over a burning fire for "sweats" for purification purposes. During the 1920s, echinacea was one of this country's most popular plant drugs. Herbalists have long appreciated the healing benefits of echinacea as an effective antiviral and as a blood purifier to cure a host of ailments, including rheumatism, psoriasis, dyspepsia, gangrene, tumors, eczema, and hemorrhoids.

Echinacea is regarded as a potent immunostimulator and as such has been used to treat such ailments as herpes, infections, *Candida*, and cancer. The herb has also been used to help restore normal immune function in cancer patients undergoing chemotherapy.

Studies have shown that echinacea prevents the formation of an enzyme that destroys a natural barrier between healthy tissue and damaging organisms, such as herpes and influenza viruses. The herb is the most popular flu and cold remedy in Germany.

Elderberry *(Sambucus canadensis)*

This herb has been intertwined with human history from the very beginning. Traces of elderberry have been found in Stone Age sites. It provided the wood for Christ's cross. Judas hung himself from an elder tree. Seventeenth-century herbalist John Evelyn so highly regarded the elderberry that he called it a remedy "against all infirmities whatever." Gypsies agreed, calling it the "healingest tree on earth." Hippocrates wrote of its value as a purgative. One of Shakespeare's characters referred to it as "the stinking elder." There is even one growing outside of Westminster Abbey, planted there for its mystical ability to ward off evil spirits and disease.

Elder was widely used by several American Indian tribes. The Houmas boiled bark for use as a wash for inflammations. The Menominees used the dried flowers to brew a tea to reduce fevers. And the Meskivakis made tea from the root bark as an expectorant and to treat headaches. Cooked elderberries were prepared as a drink by some tribes for neuralgia, sciatica, and back pain, while others used the leaves in sweat baths to induce profuse sweating, which brought relief from rheumatism pain. There is scientific evidence that a substance in elderberries does in fact stimulate perspiration.

Externally, the herb has been used to relieve skin inflammation such as burns, rashes, and eczema. Elderberries are a good source of vitamins A, B, and C plus flavonoids.

The berries are also the source of popular elderberry wine, regarded by many as a tonic, and the cooked berries are the main ingredients for pies and jams. Most recently, new evidence was found to indicate remarkable value in an elderberry extract in the treatment of the flu virus.

Ephedra *(Ephedra sinica)*

This herb goes by the American names of cowboy tea and squaw tea, reflecting its use by early pioneers and Mormon settlers, who used it primarily for asthma relief. The tea was made from powder derived from the dried green twigs of the shrub. It is also called Mormon tea, since it is brewed as a pleasant piney substitute for coffee and black tea, which Mormons avoid.

The Chinese name for ephedra is ma huang. The Chinese species of the herb grows in the Inner Mongolia region of China. Ephedra has been used in Asia for nearly five thousand years to treat asthma and upper respiratory symptoms such as coughs, as well as to reduce fevers and treat allergic skin reactions, such as hives.

Imported from China and cultivated in dry regions of North America, ephedra contains an alkaloid called ephedrine that provides effective decongestant, bronchodilator, antiasthmatic, and antiallergic functions. A synthetic version of ephedrine called pseudoephedrine is an ingredient found in many over-the-counter cold and allergy medications.

Ephedra has also been found to promote weight loss. This is due to its fat-metabolizing ability and to the fact that it suppresses appetite—an effect that is enhanced when it is combined with caffeine.

Eucalyptus *(Eucalyptus globulus)*

Native to Australia, where they account for 75 percent of the vegetation, eucalyptus trees are tall, graceful trees with slender, silvery leaves and creamy bark. Eucalyptus leaves are the dietary mainstay of koala bears, and humans have used eucalyptus oil for a wide variety of medicinal purposes.

It is the aborigines of Australia who were first to discover that eucalyptus oil possesses medicinal properties. The most popular application of eucalyptus oil is for respiratory ailments. Used in a vaporizer, it doesn't take long for the volatile oils to help you breathe more freely and relieve the symptoms of a cold, chronic bronchitis, or asthma.

Eucalyptus oil (eucalyptol) is an effective expectorant used in many commercial drops and lozenges and in liquid preparations to loosen mucus from the nose and lungs and relieve upper respiratory discomfort. Distilled from leaves, the volatile oil is also used as a germicide.

Applied to the skin, eucalyptus oil increases the flow of blood to the area, bringing warming relief from stiffness, swelling, arthritis, and rheumatism. The oil also possesses antiseptic qualities useful in the treatment of both respiratory infections and skin diseases. When aged, the oil forms ozone, a form of oxygen that will specifically destroy bacteria, fungi, and certain viruses.

Feverfew *(Chrysanthemum parthenium)*

The name of this hardy biennial or perennial herb suggests its early use to bring down a fever. The ancient Greek herbalist Dioscorides used the herb to treat arthritis and also believed that it helped regulate the uterus during childbirth.

In the lengthy history of this herb, it has been used as an aromatic to ward off disease, for toothaches, as an insect repellent, and against a variety of ailments, including kidney stones, constipation, arthritis, infant colic, and vertigo.

Perhaps the most effective modern-day application of feverfew is for headaches, but as early as 1649, herbalist Nicholas Culpeper noted that feverfew "is very effectual for all pains in the head." Later, in 1772, another famous herbalist John Hell wrote, "In the worst headache, this herb exceeds whatever else is known." But it wasn't until 1978, when British newspapers reported that a woman had cured her migraines with feverfew, that medical researchers decided to examine the medicinal value of the herb. In 1980, *The Lancet*, the highly respected British medical journal, reported that the herb shared properties with aspirin. Then in 1985, the *British Medical Journal* reported another study confirming that feverfew helps alleviate the pain of migraines. Three years later, *The Lancet* confirmed the efficacy of feverfew in treating migraines. Once again, pharmaceutical companies have worked feverishly (no pun intended) to isolate the active ingredients of feverfew and turn it into a synthetic patent medicine—but with no success. It is the synergistic combination of ingredients in the feverfew plant that brings on such effective migraine relief.

Feverfew works to inhibit the release of two inflammatory substances—serotonin and prostaglandins—both believed to contribute to the onset of migraine attacks. It also appears that compounds in feverfew serve to make muscle cells less responsive to certain chemicals in the body that trigger migraine muscle spasms. Curiously, feverfew works only for migraines and not for regular headaches.

Garlic *(Allium sativum)*

Although it is best known as a culinary herb or vampire retardant, the medicinal benefits and claims for garlic are prodigious and worthy of the appellation "wonder drug among all herbs." Throughout recorded history, garlic has been used all over the world for a wide variety of conditions. In folk medicines, it has been used for the plague, coughs, tuberculosis, and diarrhea; as an antiseptic; to promote kidney function; as a blood cleanser; to kill intestinal parasites; and to prevent heart disease and cancer. It is also used as an antibiotic and antifungal.

Garlic is noted in ancient Chinese writings, is mentioned in the Bible and in Homer's *Odyssey*, and has been found in the ancient tombs of Egypt. The Egyptians, incidentally, are said to have fed garlic to the slaves building the Pyramids to give them extra strength and nourishment.

Louis Pasteur discovered that garlic cloves would kill microorganisms in a petri dish. While working as a missionary in Africa, Dr. Albert Schweitzer used garlic to treat cholera, typhus, and amebic dysentery. During both world wars, before the advent of antibi-

otics, garlic juice was daubed on infected wounds as a disinfectant to prevent gangrene. The Soviet army relied so heavily on garlic that the herb earned the designation "Russian penicillin."

Modern-day research helps explain the broad applications of this "miracle" herb. The same component that gives garlic its strong odor is the one that destroys or inhibits various bacteria and fungi. This component is allicin, which, when garlic is crushed, combines with the enzyme allinase and results in antibacterial action equivalent to 1 percent penicillin. Garlic is reported to be even more effective than penicillin against typhus disease. It works well against both strep and staph bacteria and the organisms responsible for cholera, dysentery, and enteritis.

The irritating quality of garlic's volatile oil, readily absorbed into the bloodstream, may explain its use for respiratory problems by opening up lungs and bronchial tubes.

On top of everything else it does, this fascinating herb has been found to inhibit tumor cell formation and is under investigation by the National Cancer Institute for its cancer-inhibiting qualities.

Note that cooking garlic diminishes its potency, but several full-strength supplements and combinations of garlic are commercially available.

Ginger *(Zingiber officinale)*

It is the knotty branched root of this tropical perennial that is used for medicinal purposes as well as a pungent condiment. The Chinese have used ginger medicinally for well over two thousand years. It is primarily employed to treat gastrointestinal disorders, particularly gas, colic, and indigestion. The herb possesses the ability to calm an upset stomach and to stop gripping and cramping in the abdominal and intestinal areas.

Ginger is a very effective and safe antinauseant, preventing the symptoms of motion sickness and "morning sickness" in pregnant women, including vomiting, dizziness, and cold sweats. Drinking tea containing ginger for colds and asthma has long been a popular American remedy.

Ginger is a mild stimulant, promoting good circulation. Laboratory tests indicate that ginger will lower cholesterol levels and inhibit the clotting and aggregation of blood.

A few drops of warmed ginger oil in the ear can soothe earaches. Grated ginger mixed with a little oil and applied to the scalp helps remedy dandruff. Ginger has also been credited with relieving headache and toothache pain.

Ginkgo *(Ginkgo biloba)*

Ginkgo biloba is the earth's oldest living tree species, traced back more than two hundred million years. The tree itself can live one thousand years, reaching over 100 feet high and 4 feet in diameter. The medicinal use of this "living fossil" goes back nearly five thousand years.

An extract of ginkgo biloba offers significant benefit to people with impaired blood flow to the brain. Symptoms of this cerebral insufficiency, commonly associated with aging, include short-term memory loss, headache, tinnitus (ringing in the ears), vertigo, and depression. Due to its high flavonoid content, ginkgo also improves circulation throughout the whole body, resulting in an increase in oxygen and blood sugar utilization to all internal organ systems and lower extremities, thereby addressing problems related to poor circulation such as phlebitis. This positive vascular effect also serves to treat symptoms of underlying arterial insufficiency, providing protection against the development of Alzheimer's disease, strokes, and hearing loss. It is a valuable medicine for diabetics, who suffer from impaired circulation to the extremities.

Free-radical scavenging and antioxidant effects have been attributed to ginkgo and are credited with slowing the processes responsible for premature aging and cancer.

Hemorrhoids have been successfully treated by taking ginkgo extract. In one study, 86 percent of patients reported that bleeding and pain stopped.

The effects of ginkgo as an antiallergenic and antiasthmatic agent have been scientifically demonstrated.

Ginseng *(Panax ginseng)*

This small perennial herb is without doubt the most famous medicinal plant in China. It was the Chinese who first noted that roots of ginseng resemble the human body and interpreted this as a sign of a medicine that could enhance the whole of human health. A portion that looked like a man would bring a higher price than an entire bale of nondescript roots. The word *ginseng* literally means "root of man," and the botanical name of one type, *Panax*, is derived from "panacea."

Ginseng has been used in China for five thousand years as a tonic and rejuvenator. A Soviet scientist dubbed ginseng an "adaptogen" for its unique ability to normalize, or bring into balance, whatever is out of balance in the body. For example, if blood sugar levels are low or if blood pressure is too high, an adaptogen will bring them back to normal levels. Ginseng acts on the pituitary, helps to regulate blood sugar, supports the adrenal glands, and generally promotes physical and mental alertness, increasing energy and stamina. Diminishing fatigue is one reason athletes find particular benefit from the use of this herb.

Ginseng is believed to increase women's level of hormones and is consequently recommended for some women for menopausal symptoms.

The herb stimulates weight and tissue growth and thereby enhances the body's resistance to disease. It particularly benefits the digestive process and the lungs and therefore treats lack of appetite, chronic diarrhea, shortness of breath or wheezing, and insomnia.

Studies have shown that ginseng not only inhibits the production of cancer cells but actually converts the abnormal cells into normal ones.

The hormonelike structure found in ginseng's saponins has a stimulatory effect on sexual function in males and females, which may support the herb's reputation for enhancing sexual desire.

Goldenseal *(Hydrastis canadensis)*

Widely used by a number of Native American tribes, goldenseal is a broad-spectrum herb with a reputation for great medicinal virtuosity and as a result has been recommended for the treatment of many conditions and ailments.

An infusion of the roots is made into a wash for sore eyes and for skin diseases. Other uses of goldenseal include treatment for indigestion, loss of appetite, and liver problems. It has been available as a commercial medicine in North America and throughout Europe for well over a hundred years.

Goldenseal is primarily used to treat congestion and soothe inflammatory conditions of the mucous membranes that line the respiratory, gastrointestinal, digestive, and genitourinary tracts. Goldenseal owes its medicinal value to its high content of the alkaloids hydrastine, hydrastinine, and the better-known gerberine. These alkaloids produce a strong astringent, antibiotic, and immune-stimulating effect on mucous membranes.

Antibacterial components in goldenseal have proven effective in the treatment of diarrhea.

One experiment with goldenseal extract on laboratory animals brought about a drop in blood pressure.

Goldenseal can be used as an external application to arms and legs in the treatment of disorders of the lymphatic system and blood vessels. One folk remedy calls for rubbing goldenseal on the skin to treat eczema and ringworm.

A component of goldenseal was found to have anticonvulsive effects on the uterus. Goldenseal can also soothe irritated gums, help prevent gum disease, and treat canker sores.

The herb is commonly used for female ailments such as vaginitis, and a douche of goldenseal can help relieve fungal infections such as *Candida*.

Hawthorn *(Crataegus oxyacantha)*

The brilliant red berries of the hawthorn tree hang in dense clusters from thorny branches and remain on the tree until after the leaves drop in autumn.

Since the seventeenth century, hawthorn has had a history of use for its positive effects on the cardiovascular system. Traditionally, this herb was involved in the treatment of digestive problems, insomnia, and sore throat. Both Asian and North American cultures used hawthorn for weight loss. It also works as a diuretic, assisting the body in the elimination of excess salt and water.

Hawthorn benefits the heart in three ways: (1) Its flavonoids increase oxygen utilization by the heart; (2) it increases enzyme metabolism and acts as a mild dilator of heart muscle; and (3) it acts as a peripheral vasodilator (dilates blood vessels away from the heart), thereby lowering blood pressure and relieving the burden placed on the heart.

Specific cardiac symptoms for which hawthorn may be called for include recovery from a heart attack, cardiopulmonary disease, high blood pressure, and irregular heartbeat.

Hawthorn in combination with digitalis is given for cardiac problems such as palpitations, angina, and rapid heartbeat (tachycardia). One experiment indicated that a mixture of hawthorn and the herb motherwort might prove an effective preventive or treatment for heart disease. Components in hawthorn have been shown to lower cholesterol as well as the size of plaques in arteries.

Kava-Kava *(Piper methysticum)*

This herb, a member of the pepper family, grows as a bush in the South Pacific. The first European to discover it was Captain James Cook while he was sailing the South Seas. It was consumed during Polynesian religious rites for its ability to relax and soothe the mind.

Kava is also used for its medicinal effects as a sedative, muscle relaxant, diuretic, and remedy for nervousness and insomnia. The herb is also used as a pain reliever and can often be used instead of NSAIDs (drugs such as aspirin, acetaminophen, and ibuprofen).

Studies have shown kava to be as effective in treating anxiety and depression as the prescription antianxiety agents known as benzodiazepines (such as Valium), but without the adverse side effects. In fact, while the benzodiazepines tend to promote lethargy and mental impairment, kava has been shown to improve concentration, memory, and reaction time for people suffering from anxiety.

Lavender *(Lavandula officinalis)*

Considered by some to be the quintessential English garden herb, and highly regarded for its classic fragrance in fancy soaps, sachets, and potpourris, lavender is also important as a medicinal herb.

Traditionally, the flowers or oil from this old-fashioned herb were used to protect clothes and stored linens from hungry moths. It was also perhaps one of the first air fresheners, often found in early sickrooms. The name *lavender* is actually derived from the Latin verb "to wash," and both Greeks and Romans would scent their baths with the herb. Lavender was an ingredient of aromatic spirits of ammonia, the smelling salts that prevented or relieved fainting spells.

In China, the herb is used as a cure-all oil they call white flower oil. It is used as a medicine for hysteria, hoarseness, toothaches, colic, and skin conditions such as eczema and psoriasis. Oil distilled from the perfumy flowers of lavender has applications as a stimulant, and a tonic for headache relief and relief of intestinal gas. It has also been used to quiet coughs and was once used as a disinfectant for wounds. Applied as a compress, warm lavender tea or oil provides relief for neuralgic pains, rheumatism, sprains, and sore joints.

Licorice *(Glycyrrhiza glabra)*

We think of this plant as a candy flavoring (even though most licorice candy is actually flavored with anise oil); however, the root and constituents of this herb provide a tremendous number of valuable medicinal properties.

Two thousand years ago, the Chinese ranked licorice "superior," which meant that it could be used over a long period of time with no toxic effects. They used licorice as a tonic to combat fevers and as a remedy for infection. In fact, it is the single most used herb in Chinese medicine.

Ancient Greeks used licorice as a thirst quencher and to relieve swelling caused by water retention. The Blackfoot Indians used steeped wild licorice leaves in water as an earache remedy. Dutch physicians tested licorice as an aid for indigestion, which led to the use of the herb to treat peptic ulcers.

Other medicinal applications for licorice have included treatment of fever, menstrual and menopausal problems, influenza, arthritis, irritated urinary or bowel passages, and hypoglycemia. Additionally, it has been used as a diuretic, laxative, and antispasmodic.

The most common medical use of licorice is for treating upper respiratory ailments, including coughs, hoarseness, sore throat, and bronchitis. The rhizomes and roots in licorice have a high mucilage content, which, when mixed with water or used in cough drops or syrup, is soothing to irritated mucous membranes and contributes to its use as an expectorant.

Another component of licorice, glycyrrhizin, stimulates the secretion of the adrenal cortex hormone aldosterone and has a powerful cortisonelike effect. In fact, one study found that glycyrrhizin was as effective a cough suppressant as codeine, and safer. In Europe, this unique compound is used extensively for its anti-inflammatory properties, especially for Addison's disease and ulcers. It has exhibited antiviral activity and as a result is used in Japan to treat chronic hepatitis B.

Milk Thistle *(Silybum marianum)*

This herb is a stout annual or biennial plant, found in dry, rocky soils. One of the active principles of milk thistle is the flavonoid silymarin, which has been shown to have a direct effect on the cells of the liver, enhancing the overall function of this critical organ.

The known medicinal value of milk thistle is almost exclusively to support the liver. The liver detoxifies poisons that enter the bloodstream, such as alcohol, nicotine, heavy metals (for example, lead and mercury), and environmental pollutants such as carbon monoxide and pesticides.

To underscore the importance of the liver, it is the source of the bile necessary for the breakdown of fats. It is also where vitamins A, D, E, and K are stored. No wonder the liver is referred to as the body's "chemical factory" and that the silymarin in milk thistle is so important.

In countless scientific studies, silymarin is reported to have shown positive effects in treating nearly every known form of liver disease, including cirrhosis, hepatitis, necroses, and chemical-, drug-, and alcohol-induced liver ailments.

Silymarin's remarkable ability to prevent liver destruction and support liver function is believed to be due to its ability to inhibit the factors responsible for liver damage coupled with the fact that it works to stimulate production of new liver cells to replace the old damaged ones. In addition, silymarin acts as an antioxidant, with far greater free-radical damage control than even vitamin E in the liver.

Other studies have found that milk thistle offers some protection against the toxic side effects of the pain-relieving drug acetaminophen (Tylenol), a popular analgesic medication.

The Mints *(Mentha* spp.*)*

We're talking here about more than the mint from the garden patch used to freshen a tall glass of lemonade or a mint julep.

All mints have cool, refreshing properties, and they have been used since antiquity all over the world in cooking and for their medicinal value. There are countless varieties and species of mints, and all are generally stimulating and relieve indigestion. But three stand out in the herbal medicine cabinet: peppermint, spearmint, and pennyroyal.

Peppermint

The leaves of this perennial are a deeper, richer color than the bright, vivid green of spearmint. This species is also more stimulating to the circulation and is a stronger remedy for alleviating flatulence, heartburn, and indigestion. Rather than cool off with a cool beverage in summer, the Chinese refresh themselves with hot peppermint tea, which leaves them feeling cooler because the infusion brings more blood to the skin, causing perspiration, which then evaporates away the heat of the body. A stronger tea can be instrumental in breaking a fever. Peppermint is excellent for heartburn, stomachache, nausea, and migraines.

Among other volatile oils, peppermint contains menthol and therefore has a minor antiseptic quality and is used as a gargle for sore throats and to cleanse wounds. Have a cup of mint tea after a heavy or rich dinner, because menthol also stimulates the flow of bile to the stomach, which promotes digestion and relieves upset stomach.

A simple tea makes a good headache remedy and can be useful to relieve tension and insomnia.

Spearmint

Much like peppermint, spearmint is an aromatic stimulant used for mild indigestion and to relieve nausea, stomach spasms and bowel pains, flatulence, motion sickness, and heartburn.

Spearmint tastes different from peppermint and is also not as strong because it contains no menthol. For this reason, spearmint can be substituted for the stronger mint when small children or very old people are being treated.

Pennyroyal

This herb, referred to as the "lung mint," was used to treat coughs and colds. It promotes perspiration to the point that it helps break a fever. American Indians utilized pennyroyal to relieve menstrual cramps, and herbalists have recommended this mint to induce menstruation and treat PMS. Because of its ability to induce menstruation, pennyroyal should not be used by pregnant women. Pennyroyal oil makes an excellent insect repellent for pets.

St. John's Wort *(Hypericum perforatum)*

Squeeze the petals of the flower from this shrubby perennial and a blood-colored resin will ooze out, which may explain why, according to legend, this plant sprang from the blood of Saint John the Baptist when he was beheaded.

For centuries in Europe, St. John's wort has been utilized as a mild tranquilizer and a treatment for depression and anxiety. While synthetic psychotropic drugs manufactured to treat these symptoms are associated with significant side effects (constipation, impaired urination, drowsiness), St. John's wort extract at recommended dosages shows no adverse side effects.

St. John's wort is also a muscle relaxant and is used to treat menstrual cramps. It is widely used for insomnia, and in Europe it is a popular remedy for gastrointestinal disorders.

Externally, it is an antiseptic and painkiller for burns and other irritations of the skin. Ointments containing St. John's wort are used to treat rheumatism and sciatica.

Most recently, evidence has surfaced that components in St. John's wort may inhibit the growth of retroviruses in animals, including HIV, the AIDS virus.

Saw Palmetto *(Serenoa repens)*

Saw palmetto is a small scrubby palm tree native to the U.S. Atlantic coast from South Carolina down through Florida. The tea from the berries of saw palmetto has long been used to treat urinary conditions and has been highly regarded as a remedy for enlarged prostate for centuries. Indeed, saw palmetto was tagged the "plant catheter" due to its therapeutic effect on the neck of the bladder and the prostate in men.

An extract of the saw palmetto will decrease urinary frequency (especially during the night) due to inflammation of the bladder and enlargement of the prostate. Reduced urinary flow, dribbling, and impotence are symptomatic of an enlarged prostate or benign prostatic hyperplasia (BPH).

BPH is thought to be caused by a dysfunction of a type of the male hormone testosterone. Saw palmetto extract prevents testosterone from converting into dihydrotestosterone, the hormone thought to cause prostate cells to multiply excessively, leading to enlargement of the prostate. It is when the prostate grows abnormally that it pinches the urethra and interferes with urination. Early and effective treatment is important because when the urethra becomes completely blocked, urine can back up into the kidneys, causing severe abdominal pain that calls for immediate medical attention.

Others believe that saw palmetto stimulates and increases bladder contractions, which facilitates easier and less painful urine flow.

Preliminary evidence also suggests that saw palmetto may also aid those suffering from thyroid deficiency. Moreover, this herb is a good expectorant for use in clearing chest congestion and is used to treat coughs due to colds as well as asthma and bronchitis.

Tea Tree Oil *(Melaleuca alternifolia)*

The tea tree is a small tree native to Australia, where it is acclaimed for its broad medical applications, particularly those affecting the skin. Although used in throat lozenges and in toothpastes, the oil distilled from tea tree leaves is mostly used externally.

In 1930, a surgeon in Sydney, Australia, first noted the positive effect of tea tree oil for cleaning and healing surgical wounds. It has subsequently been determined that tea tree oil exhibits significant antiseptic and antifungal properties as well as stimulating skin rejuvenation.

The established value of tea tree oil as a disinfectant, coupled with the fact that it possesses good penetration properties and is nonirritating, makes it useful for a vast number of conditions, including acne, diaper rash, heat rash, athlete's foot, canker sores, boils, sore throat, burns, psoriasis, root canal treatment, dandruff, respiratory congestion, gingivitis, herpes, and yeast infections.

Tea tree oil is available in many products such as toothpastes, shampoos, soaps, throat lozenges, hair conditioners, and skin lotions, and it is packaged in forms such as salves, ointments, gels, and liniments. Use as directed on the label.

Uva-Ursi *(Arctostaphylos uva-ursi)*

The leaves of this perennial ground cover, also known as bearberry, have an extended record as a folk remedy, particularly in relation to urinary tract problems. It is said that the Chinese introduced Marco Polo to this herb when he was traveling in China. European herbalists in the thirteenth century recognized the healing benefits of uva-ursi.

Before the development of synthetic diuretic and urinary antiseptic drugs, uva-ursi leaves were the main medicine available for these applications. The Chinese, European, and American natives all adopted uva-ursi as an herb for healing the kidneys, using the leaves and fresh berries for treating kidney stones, bladder infections, and incontinence. Some tribes also mixed uva-ursi leaves with other herbs and honey as a longevity elixir.

The strong urinary antiseptic, diuretic, and astringent qualities of uva-ursi are attributable to the active constituents hydroquinone and arbutin, which, interestingly, possess a more potent effect working together than either acting separately.

Analysis has shown that uva-ursi contains a substance known to soothe and speed repair of irritated tissue. The herb has also exhibited antiviral, antibacterial, antifungal, and antiplaque actions.

Valerian (Valeriana officinalis)

Valerian root's relaxing effects have inspired some to call it the "Valium of the nineteenth century." Since the 1800s, it has been known to relieve anxiety, nervous tension, and panic attacks. It is a useful herb for insomnia and has also been used to relieve gas pains and stomach cramps. Valerian isn't chemically related to Valium and so poses none of the dangerous side effects of this drug. It can, however, cause feelings of weepiness, so look out for this if you use valerian.

Vitex/Chasteberry (Vitex agnus-castus)

Chasteberry (also called vitex) was at one time recommended as a means for reducing excessive sexual desire—hence the significance of the "chaste" name for the plant. It is for this alleged effect that chasteberry was also used as a spice at monasteries during the Middle Ages, where it was called "monk's pepper."

Traditionally, chasteberry was very popular in Europe as a woman's remedy for regulating the reproductive system and treating PMS and the unpleasant side effects associated with menopause, such as hot flashes.

Research has revealed the presence of a volatile oil in chasteberry that tends to balance the production of women's hormones. This oil is believed to contain a progesteronelike substance, which could explain the herb's therapeutic effect in relation to PMS symptoms such as anxiety, nervous tension, insomnia, and mood changes, as well as problems associated with menopause, such as hot flashes, vaginal dryness, dizziness, and depression. Compounds in chasteberry also produce positive results when treating endometriosis, migraines, edema in the legs, cramps, and some allergies. Chasteberry has also been used to treat irregular menstruation, heavy bleeding, and fibroid cysts.

Chasteberry extract can improve skin conditions like acne by balancing sex hormones.

White Willow Bark (Salix alba)

The white willow was introduced into the United States from Europe and is now found gracing rivers and streams throughout the country. The bark is the part of the willow used medicinally, and it is easily removed in the spring when the sap begins to flow.

Willows have been tapped since antiquity for pain relief and reduction of fever. Ancient manuscripts of Egypt, Greece, and Assyria refer to willow bark, and even Hippocrates recommended willow to counter pain.

People have chewed the leaves or the inner bark of willows in this family of plants for thousands of years, and all contain salicylic acid. This compound was originally used by the Bayer Company in Germany in the late 1890s to synthesize acetylsalicylic acid, otherwise known as aspirin.

Natural salicylic acid is nearly as potent as aspirin. However, the compound salicin from willow does not cause gastric or intestinal upset or bleeding, as aspirin can. This is because the natural product does not block prostaglandins in the stomach or intestines.

Witch Hazel (Hamamelis virginiana)

Witch hazel is a name derived from an old English word for "pliant," and the branches of this deciduous tree are in fact limber and were used as archery bows. Witch hazel is used principally as a skin liniment and astringent. Available in extract form, its anti-inflammatory action helps soothe minor scrapes, cuts, and bruises. Applied externally to varicose veins or hemorrhoids, it helps relieve the pain and itching that accompany these conditions. A decoction of the bark is used as a dandruff wash, and the extract is useful for insect bites and sunburn.

PREPARING AND TAKING HERBS

Just the slightest crush releases the wonderful aromas of plants like mint in our gardens and kitchens. This is one of the simplest ways to sample the powerful essence of herbs, one we use all the time in our kitchens. Freshly chopped mint with our potatoes or dandelion leaves in our salad are just two examples of how easily herbs end

Your Herbal First Aid Kit for the Home

Herbal Preparation	Disorder	Treatment
Arnica ointment, arnica tincture	Sprains and bruises, burns, scalds, stings, and impetigo	Rub ointment gently onto unbroken skin or apply a compress of tincture
Calendula tincture, calendula ointment	Minor cuts	Bathe with tincture and/or apply ointment to cut
Echinacea tincture	Insect bites	Apply tincture to bite and take 1 dropperful in water
Echinacea and goldenseal mixture	Infections, flu, and common cold	2 to 4 dropperfuls in water every 4 waking hours
Herbal throat spray (with echinacea, goldenseal, and licorice)	Sore throats	Spray back of throat as indicated on container
Ginger tea	Nausea	3 to 4 cups daily
Peppermint tea	Headaches	3 to 4 cups daily
Tea tree oil	Toothache, gum and fungal infections	Apply oil to affected area
Valerian root tincture	Insomnia	Take drops with water as directed on container
White willow capsules	Headaches	1 capsule as needed

up on our dinner table. Frequently, though, it's more convenient or appropriate to use an herbal preparation. Then the trick is to capture the essence in usable forms. The range of herbal preparations is wide, including, for example, ointments for external application and capsules to be swallowed.

However an herb is prepared, its effect is achieved by interaction with our body chemistry. The aim is to ensure absorption and uptake by the bloodstream. Once circulating in the blood, an herb exerts its specific influence on the body. The key to traditional use and the work of skilled herbalists has always been the use of an herb's effects to support the body's own natural efforts to recover. This is unlike the tendency of many modern drugs designed to suppress the body's response and produce short-term comfort.

This is not to say that herbs can't bring immediate relief, as anyone who has soothed sunburn with aloe or calmed a toothache with oil of cloves will tell

you. It is more that herbal treatments are gentler and aligned to the body's own processes. Treatment of illness with herbs may well require a little more time than a "knock-'em-dead" blast, say, of antibiotics, but will be without the same risk of side effects and with much more likelihood of tackling the root cause.

Different conditions suit different methods of treatment based on selection of the best route for absorption of the herb. Absorption can take place through the digestive system, the skin, the lining of the mouth, the ear, and the nose (as with inhalation of hot vapors). Herbs are widely available now in a diversity of forms. Best results are obtained from organically grown fresh herbs. They should be preserved by proper drying and storage, so always check the source and avoid pills packed with fillers.

Many preparations can also be homemade, although the strongest form, essential oils, are best bought. Review the choices and enjoy tailoring your selection to your own particular needs. Remember: Use herbs as directed, following the same precautions as with any medicine, and always consult your physician if you are already being treated for a condition.

Drops and Spoonfuls

Some of the best internal herbal preparations are liquid and include syrups and tinctures. Tinctures are preservative mixtures of the herb in alcohol and water. Alcohol not only helps herbs last longer but is also a good solvent for many of their active components. A standard ratio is 1:5 of the herb to the fluid. An example would be 7 ounces (200 g) of herbs to 4½ cups (1 L) of alcohol such as vodka, although cider vinegar can be used instead if preferred. For homemade tinctures, place the herbs in a dark, screw-top jar and cover them with the alcohol. The mixture should be shaken twice daily and stored, tightly covered, in a warm place. Use a muslin cloth to strain the residue, squeezing well, after two weeks. Tightly stoppered dark bottles help prevent evaporation and destruction of constituents by light.

Tinctures are usually taken with water and are a very concentrated way to take herbs. Some people like to add them to teas or even compresses. Mixing a tincture with a little beeswax, cocoa butter, or olive oil is also a useful way to make an ointment. And syrups? These are in fact tinctures added to sugar—a sweet way to make the herb go down!

A Nice Cup of Herb

Drinking herbal teas can be one of the most pleasurable and effective ways of getting herbs into your system, although the taste of some leaves a lot to be desired! Teas are actually infusions. Boiling water helps extract and dissolve some of the medicinal compounds of an herb. This is a particularly useful way to prepare herbs desired for their potent aromatic oils, compounds that give teas their strong aromas. Tea bags or tea leaves are made from the dried herb and are generally equivalent to three parts of the fresh plant. When no particular dose is sought, an herbal tea can become more of a tonic or included as part of a remedy rather than one on its own.

Whereas infusions mainly use the soft, aboveground parts of plants, decoctions are another method of producing drinkable herbs. Decoctions are usually made with the woodier parts of plants, like roots and bark. The chopped herb is brought to boil for 10 to 15 minutes, then strained immediately. More volatile components are lost, but decoctions capture the mineral salts and bitter principles, which can lead to some "interesting" tastes and powerful healing.

Take One As Directed

Some herbal preparations are in capsule form, as with many supplements and medicines. Gelatin containers are filled with finely powdered herbs, oils, or extracted juice, usually in a hypoallergenic form. On reaching the gut, the shell is broken down, releasing the contents for absorption.

Herbs also come in traditional pill, tablet, or lozenge form. Mucilage, gum, dry sugar, or other binders and fillers are mixed with the powdered herb or with oil to make tablets or lozenges. Lozenges can be sucked, allowing them to be taken by a small degree into the bloodstream directly through the blood vessels of the mouth, but largely, again, through the walls of the intestine.

Homeopathic and some other preparations of herbs involve solutions mixed with sugar bases to create small pills. These are then placed under the tongue where they dissolve. This is known as sublingual absorption and is useful because it bypasses the liver. Always hungry to fuel its own processes, the liver is the blood's first major "stop" on its route from the stomach, and it is sometimes helpful to direct absorption elsewhere first.

Apply with Care, Rub Gently . . .

Many conditions are relieved by direct absorption of herbs through the skin. Sometimes part of the plant itself is used, as with fresh aloe or mugwort rubbed onto skin troubled by poison oak. Tinctures in fatty or oil bases make ointments, while more fluid liniments are herb extracts mixed with oils or alcohol.

Herbs can also be wrapped in material to make poultices that are laid on the skin. You can make compresses with wads of material soaked in herb decoctions or infusions. Topical applications like these are very useful for treating localized conditions like cuts, sprains, and aches.

Expert massage can also involve specific herbal treatments with extracts of essential plant oils, as in aromatherapy. The general benefits of a good all-over rub with a perfumed oil have been recognized for centuries. There's also nothing like relaxing in a bath of herbal salts as a way to feel the benefits of herbs working from the outside in.

Great Herb Combos

On the herbalist's menu are many formulas or combinations of medicinal plants established over history as stronger or broader in their effects than treatment with a single herb. Passionflower and valerian are good examples. Both reduce tension and anxiety, and a combination produces a double action, a natural sedative for short-term use.

Scientific investigation goes on to prove the synergistic value of combining herbs, balancing or increasing their individual chemical effects. For instance, sedative herbs are often supported by more stimulating ones like damiana to enable the body chemistry to even out rather than to swing one particular way. Licorice is used with the laxatives senna and cascara. The latter can cause intestinal pain, but licorice, itself a mild laxative, contains anti-inflammatory chemicals and lowers stomach acid levels, thus protecting against the harsher effects of the other two herbs.

Herbal formulas used in this way help to achieve harmony in the body and make very effective remedies.

HEALING HERBS YOU CAN GROW IN YOUR HOME OR GARDEN

"The fresher the better" is certainly true of herbs. Gathering from the wild is still possible but should only be done with an expert guide and with care not to exhaust an area of any one plant. Indoor and outdoor cultivation at your own home can be an enjoyable and inexpensive way to create your own supply of healing and culinary herbs. Starting with seeds gives you a choice of many varieties and is much cheaper than buying the plants themselves. Several herbs make natural partners, repelling insects, for example, or promoting plant health, so be alert to opportunities for companion planting.

Remember to check if a "weed" is itself a useful herb, like dandelion, that is worth cultivating where it will not smother other plants. However, plants such as bindweed, couch grass, creeping buttercup, ground elder, and creeping thistle are all best removed as soon as they appear. They're also no good for composting.

In tending herbs, you will be following a worldwide, centuries-old tradition. With your own flowerpots or garden and rich organic soil, you can grow your own mini-pharmacy and reap the benefits of better health, not to mention more flavorful food! Try your hand with some of the herbs listed here, and consult organic gardening books for tips on organic soil preparation, pest and disease control, plant layout, and propagation.

Harvest Time

Many are the witch's brews that call for strange herbs picked at dawn or by the light of the moon. Actually, both seemingly strange practices make scientific sense, because many of the medicinal compounds found in plants are volatile. This means that they are evaporated by the sun's heat, so they are at their greatest concentration in plants before the sun is high in the sky. If you can, pick your herbs as soon as the dew has evaporated.

Pick leaves and flowers early in the morning, being careful not to bruise them. Flowers are usually best harvested as soon as possible after they have fully opened. For culinary purposes, leaves can be picked any time from a green and healthy plant. For medicinal purposes, however, leaves are usually best collected when flowers are in bud and before any have fully opened. Remember to shake off any insects.

Roots contain their greatest concentration of useful substances at the end of the growing season. Collect them at this time, discarding any that are damaged at all. Do not soak roots before drying, but wash them thoroughly to remove all soil.

Drying Herbs

Always dry your harvest in the shade to avoid extreme temperatures. Try to disturb the plants as little as possible, although herbs dried on paper or trays will need to be turned occasionally. Small quantities can be dried on sheets of paper in a well-ventilated closet or on baking trays in a cool oven with the door open. For larger amounts, a warm, airy, and shady space is needed. Herbs can be dried flat on large sheets of paper or on nets or stretched muslin. String up bunches of herbs well away from walls.

Dry small roots whole, but cut large ones into two or more pieces lengthwise. Thread root pieces on a string and hang them up to dry. Remove the outer coat of bulbs, and slice before drying. When collecting bark, scrape off the outer layer, then peel away the inner layers, which can be dried in sunlight (except black cherry, which needs shade). Temperatures should be *no higher* than 85 to 95 degrees Fahrenheit for plants and leaves, 115 degrees for roots, and 100 degrees for bulbs.

Leaves and stems are considered to be dry when they are brittle, breaking readily. Petals are ready when they rustle but do not crumble. Thick roots will chip with a small hammer, but most will snap. Three to seven days is a rough guide for most herbs, which will weigh about one-eighth of the fresh plant weight but still smell and taste very much like it.

Storing Herbs

Herbs like tarragon, marjoram, and thyme can be kept whole for bouquets garnis. Bay leaves, too, are good whole in soups and stews. Small flowers are also best kept intact, although marigold petals can be pulled off if preferred. With stalks removed, crush your dried herbs with a rolling pin or grinder or use a sieve for feathery herbs like dill.

Herbs deteriorate when exposed to oxygen and/or light. For this reason, they must be stored in airtight, opaque containers. Dark glass jars with tight-fitting lids are best. For everyday use, keep small quantities in separate containers to lessen the exposure of your main stock to air and light. Don't forget to label each container, and dating them is a good idea, too. Keep herbs in a dark, cool closet or cupboard.

Some Favorite Homegrown Healing Herbs

Aloe (Aloe spp.)

Type: Perennial. Many species.
Soil and situation: Average, well drained, full sun to light shade.
Spread/height: Up to several feet spread, up to 2 feet tall, with very long stems.
Propagation: From suckers or offshoots removed when 1 to 2 inches on indoor plant, 6 to 8 inches on outdoor plant.
Flower: Yellow/orange-red, tubular, on stalks along a stem.
Leaves: Pale, grayish green, rubbery, long, spiky.
Harvest: Older, outside leaves.

Aloe requires a minimum temperature of around 41 degrees Fahrenheit and is frequently grown as a pot plant indoors, where it can thrive for years. When propagating, it's often best to dig up the plant, remove the suckers, and then repot. Keeping a pot on the kitchen windowsill provides a simple remedy for minor burns and cuts and is always handy. Use scissors to cut off the end of a leaf, slice it down the middle, and scrape out the clear gel. The gel is wonderfully soothing and is also used to help heal sunburn, itching, and rashes. Aloe is a major constituent of many skin and hair preparations, but fresh aloe produces the best results. Josephine, wife to the emperor Napoleon, used a milk-and-aloe lotion to preserve her complexion. Indeed, aloe is said to help clear oily and acned skin. Some find aloe slightly drying, but mixing it with a little vitamin E may prevent this.

Catnip (Nepeta cataria)

Type: Perennial.
Soil and situation: Average, well drained, full sun to partial shade.
Sow: Difficult with tiny seeds—see "Propagation."
Height: 1 to 3 feet.
Propagation: 4-inch stem sections rooted in moist medium.
Flower: Small, tubular, white with purple-pink spots, massed in spikes, summer.
Leaves: Oval, tooth-edged, gray-green, with downy underside.
Harvest: Tops and leaves when in full bloom.

Cats seem to get quite a high from the aroma of this plant, but don't go looking for the same effect on yourself; our brains are wired to respond differently to the chemicals in catnip. This mild herb, listed in the *U.S. Pharmacopoeia* from 1842 to 1882, has long been used to treat illness in children. Brewed as a hot infusion, catnip promotes sweating and is good for flu. Soothing to the nervous system, it helps restless children get to sleep. This may be because the chemical structure of a major part of catnip's volatile oil is related to valepotriates, the known sedatives found in valerian. Catnip also has a calming effect on the stomach and is helpful for colic, flatulence, and diarrhea. Its sharp flavor made catnip an ingredient in Roman salads, and catnip tea was very popular in England before foreign varieties cornered the market.

Evening Primrose (Oenothera biennis)

Type: Biennial. Many other species.
Soil and situation: Stony, dry, full sun.
Sow: Late summer.
Spread/height: 2 feet by 5 feet.
Flower: Mid- to late summer, on spikes; large, bright yellow.
Leaves: Shiny, long, pointed.
Harvest: Flowers, seeds, roots.

Studies have given substantial support to the use of evening primrose in treating a number of disorders, from dry eyes and brittle nails to hyperactivity in children, premenstrual syndrome, alcoholic poisoning, acne, overweight, rheumatoid arthritis, and coronary artery disease. Evening primrose is very high in essential fatty acids, especially one called GLA, which is needed for the production of a hormonelike substance, PGE1, which has a range of beneficial effects in the body. The whole plant is edible. Try a tincture, or infusions can be made with 1 teaspoon of the plant to 1 cup of water to be taken one mouthful at a time, once a day. Exercise caution, though, as evening primrose is not recommended for epileptics, and some people have reported sensitivities to the plant.

Fennel (Foeniculum vulgare)

Type: Semi-hardy perennial.
Soil and situation: Very well drained, full sun.
Sow: Midsummer, fall.
Spread/height: 3 feet by 4 to 6 feet.
Flower: Small, yellow, on umbrella of stalks, midsummer.
Leaves: Deep green, thin, feathery, aromatic.
Harvest: Ripe seeds, young leaves, green stems.

Take care of fennel, for it is vulnerable to harm from certain plants including wormwood, which can inhibit seed germination and stunt its growth, while coriander will prevent seeds from forming. You should also make this herb a loner in your garden because it can damage other plants like bush beans, caraway, tomatoes, and kohlrabi. Fennel, with its refreshing aniselike flavor, has long been known as a digestive aid included in recipes by the Greeks, Romans, and Anglo-Saxons before spreading even further abroad. Add fennel to soups and salads. Drink fennel tea for indigestion and heartburn, and serve it to babies to relieve their colic. It's also an ancient remedy to promote the flow of milk in nursing mothers. Fennel eyewash is recommended for tired, sore eyes, and the oil is antispasmodic and antibacterial, although not recommended for those with allergies or skin sensitivities.

Garlic (Allium sativum)

Type: Perennial bulb. Many varieties.
Soil and situation: Well drained, rich to medium, full sun to partial shade.
Height: 1 foot.
Propagation: Split into cloves. Plant early spring or fall.
Flower: Very small, white to pinkish, late summer.
Leaves: Long, flat, pointed.
Harvest: Leaves, early summer; bulbs, late summer.

Many gardeners believe that roses benefit from garlic planted close by. And research shows that eating garlic protects against heart disease by lowering cholesterol and other fats and by reducing blood-clotting activity and hypertension. Garlic is also good for intestinal infections. Take grated garlic mixed with honey for coughs. Apply garlic to wounds to prevent infections. Of course, you can also enjoy garlic's unique flavor in foods.

German Chamomile (Matricaria chamomilla)

Type: Annual.
Soil and situation: Most types, especially light.
Sow: Late summer/fall.
Spread/height: 4 inches by 2 feet.
Flower: From early summer, small, daisylike.

Leaves: Feathery, bright green.
Harvest: Flowers, when fully open.

This plant is known as the "doctor's physician" and is described by Germans as "capable of anything." An aid to plants, too, German chamomile repels flying insects and even helps improve onion crop yield. Chamomile flowers contain a lovely blue volatile oil called azulene, and its many effective compounds include two powerful antiseptics. Use externally for hair care, especially fair hair, in combination with soapwort. You can also steep 3 to 4 ounces in boiling water for 1 hour to make a relaxing bath mixture. Make a tincture for washes or compresses to soothe and aid the healing of rashes, burns, and wounds.

Brew an infusion and drink chamomile as tea. This will aid nervous conditions, insomnia, and neuralgia. Chamomile has also been shown to calm restless children. In fact, chamomile was the tea served to Peter Rabbit by his mother to soothe his aching stomach! It's a famous remedy for digestive upsets, including diarrhea and flatulence, with research proving that it is both anti-inflammatory and antispasmodic. Chamomile is also used to prevent and treat ulcers.

Ginger (Zingiber officinale)

Type: Tropical biennial.
Soil and situation: Container, indoors; loam, sand, peat moss, and compost in equal parts; light shade, warmth, moisture, and humidity.
Height: 2 to 4 feet.
Propagation: From rhizome.
Flower: Rarely in cultivation; dense spikes, yellow-green, purple spotted and striped.
Leaves: Grasslike, long, pointed.
Harvest: Root, 8 to 12 months after planting.

Ginger is a commercial crop throughout the tropics, supplying an international trade in culinary spices and herbal medicines that goes back thousands of years. For your own harvest, pull the mature plant from its pot and cut off the leafstalks and thinner, fibrous roots. Cut off as much of the main root as you can store and use. The remainder can be replanted. Wrap your ginger first in a paper towel, then tightly in plastic wrap. Refrigerated, ginger will last for several months. Chew on a fresh stick to relieve a sore throat. Dry some, too, for dry ginger has slightly different chemical actions, traditionally making it more suitable for respiratory and digestive disorders.

All ginger is warming, but fresh ginger induces sweating and is said to be better for treating colds. Studies have shown that ginger provides much relief from nausea in early pregnancy at just 250 mg four times daily and also from the pain, swelling, and stiffness of both osteo- and rheumatoid arthritis, using doses of 500–4,000 mg daily. Cook Indian style and you'll soon exceed those doses! Daily amounts of 8–10 g are regularly consumed in India, where this herb continues to be very popular in both main dishes like curry and desserts such as crystallized ginger.

Lavender (Lavandula officinalis)

Type: Perennial shrub, evergreen.
Soil and situation: Light, well drained, calcareous, full sun.
Sow: Early spring or fall without heat.
Spread/height: 2 feet by 2 feet 8 inches.
Propagation: Spring, softwood cuttings; fall, hardwood cuttings.
Flower: Midsummer, mauve.
Leaves: Narrow, gray-green.
Harvest: Flowers, mid- to late summer.

Use lavender for hedging, and cut it back when it has finished flowering. Lavender takes its name from the Latin verb "to wash," and it was used by Romans and Greeks to create relaxing, scented baths. Widely known for its lovely scent, lavender is also used in steam inhalation against coughs, colds, and chest infections. Make an infusion of lavender for the same conditions as well as for tension, anxiety, stomachaches, and headaches. The oil is antibacterial, helpful for healing cuts, and one of the best remedies for stings and burns. A few drops used in massage help to relax muscles and ease pain. As with all plant oils, do not take lavender oil internally.

Lemon Balm (Melissa officinalis)

Type: Perennial, evergreen.
Soil and situation: Average, well drained, sun or semishade.

Sow: Late spring.

Spread/height: 2 feet by 2 feet 8 inches.

Propagation: In spring, layering, root division, cuttings.

Flower: Small, white to pink or yellowish, in clusters, summer.

Leaves: Broad, oval, tooth-edged, lemon fragrance.

Harvest: Leaves and stems in growing season.

Lemon balm is a good bee plant, its official name coming from the Greek word for "bees." Strangely, it is also considered a good insect repellent, used to keep flies off food and away from fires.

Harvest this herb by cutting off the entire plant 2 inches above the ground. It needs to be dried within two days of harvesting, for it can quickly turn black. A tip from Shakespeare's *Merry Wives of Windsor* is to rub lemon balm into wood, letting its fragrant oils act as a natural equivalent to lemon-scented furniture polish. You can also make a pleasant tea with this herb as a remedy for colds, flu, depression, headache, and indigestion. In fact, lemon balm has been recommended for centuries because "it makes the heart merry."

Analysis shows that the effects of the plant's volatile oils are due to antispasmodic and strong sedative properties, which also make lemon balm helpful for promoting menstrual periods and relieving menstrual cramping. Its polyphenols may be responsible for its antiviral effects, demonstrated against mumps and other viruses. Relax in a cleansing, steamy bath mixture of lemon balm, and use it as an acne rinse. Chop it up for culinary use, too, with salads, chicken, and lamb. Drink the liqueurs Benedictine and Chartreuse, and you'll be downing lemon balm, too!

Meadowsweet (Filipendula ulmaria)

Type: Perennial.

Soil and situation: Moist, rich, sun or semishade.

Sow: Spring or fall.

Spread/height: 1 foot by 2 to 3 feet.

Propagation: Divide roots in spring.

Flower: Summer, cream, clustered.

Leaves: Dark green.

Harvest: Flower heads, leaves, roots in the fall.

Meadowsweet is a good plant to grow by water. Its active compounds include aspirinlike substances, antioxidants, vitamin C, and sugar. Science shows us how meadowsweet's particular chemical package made it a safe remedy for hundreds of years for conditions like children's diarrhea, rheumatism, and fevers. Its anti-inflammatory constituents on their own could cause gastric bleeding, yet it also contains tannin and mucilage, which seem to act as buffers, preventing the adverse effect. Meadowsweet also acts as an antiseptic diuretic, aiding the excretion of uric acid. Make a hot infusion to induce sweating, an old-fashioned but useful treatment for fevers. Boil 2 tablespoons of the plant or dried rootstock in 1 cup of water and take 1 cup a day as a remedy. You can also use this decoction as a wash for wounds or sore eyes.

Parsley (Petroselinum crispum)

Type: Biennial.

Soil and situation: Rich, moist, well drained, sun to semishade.

Sow: Spring inside, warm; midsummer outside, full sun with shelter.

Spread/height: 1 foot 4 inches by 2 feet.

Propagation: Allow to self-seed.

Flower: Tiny, greenish yellow in umbrella clusters, summer.

Leaves: Dark green, feathery.

Harvest: Leaves, seeds, roots.

You may know that parsley is a useful breath sweetener, but you probably haven't heard how it used to be sprinkled on corpses as a deodorizer! Its high-chlorophyll content helps it eat up internal odors (including garlic), and its oils are naturally aromatic, leading to its popular use in bouquets garnis and as a garnish. Parsley is said to be good in a vegetable patch because it is supposed to repel some insects.

An excellent source of vitamin C, usefully packaged with iron, a nibble of parsley makes sense when you're under the weather. You'll also be taking in several B vitamins, vitamin A, calcium, manganese, and phosphorus. Its role as a nutritional minipowerhouse backs up its medicinal effects as a diuretic suitable for treating urinary infections and fluid retention. Because it helps expel uric acid, parsley is a remedy for gout, and the root has laxative properties.

Pregnant women should avoid large amounts of parsley. On the other hand, the chemistry of parsley strengthens uterine muscles and increases breast milk. Parsley is a digestive aid, and as a tincture, two to fifteen drops in water, as needed, it makes a treatment for nausea. Cosmetically, parsley infusions are soothing and cleansing and can be used as a hair rinse. Parsley oil is found in many cosmetics, shampoos, soaps, and skin lotions. If you can, freeze your parsley, as this is said to give better results than simply drying.

Rosemary (Rosmarinus officinalis)

Type: Perennial shrub; many decorative subspecies.
Soil and situation: Calcareous, well drained, full sun, sheltered from wind.
Sow: 75 to 80 degrees Fahrenheit in seed tray.
Height: 5 feet 8 inches.
Propagation: From early summer, cuttings of non-flowering shoots.
Flower: Late spring, pale to deep blue.
Leaves: Leathery, thin, gray-green, oily, aromatic.
Harvest: Leaves as needed.

Rosemary's traditional companion is sage. Plant it with carrot, too, as it repels carrot fly. It is an excellent hair tonic, and its refreshing scent leads to its use in cosmetics and perfumes. Ancient Greeks even made rosemary garlands to strengthen their memory at exam time! Medicinally, rosemary has many uses and is listed in the *U.S. Pharmacopoeia.* Even as recently as World War II, French hospitals burned juniper berries with rosemary leaves to kill germs. The oil, which, like many essential oils, is antifungal and antibacterial, is part of several liniments for rheumatism and can be applied directly to the head to relieve headaches. Enjoy rosemary with a dish of lamb, and you will be reducing flatulence and stimulating your digestion, liver, gallbladder, and circulation. Infusions of rosemary, of course, are used for the same reasons, as well as for treating painful menstruation. Use caution with rosemary, for the undiluted oil should not be taken internally.

Sage (Salvia officinalis)

Type: Perennial shrub.
Soil and situation: Well drained, calcareous, full sun.
Sow: Late spring.
Spread/height: 1 foot 8 inches by 1 to 2 feet.
Propagation: Cuttings, spring.
Flower: Tubular, purple, pink, blue, or white, early summer.
Leaves: Gray-green, velvety, aromatic.
Harvest: Leaves.

Sage is a beneficial companion plant in general and especially for rosemary and vines. In addition, it repels cabbage moths and a number of other harmful flying insects. American Indians used the fragrant, silver-green sagebrush of the American chaparral as a toothbrush, cleanser, and remedy with bear grease for skin sores, but its bitter taste rules it out of competition with the cultivated Mediterranean variety for culinary use.

Named from the Latin "to save," sage has been associated for centuries with longevity. The Chinese would even trade up to four times their fine green tea for European sage. As you stuff that turkey, you're dispensing a long-esteemed remedy for sore throats, colds, indigestion, hot flashes, and painful periods. Mix sage tea with a little cider vinegar for relief from throat disorders like tonsillitis. Use the tea as a mouthwash for infected gums and mouth ulcers. Feel its volatile oil work as it boosts digestion. It will also stop sweating and is reputed to dry up the flow of breast milk. Sage is also used for treating amenorrhea and painful periods.

This wide range of applications has its origins in the variety of substances found in sage. Besides its powerful oils, sage contains estrogenic compounds, antibacterial agents, antioxidants, and tannins. Do note, though, that sage should only be taken as a remedy for a week or two at a time, since it has another substance, thujone, which can have potentially toxic effects. But when you turn to sage in the kitchen, remember its extensive medicinal powers as you use it in dishes from soups and salads to meats, cheese, and bread.

Sweet Basil (Ocimum basilicum)

Type: Tender annual; one of many varieties.
Soil and situation: Fertile loam, sun.
Sow: Spring inside, warm; midsummer outside, full sun with shelter.

Spread/height: 1 foot by 1 to 2 feet.
Propagation: Cuttings.
Flower: Mid- to late summer, white/purplish.
Leaves: Delicate, clear green, aromatic.
Harvest: Leaves as needed, stems before flowering.

The chopped leaves of basil are famous for their distinctive flavor in dishes like pesto. Its other main use is as an insect repellent! In Europe, it is grown in pots outside doors to deter flies. Plant it near tomatoes for the same reason. Basil is also recommended for gastric disorders such as stomach cramps and constipation. Steep 1 teaspoon of dried herb in ½ cup of water. Take 1 to 1½ cups a day, one mouthful at a time. You can even do as some residents of New Mexico do and carry basil in your pockets to attract money!

AROMATHERAPY

Has a whiff of something ever sent you back to childhood, a special occasion, or the company of someone special? Such is the power of smell, harnessed even as a marketing tool, with supermarkets creating the illusion of fresh bakeries and real estate agents filling vases, heating vanilla in the oven, and brewing coffee! In plants, the source of their potent scents is essential oils. Such oils serve them as insect repellents or attractants and as antibacterial and antifungal agents, often lending them a particular character. In perfumes, ointments, and sprays, they do the same for us! Essential oils act as stimulants or relaxants to humans, frequently providing a link from the physical to the emotional as the olfactory organs connect to the parts of the brain associated with emotions. Formal research is scant, but work done at Milan University gives scientific support to the observation that plant oils can lift our spirits, relieving anxiety and depression.

As volatile substances, plant oils are extracted by distillation or soaking. The result is highly concentrated products that are absorbed through the skin or, diluted, through inhalation. Direct, external use of essential oils dates back thousands of years to ancient Egypt and Greece and the Far East. Hippocrates encouraged the burning of aromatic plants to prevent the spread of plague in ancient Athens. Gattefossé, an early French aromatherapist, recounted how, on impulse, he thrust his burned hand into a bowl of lavender essence and found that it healed extremely rapidly.

Today, we can choose an incense to burn, buy commercial vaporizers, and visit steam baths. Do-it-yourself inhalation methods include mixing one or two drops of essential oil in a bowl of steaming hot water, then placing a towel over your head and around the bowl to catch the steam. Soak in a bath, too, where five or six drops have been dissolved in warm water.

Five or six drops of oil are appropriate for massage, the oils being diluted in 2 to 5 teaspoons of a carrier oil such as almond, grapeseed, or soy. Massage with essential oils stimulates blood circulation, boosting their absorption. It also activates nerve endings, which aromatherapists believe then channel a reaction along nerves to the pituitary gland. The pituitary gland regulates the function of other glands, including the adrenals, and in this way influences whether we feel stressed or relaxed. This ties in with scientific analysis of several oils showing them to contain substances known to be stimulative or sedative in their effects.

Different oils are also reputed to produce different emotional effects, basil bringing cheer, catnip and rue inducing calm, and ylang-ylang promoting sex and love, for example. Seek out *natural* essential oils. Keep in mind that natural oils are very highly concentrated and pack the power of the plant in a way that synthetics cannot match. Choose your oil to suit, then pamper yourself with aromatherapy, one of the oldest health promotion measures known.

HERBS FOR THE BATH

For a wonderful addition to any bath, simply add a few drops of oil or a pint or so of a very strong infusion, strained, of your chosen herb to the bathwater. One of the best and simplest herbal bath remedies is eucalyptus. Just on its own, this antiseptic herb brings relief from aches and pains, clears the head and sinuses, and warms the body as it increases blood flow. You can also make an herb sachet to soak in the bath and smooth over your skin. Mix 2 cups of dried flowers, such as lime or chamomile, with 1 cup of fine oatmeal. Place them in the center of a piece of muslin about 16 inches square. Gather up the edges of the muslin, tying it up tightly with thread or string. Enjoy at least a 10-minute soak with herbal mixtures like the ones given here.

Skin Savers

To soothe dry, itchy, or inflamed skin, try a bath mixture with a cold-pressed vegetable oil base. As well as relieving symptoms and helping to protect your skin, such oils provide a natural barrier to moisture loss. Avoid using corn or cottonseed oils, as these are derived from crops usually heavily sprayed with pesticides and fungicides. Also avoid mineral oils, as they clog pores. Mix ½ cup each of almond, safflower, soy, and sesame oils. Shake all these together with a drop or two of an essential oil such as tea tree, which is a powerful skin disinfectant that penetrates and helps heal infected areas as well. Add 2 tablespoons to your bath using the full flow of the hot tap and take a luxurious soak.

Birch bark, chamomile, clover, comfrey root, marshmallow root, pansy, seaweed, white willow, and wintergreen are all recommended as calming herbs. For psoriasis, take a bath with comfrey root mixed with white willow bark.

Soak and Rejuvenate!

For an antistress bath, try a combination of comfrey leaf, linden, patchouli, sandalwood, and savory in equal parts. Comfrey works against signs of aging due to its high allantoin content. Allantoin promotes the growth of bone, cartilage, and connective tissue, the latter being essential to healthy skin. Sandalwood improves skin tone, and savory is stimulating. This is balanced by linden, a natural antiseptic and relaxant, helping to produce a fortifying, antistress, and fragrant bath.

An herbal mixture recommended especially for long-term, repeated use to keep skin young looking and firm uses 1 ounce each of aloe, comfrey root, lavender, lemon thyme, peppermint, rosemary, and fresh or dried roses. A little of this assortment works well on the body in various ways. The proven benefits of comfrey are supplemented by the cooling, healing astringency of aloe and roses. Lavender has a calming, antibacterial action, working well against acne and puffiness, and is reinforced by the roses, which also hydrate the skin. The menthol in peppermint is cooling and anesthetic as well as stimulating to the blood flow in skin. Thyme eases aches and pains and acts as a mild deodorant. Emerge from a soak in these herbs feeling fresh, clean, and alive!

MAKE YOUR OWN POTPOURRI

Forget the disinfectants and air fresheners in a can! Go for natural, environmentally friendly fragrances instead. Simply hang up bunches of herbs chosen for their scent and their effects on mood. Try your hand, too, at combining dried herbs in potpourri, following recipes like the following, or make up your own. Tip a little of each herb into a covered bowl, to be exposed when occasional scent is desired, or into an open container for continuous fragrance. Stir the herbs and other ingredients together, and sprinkle them with a few drops of an oil with a complementary odor.

Bring the scents of a flower garden indoors with 5 tablespoons of lavender flowers, 3 tablespoons each of carnations and scented rose petals, and 1½ tablespoons each of chamomile flowers, heliotrope flowers, salt, and orris root powder. A little rose oil is a nice addition.

HERBAL INSECT REPELLENTS

The single most important reason that plants contain aromatic volatile oils is to repel insects. We can take advantage of this by using aromatic oils to repel pests, instead of using the toxic petrochemical pesticides sold commercially. In fact, many of these substances can now be found at better plant and garden stores.

Pyrethrums, which come from plants in the chrysanthemum family, make potent insecticides as powder from the dried plants or spray infusions. Pyrethrum works by paralyzing insects and is so strong that prolonged contact can cause skin problems, so use it with care.

You can also make an infusion of 1 pound of elder leaves to 2 gallons of water as an effective aphid spray. And try a decoction of walnut leaves, six handfuls boiled for 20 to 30 minutes in 1 pint of water, to repel ants. Indoors, use southernwood, also known as

An Abbreviated Guide to Herbs and Illnesses

Disorder	What to Use
Allergies	Ephedra, garlic
Arthritis	Cat's claw, arnica, feverfew, licorice, evening primrose, ginger
Cholesterol too high	Garlic, ginger, hawthorn
Circulation problems	Ginkgo biloba, garlic, bilberry, calendula, ginger
Colds and flu	Echinacea, ephedra, garlic, goldenseal, elderberry
Cough	Licorice, ephedra, garlic, lavender
Depression, anxiety	Kava-kava, St. John's wort
Digestion problems	Ginger, chamomile, the mints, fennel, angelica, licorice
Headache	Feverfew (migraine only), white willow bark, ginger, ginkgo, lavender, the mints
Heartburn	Licorice, the mints, fennel
Heart problems	Hawthorn berries, garlic, dong quai
Immune deficiency	Echinacea, garlic, ginseng, angelica, cat's claw, goldenseal
Liver problems	Milk thistle
Lung ailments	Licorice, eucalyptus, garlic, ginseng, pennyroyal
Memory problems	Ginkgo biloba, kava-kava
Menopause	Dong quai, vitex/chasteberry, angelica, licorice, ginseng
Pain	White willow bark, feverfew, arnica, licorice, aloe, calendula, cat's claw, echinacea, elderberry, kava-kava, lavender
PMS	Vitex, dong quai, pennyroyal
Prostate problems	Saw palmetto
Sores, wounds, cuts, bruises, stings, bites, and itches	Witch hazel, aloe vera, arnica, calendula
Urinary tract problems	Uva-ursi, saw palmetto
Vision problems	Bilberry

garderobe (clothesguard), between sheets of tissue lain among clothes to keep moths away. Hanging bunches of herbs such as pennyroyal, rosemary, rue, and tansy adds lovely scents to the summer air as they keep insects out of the house on summer evenings.

Venture out to flea-ridden grasses and the muggiest swamps wearing some of nature's own bug repellents! A short-term mosquito repellent is fresh elder. Simply rub the leaves on exposed parts, but be prepared to do this every 20 minutes. You can also make strong infusions of elder or chamomile to dab on frequently.

Citronella oil, made from the stone root plant, is a well-known and longer-lasting bug deterrent. It also has a pleasant fragrance and is much more effective and easier to apply than most store-bought insect repellents. Lavender oil is reputed to be similarly useful and has its own well-loved scent. Any of the plants with aromatic essential oils, but especially pennyroyal, can also be used as insect repellents.

Armed against bugs and perfumed as well—yet another typically effective, gentle, and enjoyable result of using herbs!

5 FIBER AND DIGESTION ~

A HEALTHY DIGESTIVE SYSTEM IS THE FOUNDATION OF GOOD HEALTH

In this chapter, we're going to explore the primary organs of the digestive system. In the course of our exploration, I'm going to tell you that heartburn is usually caused by too little stomach acid; that your arthritis may be caused by microscopic holes in your intestines; and that your gas and bloating may have been caused by the antibiotics you took last spring. We're going to explore the stomach, its hydrochloric acid, and how to prevent heartburn; the small intestine and its digestive enzymes; the large intestine, its beneficial bacteria, and *Candida* yeast infections; and food allergies, which affect the entire digestive system.

My approach to preventing and treating digestive difficulties may be completely new to you because the information you get from your doctor, from magazines, and from TV about your digestive system tends to be dictated by large companies trying to sell you drugs rather than by the facts. Information based on advertising and marketing has very little to do with what's really going on in there!

This is why even though H2 blockers such as Tagamet and Pepcid are some of the best-selling drugs in the United States, digestive problems remain one of the most persistent and bothersome of all American illnesses. If these drugs were working, wouldn't they be making you better? Instead, they cause a reliance on the drug to suppress symptoms. Taking H2 blockers does absolutely nothing to treat the *source* of indigestion; they only treat symptoms and in the long run tend to make the problem worse and create dependencies and troublesome side effects.

Your dependency on their drug just makes profit margins higher, and the side effects will be treated with yet another drug.

Poor digestion has repercussions in every other part of the body because it causes poor absorption of nutrients and puts stress on all the other organs of the body as well as on the blood, the lymphatic system, the muscles, the ligaments, and the bones. It's amazing how many minor complaints, aches, and pains will clear up when digestion is cleared up.

Your key to good digestion is like the key to much else in life: moderation, balance, variety, and avoiding what is packaged in plastic. Overwork, overeating, underexercising, overmedicating, and overconsumption of junk foods (which in my book includes nearly all processed foods) are some typical examples of imbalances that can lead to indigestion. Millions of Americans are plagued by indigestion, and yet good digestion and absorption of nutrients is one of the great keys to vibrant good health, clear-headedness, and longevity. Take it from me—if your digestion isn't good, nothing else will be, either. You can eat the most nutritious diet possible, but if your body isn't absorbing the nutrients, it won't do you a bit of good.

I believe that delayed food allergies (also called food sensitivities or food intolerances) that damage the small intestine and an overgrowth of *Candida* bacteria in the colon rank among the leading causes of (or contributors to) such common chronic American illnesses as indigestion, hay fever, arthritis, headaches, fatigue, skin problems, and autoimmune diseases. But most American doctors don't even acknowledge the existence of delayed food allergies or *Candida* overgrowth, let alone treat them. Why should they? They can't be quickly treated with a drug prescription, and they don't fit a neat pattern of cause and effect.

I have devoted the final section of the chapter to fiber. Why so much attention to a nonnutritional food substance? Because a lack of it can contribute to constipation, diarrhea, Crohn's disease, irritable bowel syndrome, colon cancer, varicose veins, excess estrogen, and more! You'll find out how fiber does its job and how you can put more fiber into your life.

Stick with me as we take this journey through your wondrous digestive system. Implement my strategies for balancing it, system by system, and I can almost guarantee that you'll achieve more energy, better memory, clearer thinking, and better overall health. You'll look better, feel better, and do better. You'll also enjoy life more if you're not suffering from stomach cramps, bloating, gas, and heartburn. Enough said!

A QUICK TOUR OF THE DIGESTIVE SYSTEM

Digestion doesn't really begin in the stomach. It begins when you smell food or anticipate it. Those signals from your nose and your imagination stimulate the brain to send signals to the mouth and stomach to start producing digestive juices. Those in turn stimulate the pancreas and gallbladder, and thus the complex process of extracting nutrition from plants and animals begins.

Your mouth "waters" in preparation for eating, and when that saliva mixes with the food you're chewing, salivary enzymes begin the process of breaking down the food. The most important of these is the enzyme amylase, which breaks down starches.

While you're chewing, you're absorbing some fat-soluble nutrients through the mucous membranes in your mouth. These send further signals ahead to the digestive system about what types of digestive juices and enzymes to churn out. The better you chew your food, the more you're assisting the process of breaking it down into absorbable bits and pieces. (However, moderation being a key to good health, I don't recommend that you chew each mouthful of food one hundred times, as was advocated by a nutritionist in the 1950s. That's overdoing it!)

The esophagus is where peristalsis begins. This is the movement of special muscles that resembles kneading or milking—a constriction and relaxation that propels material through the digestive system.

Looked at simplistically, your digestive system is one long tube, starting at your mouth and ending at your anus. The picture becomes more complex because each section of the digestive system is separated from its neighbor by a sphincter, or one-way valve. Your esophagus is separated from your stomach by the esophageal sphincter, which is opened by the action of swallowing a mouthful of food. Your stomach is separated from your small intestine by the pyloric sphincter, which allows just enough food through at a time to fill the duodenum, a sort of holding area between the stomach and small intestine. The esophageal sphincter and pyloric sphincter both protect delicate tissues from the stomach's powerful acid. In turn, the pyloric sphincter protects the stomach from the alkaline contents of the small intestine. Moving on down the line, the ileocecal sphincter separates the small intestine from the colon, protecting the small intestine from the bacteria of the colon. At the end of the colon, yet another sphincter separates the colon from the outside world.

In the following sections, we're going to take a closer look at each of the digestive areas separated by sphincters—the stomach, the small intestine, and the colon—because each has a distinct job to perform in moving food on its journey through the body.

THE STOMACH

The stomach is the biggest bulge in the tube that is the digestive tract, as most of us are well aware. But it is located higher than you might think, lying mainly behind the lower ribs, not under the navel, and it does not occupy the belly. It is a flexible bag enclosed by restless muscles, constantly changing form.

Virtually nothing is absorbed through the stomach walls except alcohol. An ordinary meal leaves the stomach in 3 to 5 hours. Watery substances, such as soup, leave the stomach quite rapidly. Fats take much longer to move through. Special glands and cells lining the stomach walls produce mucus, enzymes, and hydrochloric acid, a substance that enables vitamin B_{12} to be dissolved through intestinal walls into the circulation. A normal stomach is quite acidic, and gastric juice contains many substances.

Every day your stomach secretes hydrochloric acid (HCl) by the quart, along with an enzyme called pepsin that breaks down proteins. These secretions are stimulated by a hormone called gastrin, which is released in the stomach in response to food. HCl is a potent acid, with the power to turn your steamed broccoli and grilled chicken into a wicked semiliquid brew called chyme. HCl doesn't just break down foods; it also kills bacteria and parasites, allows the body to absorb minerals, and sets the stage for the absorption of B_{12} and folic acid in the small intestine. If the stomach doesn't contain enough hydrochloric acid, the pyloric valve into the small intestine won't open properly, causing food to sit in the stomach for hours and setting the stage for heartburn.

Stomach Acid Is a Friend, Not a Foe

If stomach acid is a friend of good digestion, why are we spending billions of dollars every year on antacids and H2 blockers such as Tagamet, Pepcid, and Zantac, which block hydrochloric acid? Why do advertisements for these products blame all indigestion on stomach acid? It's because if your foods sit undigested in your stomach for hours, marinating in insufficient stomach acid, it can cause pain not only in the stomach but from "reflux," or burping up the contents of the stomach, which burns the lining of the esophagus—otherwise known as heartburn. Antacids and H2 blockers will temporarily block those symptoms but in the long run will only make digestion more problematic and block the absorption of minerals and some B vitamins.

Most people with chronic indigestion or heartburn, and especially those over the age of fifty, have low levels of HCl. One way to stimulate your digestive juices is to drink a glass of lukewarm water half an hour before eating. (Cold water suppresses digestive juices.) Other people swear by a tablespoon of apple cider vinegar in a glass of water before a meal.

Vinegar is highly acidic and may provide your stomach with enough acidity for quicker, easier digestion. Instead of vinegar, you can try some type of bitters, such as the herb gentian or Angostura bitters, with warm water. A walk after a meal will also help stimulate your digestive juices.

The most common symptoms of a stomach acid deficiency show up after eating in the form of heartburn, belching, bloating, or a heavy feeling. If you can feel that most of your meal is still in your stomach more than 45 minutes after eating a normal meal, your stomach is working inefficiently.

If you suspect that your stomach acid isn't up to par, and the other solutions I've given you aren't working, try taking betaine hydrochloride supplements. (Don't take vinegar or start HCl supplements while you have an active case of heartburn. This will only irritate things even more.) Try taking one tablet of around 300 mg with food. You can increase your dose to two or more tablets per meal, but if you get a burning feeling in your stomach, you're taking too much. (Some betaine hydrochloride supplements add pepsin, which is fine.)

A Hot Remedy for Sluggish Digestion

Capsicum peppers—chili peppers and cayenne peppers—are some of the most versatile and powerful healing condiments known. The ingredient in peppers that makes them hot, capsaicin, is widely used in alternative medicine and in Asian medicine.

The hot-to-the-taste quality of peppers will initially produce a burning feeling in the mouth and sometimes on the skin, but the body then responds by blocking nerve pain transmissions, producing a pain-relieving effect.

Cayenne aids digestion by stimulating the production of stomach acid and increasing circulation in the gut.

There are many anecdotal reports of taking cayenne internally to stop internal bleeding and to treat ulcers. If you use cayenne to treat an ulcer, be careful not to take too much, and don't use it when the ulcer is inflamed. In fact, if you are taking cayenne to treat an ulcer, you should probably do so under the supervision of a health care professional.

You can use cayenne and chili peppers in your food, or you can take them in capsules, which you can find at your health food store.

My Favorite Remedy for Nausea

Ginger *(Zingiber officinale)* is one of my favorite healing spices. The root of this plant has been used both as a food and as a medicine for thousands of years.

Ginger is best known for its effectiveness in relieving indigestion and most types of nausea, including morning sickness and motion sickness. In studies, ginger has been shown to be more effective than dimenhydrinate (Dramamine) in relieving motion sickness. Researchers believe that it is ginger's mild suppressing effect on the central nervous system that prevents nausea.

A substance in ginger called zingibain, which acts as a digestive enzyme, contributes to its ability to aid digestion and relieve gas. Ginger also stimulates the gallbladder to release bile, helping with the digestion of fats. And if that isn't enough, ginger may also help protect against ulcers by stimulating the production of protective mucus in the stomach. Ginger contains antioxidants as well as anti-inflammatory and anti-bacterial substances.

As well as using fresh gingerroot, you can also take it in a powdered form in capsules, which you can find at your health food store.

The Real Cause of Ulcers

For years, mainstream medicine claimed that stress and excess stomach acid caused ulcers. Although stress can contribute to ulcers by either suppressing stomach acid or causing an oversecretion of it, we now know that the real culprit is a nasty spiral-shaped bacteria called *Helicobacter pylori*, which lives in the stomach lining. This destructive little stowaway suppresses the production of hydrochloric acid, causes inflammation, reduces the protective mucous coating in the stomach, and creates holes in the lining of the stomach, which allows the stomach acid to burn it and cause ulcers. It may be that in many people, *Helicobacter* doesn't create enough damage to cause ulcers but does suppress stomach acid enough to cause chronic indigestion and heartburn.

The standard medical treatment for *Helicobacter* infection is one or two antibiotics, usually tetracycline and amoxicillin, combined with a bismuth agent such as Pepto-Bismol, for a week to ten days. However, if you want to avoid antibiotics, you can try a combination of garlic capsules to kill the bacteria (one or two capsules with meals); licorice root tincture or capsules to aid in healing and protecting the stomach lining; and cabbage juice to speed up healing.

Ulcers are also commonly caused by NSAIDs (nonsteroidal anti-inflammatory drugs), such as aspirin and ibuprofen. I encourage you to avoid them, especially if you're having stomach pains.

The Natural Way to Prevent Heartburn

If *Helicobacter* or low stomach acid isn't the cause of your heartburn, it most likely has a very simple cause. Most cases of heartburn have simple, easy-to-explain causes and do not require any supplements or drugs. Here are some of the most common causes of heartburn:

- Eating in a hurry
- Eating too much
- Eating a lot of fried and fatty foods
- Eating a lot of spicy foods
- Eating foods that contain nitrates and nitrites
- Eating citrus fruits (oranges, lemons, grapefruit)
- Drinking a lot of coffee
- Eating a lot of chocolate
- Drinking ice-cold liquids before or with meals
- Not chewing food thoroughly
- Wearing tight clothing, which constricts the stomach
- Lying down after a meal, which irritates the esophageal sphincter

Once you get chronic heartburn, it tends to stay with you for the rest of your life. That's the bad news. The good news is that it can be managed by changing your lifestyle. Consider the following homespun tips for preventing heartburn.

Because your stomach has to work much harder to digest fat, it's important to avoid fried foods and stick to healthy oils, such as olive oil and canola oil.

Eating small meals and chewing your food thoroughly is the next best prevention. Overeating and eating on the run are two of the most common causes of heartburn.

If you're overweight, losing some poundage could be your ticket to digestive happiness (not to mention better overall health).

If you drink a lot of alcohol, cutting down (no more than two drinks daily) will almost certainly help long-term, and abstaining while you have symptoms will make healing much faster.

Are you one of those people whose stomach clutches when you're stressed? Try meditation, yoga, chi gong, tai chi, a hot bath, or any form of relaxing exercise. (Flopping down on the sofa in front of the TV with a drink does *not* count as relaxation. Lying down will make it worse, alcohol will aggravate it, and TV is not deeply relaxing.)

Stop smoking, and your heartburn may disappear. Nicotine relaxes the sphincter muscle that separates the esophagus from the stomach, allowing stomach acid to reflux (burp) up.

Home Remedies for Heartburn

If you are suffering from heartburn, aloe vera juice and papaya are both effective heartburn remedies. You can find both, separately and in digestive formulas, at your health food store. My grandmother drank a little potato juice for heartburn and swore by it.

At the first sign of heartburn, drink an 8-ounce glass of room-temperature water to rinse the esophagus of its acid bath and dilute your stomach acid if more comes up. (Ice-cold water interferes with digestion.)

Aloe vera gel soothes the esophagus and the digestive tract. It tastes bitter but works well. Take 1 teaspoonful before a meal and 1 teaspoonful after a meal.

If you get heartburn at night when you're sleeping or are waking up with it, try putting a 2-inch block of wood under each leg at the head of your bed. This will raise your chest slightly higher than your feet. If that's not practical, try sleeping on a wedge-shaped foam rubber pillow. Midnight heartburn happens because when you lie down and sleep, the

sphincter muscle between the esophagus and stomach relaxes. If you have undigested food in your stomach, it's more likely to escape back up into the esophagus.

Baking soda will neutralize your stomach acid, temporarily relieving symptoms. Because this is a form of sodium, it's not recommended for those on a low-sodium diet or for regular long-term use.

Herbal teas that can help relieve heartburn include fenugreek, slippery elm, comfrey, licorice, and meadowsweet. They are all soothing to mucous membranes and will help your esophagus heal. Drink these teas lukewarm, with no lemon. (High doses of comfrey tea used over a long period of time may cause liver damage, but I don't expect you to drink gallons of the stuff every day, and it's one of nature's most soothing and healing substances.)

Herbal bitters are widely used in Europe as a digestive aid. The bitters stimulate the digestive juices. Europeans also eat a lot of the bitters, such as endive and dandelion greens, in their salads. Gentian root is the best-known bitter herb. Chamomile is also a "bitter" tea, although it doesn't have a bitter taste.

Antacids Will Only Make It Worse in the Long Run

Although antacids such as Mylanta, Rolaids, and Tums can temporarily suppress the symptoms of heartburn, in the long run they'll do you more harm than good. You may even become dependent on them. These over-the-counter medications help neutralize the acid in your stomach for up to an hour. That's fine for the moment, but your stomach may respond an hour later by producing even more acid to make up for what was neutralized, causing you to reach for more antacids. They also contain aluminum, silicone, sugar, and a long list of dyes and preservatives. Your stomach acid is also one of your frontline defenses against harmful bacteria. Suppress it and the rest of your systems have to work overtime to protect you.

Drugs That Can Cause Heartburn

Many prescription and over-the-counter drugs can cause or aggravate heartburn. Drugs that specifically relax the esophageal sphincter muscle, allowing stomach acid to reflux up, include anticholinergics (such as drugs to treat Parkinson's), calcium channel blockers (antiangina drugs), nicotine, and beta-blockers (drugs that lower blood pressure and prevent spasms in the heart muscle).

Drugs That Can Cause Heartburn

- Antibiotics
- Cholesterol-lowering drugs
- Blood pressure–lowering drugs
- Asthma drugs
- Corticosteroids
- Antidepressants
- Painkillers
- Chemotherapy drugs
- Tranquilizers
- Barbiturates
- Synthetic estrogens and progestins, such as Provera and Premarin

---

THE SMALL INTESTINE AND ACCESSORY ORGANS

The small intestine is where most absorption of nutrients takes place. This is where the digestive system moves into high-performance mode, breaking down foods with digestive enzymes, extracting thousands of nutrients from the foods you eat, and sending them off to the liver for processing, which then sends them off to perform millions of jobs throughout your body.

Unlike the stomach, which has an acidic environment, the small intestine has an alkaline environment, created by secretion of bicarbonate (like baking soda) from the pancreas. This alkalinity then stimulates the pancreas to secrete digestive enzymes. Meanwhile, the gallbladder releases bile, which aids in the breakdown of fats.

The Small Intestine

The health of the small intestine is so important to your overall health that naturopathic doctors estimate that some 60 percent of the patients they see with previously unidentified symptoms (that is, those that mainstream medicine could not help) are suffering, underneath all their other symptoms, from a dysfunctional gastrointestinal system.

Impossible as it may seem, you have about 22 feet of small intestine inside you, with more than 2,000 square feet of surface area—that's about the square footage of an average two- or three-bedroom house! This relatively huge surface area is created by villi, tiny fingerlike protrusions that interface between the small intestine and the rest of the body, absorbing nutrients and sending them into the bloodstream, where they are processed by the liver. When the small intestine is damaged, the villi are damaged, paving the way for poor absorption of foods.

Are You Getting Your Vitamin B_{12}?

While we're on the subject of absorbing nutrients, I want to briefly touch on a very important topic—the absorption of vitamin B_{12}—which happens at the end of the small intestine, in the ileum. A deficiency of vitamin B_{12} can actually cause the symptoms of senility and aging, such as an unsteady gait, memory loss, weakness, shortness of breath, indigestion, poor appetite, and, for many, personality changes that include irritability, anxiety, depression, and listlessness.

Most mainstream medical doctors will tell you that we get our vitamin B_{12} mainly from meat and dairy products, that it's stored in the liver for future use, that we need only a tiny amount to last us for years and years, and that it's therefore almost impossible to have a B_{12} deficiency, so B_{12} shots are a waste of money. They'll tell you that the only disease related to B_{12} deficiency is pernicious anemia, caused by a deficiency of intrinsic factor in the stomach. Unfortunately, by the time pernicious anemia shows up, a lot of damage has been done.

While it is true that we can store up to six years' worth of B_{12} in the liver and that most Americans get plenty of B_{12} in their diet, it's also true that as we age, our ability to absorb B_{12} can become so impaired that we do become deficient.

Without good digestion, it's difficult to absorb B_{12}, which is a complex process beginning in the stomach. There, parietal cells secrete hydrochloric acid, which releases the vitamin B_{12} from food, and they secrete a substance called intrinsic factor, which, with the aid of the pancreatic enzyme trypsin, binds to B_{12} in the ileum to carry it through the intestinal wall and into the rest of the body.

In other words, if your parietal cells are blocked and your pancreas isn't secreting adequate digestive enzymes, your ability to absorb B_{12} can be greatly impaired. The process of aging tends to slow the action of parietal cells, but even bigger enemies of good digestion and absorption are a poor diet, antacid medicines, and H2 blockers such as Tagamet, Pepcid, and Zantac. Please throw away these medications! They may temporarily improve symptoms, but in the long run they will only hurt you.

The symptoms of B_{12} deficiency can begin showing up long before a blood test will show a deficiency. However, since the neurological damage done by a true B_{12} deficiency seems to be largely irreversible, it's not worth waiting around for it to show up that way. In a Dutch study of sixteen older people with dementia, nine had normal blood serum levels of B_{12}, but twelve had abnormally low levels of B_{12} in their cerebrospinal fluid (in the brain and spinal column). All of these patients improved significantly after receiving B_{12} injections.

If you or a loved one is showing symptoms of a B_{12} deficiency, find a health care professional who will give you four to eight weeks of B_{12} injections to see if the symptoms improve. In the meantime, start taking vitamin B_{12}. It is not well absorbed when taken orally, so it's best to take it as a nasal gel or sublingually (under the tongue).

The Accessory Organs

The liver, the gallbladder, and the pancreas play an important role in the digestion of foods, so let's take a closer look at how they work.

The Liver

The liver is the main storage organ for fat-soluble vitamins, such as vitamins A, D, and E, and is also largely responsible for ridding the body of toxins. It is the largest solid organ of the body and weighs about 4 pounds. It is an incomparable chemical plant.

It can modify almost any chemical structure for the body to use or eliminate. It is a powerful detoxifying organ, breaking down a variety of toxic molecules and rendering them harmless. It is also a blood reservoir and a storage organ for those fat-soluble vitamins and for digested carbohydrate (glycogen), which is released to sustain blood sugar levels. It manufactures enzymes, cholesterol, proteins, vitamin A (from carotene), and blood coagulation factors.

One of the prime functions of the liver is to produce bile. Bile contains salts that promote efficient digestion of fats by detergent action, emulsifying fatty materials much as soap disperses grease when you're washing dishes.

The Gallbladder

This is a saclike storage organ about 3 inches long. It holds bile, modifies it chemically, and concentrates it tenfold. The taste or sometimes even the smell or sight of food may be sufficient to empty it out. Constituents of gallbladder fluids sometimes crystallize and form gallstones. One of the best ways to keep your gallbladder healthy is to eat plenty of fiber.

The Pancreas

The pancreas provides important enzymes to the body. This gland is about 6 inches long and is nestled in the duodenum. It secretes insulin, which ushers sugar from the bloodstream into the cells. (Insulin is secreted into the blood, not the digestive tract.) The larger part of the pancreas manufactures and secretes pancreatic juices, which contain some of the body's most important digestive enzymes, and bicarbonate, which neutralizes stomach acid.

DIGESTIVE ENZYMES

Most enzymes are extremely tiny and found in very small quantities in the body. They work in organs, blood, and tissue. The digestive enzymes, however, are a different story. Although you still need a microscope to see them, they are much larger than most other enzymes and are present in the digestive system in large amounts.

Digestive enzymes are the catalysts in digestion and absorption, speeding up and enhancing the breakdown of foods. In one of those small miracles of biochemistry, the digestive enzymes cause biological reactions in our digestive systems without themselves being changed.

Fats, starches, sugars, amino acids, vitamins, minerals, and thousands of other nutrients each have their own enzyme catalysts. Until enzymes break them down, these nutrients can't be used by the body. A shortage or absence of even a single enzyme can make all the difference between health and sickness.

We can also look at enzymes as the guide that shows the vitamin or mineral or fat the way into the cell. Without the introduction by the enzyme, the cell might never know the identity of the nutrient.

According to Ann Louise Gittleman, author of *Guess What Came to Dinner: Parasites and Your Health* (Avery Publishing, 1993), a lack of digestive enzymes also creates an ideal breeding ground for parasites. She explains that undigested food tends to rot and ferment in the intestines, which is the perfect environment for parasites.

The Digestive Enzymes— Nature's Wonder Workers

Enzymes are the catalysts in the digestive process. Food only becomes useful to the body after it has been converted to its component carbohydrates, proteins, and fats in the digestive process. Only after digestion can valuable vitamins, minerals, and amino acids be released to keep us alive and healthy. Because each digestive enzyme works with a specific type of food, a shortage or absence of even a single enzyme can make all the difference between health and sickness.

Digestive enzymes are named after the food substance they act on. For example, the enzyme that acts on phosphorus is named phosphatase; one of the enzymes that works on sugar (sucrose) is called sucrase.

As nutrients move through the digestive system and into the cells, they are helped along by at least one enzyme. Although an enzyme is a protein, in order for it to work properly, it needs an amino acid

and a coenzyme. Most coenzymes are vitamins and minerals. Two of the most important coenzymes are magnesium and zinc. Magnesium alone is an essential cofactor (meaning the enzyme won't work without the magnesium present) for more than three hundred different enzymes. Other mineral coenzymes include iron, copper, manganese, selenium, and molybdenum. The B vitamins thiamin, riboflavin, pantothenic acid, and biotin are all coenzymes that help us digest starches, fats, and proteins.

Getting to Know Your Enzymes

There are far too many enzymes involved in breaking down nutrients for me to list them all here. The most important ones for digestion are those that break down proteins, fats, starches, and roughage (cellulose). Enzymes that break down proteins are called protease enzymes or proteolytic enzymes. Lipase breaks down fats, cellulase breaks down cellulose, and amylase breaks down starches. Trypsin and chymotrypsin, produced by the pancreas, break down proteins.

The enzyme renin causes milk to coagulate, changing its protein, casein, into a form the body can use. Renin also releases important minerals from milk, such as calcium, phosphorus, potassium, and iron. Lactase is the enzyme that breaks down the milk sugar lactose. An absence of lactase is what causes many delayed allergies to milk.

How Lipase Works

Enzymes that break down fat are especially important in Western cultures, where people tend to eat more fats than the body needs. Inadequate digestion of fat can cause stress in the entire digestive system, contributing to its chronic diseases.

Lipase and phospholipase break down fats in many stages, beginning with the upper portion of the stomach, called the cardial region. Here the lipase enzymes work in the acidic environment of the stomach to produce specific breakdown substances. If we aren't supplying enough enzymes here and in the main portion of the stomach to break down the fat we eat, when it reaches the small intestine it puts a much bigger load on the pancreas and gallbladder.

The lipases supplied by the pancreas only work in the alkalinity of the small intestine, producing a whole different set of fat breakdown products than the acidic environment of the stomach. An enzyme supplement can greatly aid the digestive system by making sure that the fats we eat are well down the road to digestion by the time they reach the small intestine.

Enzyme Partners

Although a digestive enzyme is a protein, it needs an amino acid and a cofactor, usually a vitamin or mineral, to work properly. One study showed that taking a B-complex vitamin supplement increased the activity of one enzyme by 25 percent!

Unlike the enzymes, the coenzymes are destroyed as they work with the enzymes. Thus, we need to replace our minerals and vitamins through what we eat. This is an important reason to take a good multivitamin every day (see chapter 1).

Keeping Your Enzyme Tank Full

Many stresses of modern life can contribute to the destruction of enzymes, and these include toxins and pollutants; mental, emotional, and physical stress; yo-yo dieting; drug and alcohol abuse; improper nutrition; and allergies. Some substances, such as fluoride, are necessary in extremely tiny amounts as enzyme cofactors, but in larger amounts they actually begin to destroy enzymes. Cadmium is found naturally with zinc, but when we get too much, it replaces zinc in the enzyme pathways and then can't finish the job, wreaking havoc on our cell membranes.

Some of the best food sources of enzymes are avocados, bananas, papayas, mangoes, pineapples, sprouts, and the aspergillus plant.

Digestive enzyme supplements can work wonders for those who need a little extra help with digestion. If you have symptoms of indigestion, such as gas, bloating, and cramping, or if you suspect that you have food allergies, digestive enzyme supplements can help speed up the digestion process.

There are two sources of enzyme supplements: plants and animals. The most common sources of plant enzymes are papaya, from which papain is extracted, and pineapple, from which bromelain is extracted. Both papain and bromelain are proteases, or protein-digesting enzymes. I recommend that you use plant-based enzymes.

When you take a digestive enzyme, be sure that it includes the three major types of enzymes: amylase, protease (or proteolytic enzymes), and lipase. If you eat dairy products and want some help digesting the lactose in them, get an enzyme supplement that contains lactase. Take the supplement just before or with meals.

Enzymes and Pain

There are new clinical studies showing that supplemental digestive enzymes help reduce inflammation caused by arthritis and injuries to joints and other connective tissues, such as muscle sprains, and can even relieve back pain. Enzymes tend to speed up the rate at which many bodily processes work, and injuries are no exception. Enzymes working at the site of an injury go to work to remove damaged tissues, which reduces swelling, and to help the body repair itself. As the enzymes do their work, they also become an effective pain reliever. The enzymes trypsin, chymotrypsin, papain, and bromelain have been most commonly used in the studies of enzymes and pain relief.

The Four Basic Types of Digestive Enzymes

1. Amylases, or amylolytic enzymes, are found in the saliva, pancreas, and small intestine. They aid in the breakdown of carbohydrates.
2. Proteases, or proteolytic enzymes, are found in the stomach, pancreas, and small intestine. They aid in the breakdown of proteins.
3. Lipases, or lipolytic enzymes, aid in the breakdown of fats.
4. Cellulase aids in breaking down cellulose.

Amylase Enzymes Digest Starch

1. Alpha-amylase is found in saliva and in the pancreas. It helps break down starches into sugars.
2. Beta-amylase is found in raw, unprocessed grains and vegetables and also helps break down starch into sugar.
3. Mylase and glucomylase are starch-digesting enzymes capable of dissolving thousands of times their own weight in starches in the small intestine.

Protease Enzymes Digest Proteins

1. Prolase is a concentrated protein-digesting enzyme derived from papain, which is extracted from papaya.
2. Protease is also extracted from papaya.
3. Bromelain is a digestive enzyme derived from pineapple.
4. Pepsin is released in the stomach and splits protein into amino acids. In supplements, pepsin is made from animal enzymes.
5. Trypsin and chymotrypsin, produced by the pancreas, break down proteins.
6. Renin causes milk to coagulate, changing its protein, casein, into a form the body can use. Renin also releases certain minerals from milk, such as calcium, phosphorus, potassium, and iron.
7. Pancreatin is an enzyme found in the pancreas. This enzyme functions best in the small intestine.

THE LARGE INTESTINE

Your large intestine, also called the colon, is the waste disposal system of the digestive tract. The small intestine ends in a section called the ileum. This is where the body absorbs vitamin B_{12} and some of the fat-soluble vitamins, including A and E.

The colon is located in the navel area and is shaped something like an upside-down U, with the small intestine ending at the bottom of the left side of the U. The ileocecal valve, a one-way sphincter, separates the small intestine from the large intestine. After food has moved through the small intestine, giving up its nutrients to the bloodstream, what's left is water, fiber, and waste material such as bacteria, excess nutrients, and undigested food. The ileocecal valve allows this material into a sac in the bottom of the colon called the cecum. Here the colon begins the process of pulling water and electrolytes (minerals) out of the waste material. The process continues as the material moves up the ascending colon and across the top part, called the transverse colon. As it moves down the descending colon, the material is formed into a more solid mass that is excreted through the rectum and anus as feces.

In a healthy body, it takes 12 to 14 hours for waste material to make the circuit of the large intestine. Any material leaving the ileum and entering the cecum (where the small and large intestines join) should be quite watery. (If it isn't, you will be constipated!)

Keeping Your Good Bacteria Healthy Will Keep You Healthy

The colon, in contrast to the germ-free stomach, is lavishly populated with bacteria, which are normal intestinal flora. These bacteria, also called probiotics, are also found in the mouth, the urinary tract, and the vagina. There are about one hundred trillion of these bacteria living in our bodies, and over four hundred species. In a healthy body, the "good" bacteria run the show, and the bad bacteria are kept to a minimum.

When the bad bacteria outweigh the good bacteria, the result is often an overgrowth of bad bacteria (actually a fungal yeast) called *Candida albicans*. Women are familiar with the yeast infections that can occur in the vagina, but these infections can also happen elsewhere in the body, including the intestines. An overgrowth of yeast in the intestines can cause fatigue, bloating, gas, diarrhea, constipation, and a long list of secondary symptoms, such as headaches, mental fogginess, and pollen allergies.

Probiotics are the "good" bacteria. Your overall health is closely tied to the health of these bacteria. If they are sick, often so are you. They play a major role, along with our digestive enzymes, in digesting food and moving it out of the body.

The three most common families of friendly bacteria are called *Lactobacillus acidophilus, Lactobacillus bulgaricus,* and *Bifidobacterium bifidum.* These versatile bugs change and adapt rapidly, depending on geographical location, individual biochemistry, and what types of unfriendly bacteria are invading the body at the moment. Probiotics are the ultimate antibiotics, elegantly crafted by nature to fight off unfriendly bacteria without killing the friendly ones. It's simple: Take care of your friendly bacteria, and they will take care of you.

Probiotics play other roles as well: Your immune system depends on them; they manufacture the B vitamins and vitamin K; they reduce cholesterol; and they help keep hormones in balance. A deficiency of probiotics can cause allergies, arthritis, skin problems, and *Candida* and may sabotage the role of your body's defense system in keeping cancer at bay.

The most common cause of a *Candida* overgrowth is taking antibiotics, which kill the friendly bacteria right along with the unfriendly ones but don't seem to bother *Candida.* Always follow antibiotic treatment with at least two weeks of probiotics.

Steroids such as prednisone and cortisone can also upset the balance of intestinal flora. Other factors are a poor diet, stress, and poor digestion in the stomach and small intestine. Your friendly bacteria do better on the same diet that you do better on. (Hmm, what a coincidence.) They like complex carbohydrates, such as whole grains and beans, and they like fresh vegetables, and they don't like a lot of sugar, refined flour, and dairy products.

Probiotics also decline as we age, so it's important to add probiotic supplements to your diet or eat unsweetened yogurt with live cultures (check the label) daily.

Many supermarkets and health food stores also sell "acidophilus," a milk product containing live cultures. Probiotic supplements are "alive" and have a relatively short shelf life of a few months. If you want to try probiotic supplements, stick to the refrigerated capsules and reputable brands.

Preventing Colon Cancer

Colon cancer is a topic most people prefer to avoid, but fifty-seven thousand people will die of it this year. This is tragic, because all colon cancers can be prevented so easily. We know that there may be a genetic predisposition to get colon cancer, and we also know some major factors that can cause colon cancer:

- There are a lot of toxic substances passing through your system that will harm your bowel and possibly create cancerous cells if they sit there for very long.
- Many studies have linked a high-fat diet to colon cancer. Fat stimulates your gallbladder to produce bile, which is one of those toxic substances that shouldn't sit there. Also, the high temperatures needed to cook fat can produce potentially cancer-causing substances in your food.
- Low levels of the mineral selenium have been repeatedly linked to colon cancer.

Fortunately, by following these four dietary guidelines, you can dramatically lower your risk of developing colon cancer:

1. *Keep things moving through your bowels.* Chow down on vegetables such as broccoli, kale, carrots, onions, cabbage, collards, peas, potatoes, and all dark green, yellow, and orange vegetables. Why? They're high in fiber, so they keep your bowels moving, but that's not all. Vegetables contain substances that take toxins through your intestines quickly and harmlessly. And don't forget the wheat bran for more fiber. There is some evidence that fiber may even reverse the growth of precancerous polyps (bumps in the lining of your intestines).
2. *Cut down on the saturated fat you're eating.* Saturated fat is usually solid at room temperature. Examples are butter, the marbled fat in meat, the fat from fried foods, and hydrogenated

oils. Your fat calories should be no more than 25 percent of your diet, and of that, 10 percent or less should come from saturated fat.

3. *Get your calcium.* Calcium is paramount in the prevention of colon cancer. The French eat five to six servings of yogurt daily, and even though they consume as much fat as most North Americans, their rate of colon cancer is much lower.

4. *Say yes to selenium!* Over the past few years, a number of studies have linked low selenium levels with colon cancer. In a study at the University of Arizona, it was found that people with high levels of selenium in their blood had fewer colon polyps, which are often precancerous. Selenium is an important part of an antioxidant enzyme called glutathione peroxidase. This enzyme may prevent damage to cells. Some studies show that it plays a role in the repair of DNA and helps activate the immune system. Onion and garlic are rich sources of selenium. Other great sources are brown rice, seafood, kidney, liver, wheat germ, bran, tuna fish, tomatoes, and broccoli. You can take 100–200 mcg of selenium daily.

Relieving Constipation Naturally

Constipation occurs when the contents of the bowels become hard and compact and bowel movements are infrequent. If you aren't constipated yourself, you probably know someone who is. About thirty million Americans are afflicted with this uncomfortable and unhealthy problem.

So why aren't America's bowels moving? We need to eat more fiber, drink more water, and get more exercise. Whatever you do, avoid those habit-forming over-the-counter laxatives.

When I was a kid and looking for something to do on a rainy day, my mother would sometimes give me some construction paper and scissors, and then she would make me a paste out of white flour and water. It works pretty well to stick things together. Well, that's just about what white flour does in your gut. It sticks to your ribs, all right! If you don't believe me, get some white flour and add water until you get a nice gluelike paste. Your bowels need the fiber nat-urally found in whole grains, fruits, and vegetables to function properly. The real secret to ending consti-pation is fiber, which you'll read a lot more about later in this chapter.

If you don't drink enough water, your body won't have any to spare when it comes to making stools, and the stools will be hard and dry. This is painful and can cause bleeding and hemorrhoids. Exercise helps move the bowels. (Just remember that moving your body will move your bowels!)

It's also important to have a bowel movement when you have the urge to have one. Chronically hold-ing back bowel movements can cause constipation.

Age can play a factor in constipation. The muscles you use to have a bowel movement can simply become weaker with time, especially if you've been stressing and straining them for a lifetime. Bran and prunes become a staple in the diet of many older people.

Some pharmaceutical drugs cause constipation, including painkillers, decongestants, narcotics, anti-histamines, antidepressants, and tranquilizers. Iron tablets can also cause constipation. And dairy products—cheese in particular—can cause constipation in some people.

Many of us become constipated when we travel. Long hours of sitting, changes in diet and water, and changes in our daily routine can make us "irregular." Pack prunes or bran.

If all these remedies don't work to relieve your constipation, try psyllium powder. It's made from a fibrous plant that can help give your stools more bulk. It's the main ingredient in products such as Metamucil and Correctol, but you can get it in a much purer and cheaper form at your local health food store. Mix about a teaspoon with 8 ounces of water or juice and drink it right away. It's very important to drink plenty of fluids when you're using a bulk-forming laxative such as psyllium.

Herbs such as cascara sagrada and senna can relieve constipation by stimulating the bowels. In general I don't recommend them because they can become habit-forming, but once in awhile they are fine. Cascara sagrada is made from the bark of a tree and is fairly gentle. It is found in some over-the-counter laxatives, but I suggest you get it in capsule form at your local health food store. Senna is another plant laxative. It is a more powerful bowel-stimulating laxative that has been used for centuries. Stimulating laxatives become habit forming if your bowels lose their natural ability to be stimulated, so use them only when absolutely necessary.

Magnesium can cause diarrhea, and thus can also be a remedy for constipation. This is particularly true when pregnancy is causing constipation. Taking 300 mg of magnesium is a safe and nutritional way to combat constipation. However, if you have chronic constipation, it's important to get to the cause and treat that.

My grandmother used to drink a glass of warm water before she went to bed at night. This makes sense, because many people are constipated simply because they don't drink enough water. Water naturally softens stools. If you are taking a diuretic medicine, it will tend to pull water out of your bowels, which in turn can cause constipation. My advice? Drink six to eight glasses of clean water every day.

Coffee can help move your bowels unless you overdo it. Drink too much coffee and you may end up constipated. I'm not a big fan of coffee, and I certainly don't want you to make it a daily habit, but if you find yourself constipated and without a handy remedy, you can almost always find a cup of coffee.

Natural Remedies for Diarrhea

Diarrhea is loose, unformed, watery stools that tend to come frequently. Diarrhea is very common, especially in children. It can be caused by bacteria, such as in bad food; by a cold or flu virus; by parasites; by stress; and by antibiotics and other prescription drugs. Chronic diarrhea or diarrhea with blood or pus can be a symptom of a more serious illness and should be checked out by a health care professional.

In the United States, we talk about getting "Montezuma's revenge," or diarrhea caused by drinking the water in a foreign country. However, when people from other countries come to the United States, they also tend to get diarrhea because they aren't used to our bacteria, either! Any time you travel, it's important to stick to bottled water and eat plenty of yogurt to keep the colon healthy.

Here are some natural remedies for diarrhea.

Add More Fiber

This may sound strange, but sometimes the cure for diarrhea is the same as the cure for constipation: fiber. Adding more bulk to your stools can give watery stools more firmness. Some people simply tend to have watery stools, and fiber is a good solution in that case.

Take Garlic

Studies have been done comparing garlic and drugs in their effectiveness for killing diarrhea-causing bugs. The garlic either wins or comes out performing as well as the drugs. It's cheaper than drugs, doesn't have any side effects, and will also clean up parasites as it moves through. If you're using garlic to treat diarrhea that you suspect is caused by a bug, it's best to take it in capsules so you don't further irritate your digestive tract. You can find many types of garlic supplements at your health food store.

Eat Bland Foods

It's important to eat simple, bland foods when you have diarrhea. In fact, this is the one time when I would recommend white rice or white flour, because it is binding. Apples and bland cheeses also tend to be binding. Plain yogurt will help repopulate the friendly bacteria in the colon.

ARE YOU ALLERGIC TO YOUR FOOD?

An estimated one in three people suffer from allergies of some kind. Allergies to pollen, dust, pets, synthetic chemicals, and food are the most common. One of the most common sources of digestive ailments is food allergies.

Before we go any further, let's qualify what I mean by food allergies. Allergy specialists love to argue about the definition of food allergies versus food intolerances or food sensitivities. For the purpose of simplicity, I divide all negative reactions to foods into two groups: immediate allergies and delayed allergies. This is easy because the treatment for delayed food allergies is the same, whether they are, strictly speaking, intolerances, sensitivities, or allergies.

Immediate allergies cause symptoms such as hives, asthma, sneezing, watery and itchy eyes and nose, and even anaphylactic shock. Children suffer most from immediate allergies and normally outgrow them, though a sudden stress combined with eating a childhood food allergen can bring it all back. Only 1 percent of the adult population is estimated to suffer from immediate allergies to foods. Seafood, strawberries, milk, and beans are some of the more common foods that can produce immediate allergic reactions.

Delayed allergic reactions to food, also called food intolerances or food sensitivities, are far more common than immediate allergies. These symptoms may not show up for hours or days and can vary considerably. Many of our chronic complaints, such as headaches, immediate allergies to pollen and chemicals, indigestion, stiff and achy joints, and fatigue can all be symptoms of a delayed food allergy and the damage it does to the intestines.

When digestion becomes problematic due to chronic delayed food allergies, the rest of the body is more vulnerable to illness. For example, the inability to absorb nutrients can cause low-grade, generalized symptoms of malnutrition and essential fatty acid deficiency, such as dull hair, dry skin, and weak nails. Constipation can allow estrogen in the large intestine to be reabsorbed, causing PMS. The immune system becomes constantly stressed, causing greater susceptibility to colds and flu.

Many mainstream doctors do not even acknowledge the existence of delayed food allergies, but then again, they are unable to successfully treat many of the diseases caused or aggravated by them, such as Crohn's disease, psoriasis, irritable bowel syndrome (IBS), and arthritis and other autoimmune diseases. Your best bet, if you have any of these illnesses, is to go to a health care professional who is able to recognize and treat them.

For most people, a delayed food allergy causes low-level chronic symptoms that worsen with age or under stress. Your energy may be low, and you may

have skin, hair, and nail problems, minor aches and pains, headaches, various forms of indigestion, hay fever, stiffness in the joints, muscle weakness, and frequent colds. Many people think that it's normal to walk around feeling like this, but if you fall into this category, removing one or two foods from your diet may change your life.

What Causes Delayed Food Allergies?

The root causes of food allergies are interwoven with the root causes of intestinal damage. It's difficult to know whether intestinal damage causes allergies, or allergies cause intestinal damage. For example, if the stomach doesn't secrete enough hydrochloric acid or if the pancreas is unable to release adequate digestive enzymes, foods won't be broken down properly, which can damage the intestinal walls. This damage in turn reduces the absorption of nutrients and allows large, unidentified food particles to escape into the bloodstream, causing the immune system to react with inflammation (in effect, an allergy) somewhere in the body. In that case, the intestinal damage is causing the food allergy.

But suppose you have an inherited sensitivity to yeast, so that every time you eat bread, crackers, vinegar, beer, and many other foods, your immune system responds with alarm as the yeast enters your bloodstream. This may set up inflammatory reactions in the intestines, causing intestinal damage. In that case, the allergy has caused the intestinal damage. Fortunately, the treatment is the same, although if you have underlying genetic susceptibilities to allergies, you may want to focus more on strengthening your immune system and reducing inflammatory reactions. (For more on strengthening the immune system, see chapter 9.)

I believe that much of what we call hyperactivity and treat with the drug Ritalin (one in twenty boys at last count—a national scandal) is really delayed allergic reactions to foods, especially food dyes and preservatives. Those children are set up for this by being on antibiotics for most of their toddler years, which severely suppresses the immune system as well as all the friendly bacteria in the large intestine.

By the time many children are introduced to solid foods, their immune system and digestive tract have been damaged by antibiotics, and their liver has been damaged by acetaminophen (children's Tylenol). This is a triple whammy! No wonder they're hypersensitive! Add to this an almost constant exposure to environmental estrogens, known as xenoestrogens, through pesticide-sprayed fruits and vegetables, hormone-laced meat, and air pollution. Excessive estrogens cause sodium and water retention (which affects the brain, especially in children), inflammation, suppression of thyroid function, excess copper, and many more unpleasant symptoms. A healthy digestive system might be able to excrete excess estrogen, but a damaged and constantly stressed digestive system will barely be delivering the necessary nutrients for growth and development.

Children who aren't breast-fed (which would give them needed immunities) and who are introduced to hard-to-digest grains and other solid foods too early tend to have more food allergies. Throughout our lives, but especially in childhood, the digestive system and immune system are busily sorting out what's friend and what's foe, what's a nutritious food and what's a bacterial or viral enemy. Foods for which a child isn't prepared or maybe even has a genetic susceptibility can be mistaken for an enemy, causing diarrhea, vomiting, asthma, fatigue, poor absorption, or some type of inflammatory reaction, such as eczema.

In adults, there are many potential underlying causes of food allergies, including chronic stress (which shuts down the secretion of digestive juices), alcoholism, poor diet, and the many outside environmental factors that damage the intestines, such as pesticides, parasites, heavy metals such as lead and mercury, food additives, and especially drugs such as antibiotics and NSAIDs (nonsteroidal anti-inflammatory drugs), which damage the intestines.

Identifying the Most Common Food Allergen Culprits

The common delayed food allergens are wheat, corn, dairy products, soy, citrus fruit, the nightshade family of vegetables (potatoes, tomatoes, eggplant, red and green peppers, and cayenne), peanuts (often caused by aflatoxins, a fungus found in most peanuts), eggs, beef, and coffee—but we can become allergic to almost anything.

Irritable bowel syndrome (IBS) is often a delayed food allergy to dairy products. People with an allergy to gluten, known as celiac sprue, are allergic to all grains that contain gluten, including wheat, rye, barley, and oats. Some of the worst and most insidious culprits, because they are hidden in processed foods, are food additives such as food colorings (especially red and yellow dye), BHT, BHA, MSG, benzoates, nitrates, and sulfites—yet another great reason to avoid processed foods.

The most common symptom of parasites, another cause of damaged intestines, are diarrhea and cramping. If you suspect that you have parasites, which many people do after traveling in a foreign country, see a health care professional for testing and treatment.

Leaky Gut Syndrome

Leaky gut syndrome occurs when the villi that line the small intestine become damaged. The damage creates microscopic holes in the intestine, through which relatively large, partially digested food particles escape into the bloodstream. Bacteria and other microorganisms are also able to pass through the intestinal wall. The immune system detects these foreign invaders and sends out the troops to get rid of them. If this is happening constantly, such as every time you eat, the immune system becomes overstressed and inflammation sets in.

Foreign particles in the bloodstream may migrate almost anywhere in the body, often to the place of greatest vulnerability, such as the joints, where an inflammation reaction causes arthritic symptoms. A high percentage of arthritic symptoms can be effectively cleared up just by removing food allergens from the diet and healing the intestinal tract.

A leaky gut also interferes with the body's system for distinguishing safe and needed nutrients from foreign invaders. When digestion is proceeding normally, our foods are broken down into usable nutrients. As digestion moves along, special areas along the digestive tract identify the food and "tag" it as a friend, thus desensitizing the immune system to that food. However, when the intestines are damaged, the tagging process starts to break down. When untagged food particles move into the bloodstream and run into the body's immune system, antibodies are made to fight them and get rid of them.

So here we have the immune system on overtime trying to handle genuine foreign invaders such as bacteria and viruses. Meanwhile, it's constantly going after large, partially digested food particles. And on top of it all, it's reacting to necessary nutrients as if they, too, were enemies!

Meanwhile, the liver, our most important detoxification organ, which is already very busy shunting nutrients off to the rest of the body, is forced to work overtime to detoxify what the small intestine was unable to take care of.

Preventing Leaky Gut Syndrome and Food Allergies

Probably the single best way you can prevent leaky gut syndrome and food allergies is by avoiding anti-inflammatory drugs. My guess is that aspirin, ibuprofen, and similar anti-inflammatory drugs cause the vast majority of intestinal damage, which then causes delayed food allergies. We take these drugs casually, as if they are perfectly safe, but they really aren't. Aspirin alone is responsible for some ten thousand deaths and tens of thousands of hospitalizations every year due to intestinal bleeding. As a pharmacist, my advice to you is to take drugs only when you really need them, and then for as short a time as possible and in as small a dose as possible. That advice alone could spare you a lifetime of illness!

Avoiding antibiotics whenever possible will also help prevent leaky gut syndrome and food allergies. As important as these miracle drugs are for treating life-threatening infections, they have serious side effects that have been largely ignored by mainstream medicine. Antibiotics suppress the immune system, and they kill both good and bad intestinal bacteria. As discussed in the section on the large intestine, we need to keep our friendly bacteria healthy if we are going to stay healthy.

Fundamental to a healthy digestive system are my basic tenets for staying healthy: eating a wholesome, balanced diet free of processed foods; drinking six to eight glasses of clean water every day; getting some exercise at least three or four times a week; and

taking a multivitamin every day. It is also important that you avoid drugs, because many of them are very hard on the liver, which only adds to the burden on the immune system. It's best to use natural alternatives to prescription drugs whenever possible.

Leaky gut syndrome can be made much worse when we aren't producing enough digestive enzymes to break down food particles sufficiently. Starting with the enzymes in the upper stomach, a snowballing effect can be produced, where food not digested properly at one stage puts a bigger load on the enzymes at the next stage, and so forth. One research study showed that 90 percent of people with gastric disturbances were not producing enough of one specific digestive enzyme, as compared to only 20 percent of a group of healthy people.

One of the best ways to combat leaky gut syndrome is to take digestive enzyme supplements when you eat. These will help the digestive system break down the food particles better. Taking digestive enzymes can significantly increase the digestion of food and greatly reduce symptoms of food allergies.

Treating Leaky Gut Syndrome and Food Allergies

To treat leaky gut syndrome, you need to identify food allergens and take supplements to heal the intestinal tract. It's also important to avoid large amounts of alcohol and prescription drugs, which stress the liver. To support the liver, you can take the herb milk thistle (silymarin), which you can find where you buy your other supplements.

Some health professionals will test for leaky gut syndrome with a test called the lactulose/mannitol absorption test. The test measures levels of lactulose, which is made of very large molecules that normally don't enter the body. If the test shows elevated levels of lactulose, then large molecules are being allowed through the intestines.

An Elimination Diet May Be Your Ticket to Better Health

Tests that identify food allergens vary in expense and reliability. The least expensive and in some ways the most accurate way to identify problem foods is to go on an elimination diet. If your self-discipline and your ability to track your symptoms every day are very good, you can try this on your own. Otherwise, I recommend that you do it with the support of a health care professional. I also recommend the book *Optimal Wellness* by Ralph Golan, MD (Ballantine Books, 1995), which contains a very thorough and detailed chapter on food allergies and elimination diets.

The basic principle of the elimination diet is to follow a specially limited diet for two weeks and then reintroduce foods that you suspect of being allergens one day at a time, while closely observing how your body responds. Your body will tend to have a strong response to an offending food after a few days of being off it. Conversely, if you eliminate the offending foods during your two weeks, many of your chronic symptoms will disappear and you'll notice increased energy.

But before you start an elimination diet, it's important to spend ten days keeping a daily journal of *everything* you eat and drink. That means food and drink, snacks and meals, eating in and eating out. At the end of the ten days, make a list of all the foods that you ate more than five times in that ten-day period. Odd as it may sound, the foods you ate every day are most likely the culprits. It may seem as if the foods you like best are those that make you feel best, but we tend to become addicted to the foods we are allergic to. You should be able to reintroduce most of your favorite foods back into your diet very gradually, although I don't recommend that you eat them every day.

Ideally, you will eliminate both the daily foods and the "more than five times" foods from your diet for at least two weeks. If you suspect other foods of being allergens, also eliminate those. Sometimes supplements contain fillers and binders that are allergens, so eliminate those, too, for two weeks if they are suspect. (The label should identify all fillers and binders or say that there aren't any. If it doesn't, don't buy that supplement.)

During the two weeks you are off your suspect food allergens, be sure to keep a journal of the foods you're eating. People who are allergic to foods find that they tend to become allergic to almost *anything* they eat every day. This makes it important to ro-

tate the foods you do eat so that if at all possible, you're not eating any one food more than every other day.

When you eliminate suspect foods, you must not eat even a tiny amount of them or you'll throw off your test. Wheat, corn, dairy products, and eggs are hidden in many processed foods, so if you're not familiar with something on a label, skip that food item. Your best bet is to eat whole, fresh foods that don't need a label!

If food allergy and a leaky gut are at the root of your problem, you should see a significant change in your health within the two-week period. Symptoms such as diarrhea and skin rashes should clear up within a week or so. Children tend to recover especially quickly from the symptoms of food allergies when they are put on an elimination diet.

People who have spent years with chronic low-grade health problems caused by food allergies and leaky gut syndrome are likely to be suffering from other problems as well, such as *Candida* overgrowth, arthritis, autoimmune diseases, and hay fever. In this case, it's important to work with a health care professional who can help you heal your whole body and bring it back into balance.

After two weeks, begin reintroducing foods, one every 24 hours. Keep a meticulous journal of symptoms. If you have any symptoms such as a faster pulse, rapid or irregular heartbeat, sudden fatigue, a feeling of heaviness or sleepiness, stomach cramps, bloating, gas, diarrhea, constipation, headache, dizziness, chills, sweats, flushing, skin rash, runny or itchy eyes or nose, stiffness, achiness, muscle weakness, or any other unusual physical symptom, you are most likely sensitive to that food. Eliminate that food completely from your diet for two months and then try reintroducing it again. If you are still sensitive to it, eliminate it for six months and try again.

Some foods may always be allergens for you, but if you're taking good care of yourself and your digestive system, you should be able to safely reintroduce food allergens into your diet. But if you start eating them every day, you'll probably become allergic to them again. Children may have to outgrow a food allergy, which can be hard for everyone if it's a common food like wheat or dairy products.

Supplements for Healing Your Intestines

Glutamine

Glutamine is an amino acid that is found in very high concentrations in the small intestine, and plays an important role in maintaining gut mucosa. Your body needs manganese to make glutamine, and it needs glutamine and tryptophan to make niacin.

Glutamine may be a food for cancer tumors, so don't take this as a supplement if you have cancer. I recommend 500 mg of glutamine taken three times daily with meals when you're working on healing your intestinal tract.

Essential Fatty Acids

Essential fatty acids, and particularly GLA (gamma-linolenic acid) from borage oil or evening primrose oil, help prevent inflammatory reactions throughout the body and specifically in the gut. GLA is an omega-6 fatty acid normally made in the body from the essential fatty acid linoleic acid.

The best way to ensure that your GLA levels stay high and in balance with the other fatty acids is to avoid those things that deplete GLA. The biggest offender is the *trans*-fatty acids found in hydrogenated oils used in margarine and nearly all processed foods. These "fake" oils rob the body of GLA. The second biggest offender in depleting GLA is processed foods depleted of GLA. Whole grains, particularly oatmeal, as well as many nuts and seeds contain small amounts of GLA.

Taking too much alpha-linolenic acid, the omega-3 fatty acid found in flaxseed oil, is another way to suppress GLA production. Flaxseed oil is something of a nutritional fad right now, but I don't recommend you take large amounts of it long-term, as it is a highly unstable unsaturated oil that can do just as much harm as good if it's rancid or taken in excess.

You can also take GLA in the form of a supplement of evening primrose oil or borage oil. Follow the directions on the container.

It's also important to get plenty of omega-3 fatty acids, which are mainly found in fish oils. Eicosapentaenoic acid (EPA), found in fish oil, will also inhibit inflammation. This is why I encourage you to eat cold-water, deep-sea fish such as salmon, cod, sardines, and flounder at least twice a week.

You should be taking fifty to a hundred times more EPA than GLA oils. You need only 1–2 mg of GLA and 50–100 mg of EPA.

If you'd like a clearly written, well-researched book on prostaglandins and essential fatty acids, try *Enter the Zone*, by Barry Sears (Regan Books, 1995).

Herbs for Healing the Gut

Licorice

You probably think of licorice as a candy because its distinctive flavor and sweetness make it a great sweet treat, especially for diabetics. It is commonly used in throat lozenges, and the Chinese give it to teething babies to help relieve pain and to young children to promote the growth of muscle and bones. Licorice is fifty times sweeter than sugar, but it is also a powerful medicine, with literally hundreds of studies backing up its effectiveness.

Glycyrrhiza glabra (the Latin name for licorice) contains a chemical called glycyrrhizin that stimulates the secretion of the adrenal cortex hormone aldosterone and has a powerful cortisonelike effect. This makes it a useful anti-inflammatory. However, glycyrrhizin can cause high blood pressure, potassium loss, and edema (swelling or water retention) due to sodium retention when it is used in high doses for many months. To avoid this effect, some licorice preparations are deglycyrrhizinized and known as DGL, which comes in lozenge form because it needs to be chewed to be most effective.

The antiulcer effects of licorice are due to its ability to increase beneficial prostaglandins (hormonelike substances that regulate many bodily functions, including inflammation) that promote mucus secretion and the healing process in the stomach. According to a study cited by herbalist Donald Brown, licorice root, which stimulates growth of the surface layers of intestinal mucous lining, works even better when combined with ginger, which stimulates deeper layers of mucosal healing. In Europe, licorice is often combined with the herb chamomile for treating stomach problems.

You can take licorice root in lozenges, capsules, or tincture form for up to two weeks, following the directions on the container. DGL lozenges are fine to take long-term. They should contain 250–500 mg of licorice, and one to three lozenges should be chewed 15 minutes to half an hour before meals.

California Black Walnut and Yellow Dock

According to herbalist Michael Moore, the dried leaves of the California black walnut tree (*Juglans californica, J. hindsii*), which is found throughout the United States, can be made into a tea that is a wonderful healing agent to the small intestine. It acts as an astringent and tonic and improves mucous membrane absorption and reduces inflammation. According to Moore, you can use one part leaves to two parts water. Drink 2 cups of the tea daily.

For an even more effective remedy, add yellow dock (*Rumex crispus*) root, which you can find in tincture or capsule form at your health food store. Follow dosage instructions on the container.

FIBER AND YOUR HEALTH

For twenty years I have been telling people that if they would include more fiber in their diet, a lot of their health problems would clear up. Cultures with plenty of fiber in their diet have virtually no constipation, no colon cancer, no varicose veins, no hemorrhoids, and on and on. Cultures that emphasize fiber-free refined grains and processed foods have all those illnesses and more. Americans seem to have to work to include 30 g of fiber in their daily diet. Members of cultures whose diet contains a lot of fiber may eat as much as 150 g in a day. That's a big difference! The average American consumes 10–15 g of fiber daily. I don't want you to try to eat 150 g of fiber a day—that's overdoing it—but I do want you to try to get 30–45 g daily.

My grandmother used to tell me that I needed "roughage," but then it somehow fell out of favor and was just seen as a nutritionally unnecessary filler. But lately, fiber has become nutritionally chic. Mainstream medicine is catching on and catching up, and fiber is now recommended by doctors and dieti-

tians alike. It has finally dawned on our collective consciousness that our white flour, white rice, and all the other white, refined foods in our diet are killing us, not just because they are nutrition free, but because they gum up the system. Fiber plays an absolutely essential role in good health, and that's what the remainder of this chapter is about.

What Is Fiber?

Fiber is what gives plants their structure. It is the part of the food we eat that is not digested, passing through all the various chemical baths and enzymes of the gastrointestinal system untouched. It has virtually no calories but provides bulk for digesting food and especially for stools. Meat, eggs, and dairy products do not contain any fiber.

Although fiber comes packaged in many different types of plants and their fruits, seeds, and nuts, the actual fiber itself can be divided into two types, soluble and insoluble. Soluble fiber becomes gummy in water, and insoluble fiber isn't changed in water. It is the insoluble fiber that passes through the digestive

---

Soluble Fiber

Sources: Vegetables (especially onions), fruits, oat bran, gums from nuts, seeds, and beans.

Benefits: Stabilizes blood sugar, lowers cholesterol and blood pressure, and provides a friendly environment for "good" bacteria.

Insoluble Fiber

Sources: Whole grains (wheat, barley, rye, for example), vegetables, and beans.

Benefits: Adds bulk to the stools, prevents constipation, helps remove toxins from the bowel, and keeps the intestines clean by having a scrubbing action.

All Fiber

Reduces fat intake by increasing volume of food and giving a full feeling. Speeds up transit time.

system unchanged, while soluble fiber has turned into a gum or jelly by the time it reaches the large intestine. Nature packages itself well when it comes to human health benefits, and fiber is no exception, since most fruits and vegetables come with both types of fiber.

Both soluble fiber and insoluble fiber have many benefits. Soluble types of fiber, including gums, pectins, and mucilages, tend to stabilize blood sugar, reduce cholesterol and blood pressure, and provide a friendly environment for "good" colon bacteria. Insoluble types of fiber, which include cellulose, hemicellulose, and lignin, add bulk to the stools, prevent constipation, help remove toxins from the bowel, and keep the intestines clean by their scrubbing action.

Fighting Disease with Fiber

You already know that fiber increases the bulk of stool, which helps relieve constipation, but it can also decrease transit time, which is the amount of time it takes for food to go through the entire digestive process. Transit time will vary a lot from person to person, based on genetics, environment, and personality, but the amount of fiber in the diet also plays a significant role. Cultures that eat a lot of fiber tend to have much faster transit times than cultures with a low fiber intake. And soluble fiber eaten without insoluble fiber may speed up transit time, which for most Americans is a positive benefit. However, if you are one of those people with too fast a transit time (which tends to come with loose, watery, unformed stools), then fiber may also normalize your transit time by adding bulk to the stools and absorbing water.

Ideally, transit time should vary from 12 to 18 hours. For most Americans, however, transit time is 50 to 60 hours. You can find out what your transit time is by eating some corn or swallowing three or four 10-grain charcoal tablets (found at your local pharmacy) and tracking how long these substances take to show up at the other end. Corn tends to show up in feces unchanged, and charcoal will turn the stools black.

Oral contraceptives tend to slow transit time, and excess alcohol consumption speeds transit time.

Constipation

Clearly one of the biggest benefits of eating a high-fiber diet or taking fiber supplements is relief from constipation. Fiber is by far the best remedy for this common affliction. However, if you increase your fiber up to 30–35 g daily and you still have constipation, see a health care professional to make sure there isn't something more serious going on.

Diverticulitis/Diverticulosis

Diverticula are pouches in the wall of the large intestine. Constipation and straining can force fecal matter into these pockets, causing them to enlarge, to become inflamed, and to leak digestive matter into the surrounding tissues. This is what we call diverticulitis. Since whatever is in the large intestine is full of noxious bacteria and waste matter, this causes infections and abscesses in the tissues surrounding the leaky diverticula.

Digestive matter that gets caught in the diverticula sits there and ferments, rots, and becomes toxic to your system. Environmental toxins and waste products can also accumulate.

In diverticulosis, the diverticula bulge outward from the intestine, but there isn't inflammation. This is a common ailment of older people and can cause gas, pain in the navel area, especially on the left side, and sometimes bleeding. Diverticulosis, if left untreated, can lead to diverticulitis.

The best remedy for diverticulosis is to avoid processed foods and make fiber-rich foods a staple of the diet. The best type of supplemental fiber to take for diverticulosis is psyllium, since it has a fairly gentle action on the bowel but adds plenty of bulk.

Diseases of Excess Estrogen

The ailments caused by excessive estrogen, coined "estrogen dominance" by John R. Lee, MD, author of *What Your Doctor May Not Tell You About Menopause* (Warner Books, 1996), are many. I'm going to mention some of the most common here, but I recommend that if you're a woman over the age of forty, you read Lee's book. It's a real eye-opener.

Excess estrogen can contribute to insulin resistance, block thyroid function, and lower zinc levels, which impairs immune system function. This is a good hormone to have in balance!

Lack of fiber causes excess estrogen to be recycled back into the body through the large intestine. A diet with plenty of fiber will soak up excess estrogen and other waste material in the large intestine, and from there the excess estrogen will be excreted. When there isn't enough fiber to act like a sponge for the waste matter, or when there is constipation and the waste matter has to sit in the bowel for longer than it should, estrogen gets recycled back into the system rather than being excreted.

Another benefit of eating plenty of fiber-rich vegetables is that many of them have phytohormones that take up estrogen receptor sites on cells, in effect blocking the action of the estrogen and lowering its levels in the body.

There have been many studies showing that fiber lowers estrogen levels. In one study, twelve premenopausal women ate a daily diet consisting of 30 percent of calories from fat and 15–25 g of fiber for one month. Then, for two months, they ate a daily diet consisting of only 10 percent fat and 20–35 g of fiber. At the end of the very-low-fat, high-fiber diet, estrogen levels had fallen significantly. (By the way, I do not recommend that you reduce your fat to 10 percent of calories. That's too low, and it's not healthy. A more gradual approach of 20 to 25 percent calories from fat and 30–35 g of fiber daily will achieve the same result over a longer period of time.)

PMS (premenstrual syndrome). PMS tends to have multiple causes, but balancing excess estrogen can bring quite a lot of relief to many women. The hormone progesterone balances, or opposes, estrogen. If a woman is deficient in progesterone at the end of her cycle, which may happen if she doesn't ovulate, she will have too much estrogen relative to progesterone and will have estrogen dominance symptoms, such as water retention, irritability, sore breasts, headaches, and fatigue. Adding supplemental fiber to the diet at the end of the menstrual cycle can help greatly to reduce estrogen levels and thus PMS symptoms.

Breast cancer. Breast cancer is an estrogen-driven cancer, and women at risk for it should strive to keep their estrogen levels in balance. Getting plenty of fiber is an essential part of a breast cancer prevention plan. A study in which women with benign breast tumors were compared with healthy women found that the women without breast tumors ate significantly more fiber.

Menopause symptoms. Menopause is not an estrogen deficiency disease, and adding estrogen to the body of a menopausal woman, especially one who is overweight, is asking for problems. Again, I recommend Dr. Lee's book, and that you keep your fiber high when you are menopausal, to keep your hormones in balance.

High Cholesterol and High Blood Pressure

Although high cholesterol is vastly overrated as a risk factor for dying from heart disease, it is a good idea to keep it under control. You don't want sky-high cholesterol because that's a sign that something is not working right in your cardiovascular system.

We know from many scientific studies that fiber plays a direct and substantial role in lowering cholesterol. Soluble fiber in particular seems to keep cholesterol levels in the healthy range.

The Johns Hopkins Medical Institutions did a study of fiber and cholesterol in China and showed that eating oatmeal or buckwheat not only lowers cholesterol but also lowers blood pressure. An amount as small as a 1-ounce serving eaten daily can give the blood pressure–lowering effect. That sure beats beta-blockers!

Another study of sixty people with moderately high cholesterol who ate just 20 g of fiber a day for nine months found that their ratio of LDL ("bad") to HDL ("good") cholesterol improved by 11 percent, and the LDL cholesterol dropped 9 percent. Best of all, these changes started showing up after only three weeks of adding fiber to the diet.

Heart Disease

We know that fiber lowers high cholesterol and high blood pressure, both risk factors for heart disease.

But a high-fiber diet seems to protect against heart disease even without factoring in blood pressure and cholesterol levels.

One major study kept track of more than forty-three thousand male health professionals between forty and seventy-five years of age for six years. Those who had the most fiber in their diets had half as many heart attacks as those who had the least amount of fiber in their diets, regardless of their fat intake, exercise, and smoking. That's some potent medicine! I don't know of any prescription drug that even comes close to that kind of track record for preventing heart disease. Although all types of fiber were protective, those from breakfast cereals were the most beneficial.

Colorectal Cancer

Fiber so clearly prevents colon cancer that every box of bran cereal should be able to make that claim in big bold letters. A study published in the *Journal of the National Cancer Institute* put 411 patients who had benign tumors in their colon on a diet that reduced fat by 25 percent and added 25 g of wheat bran every day, as well as 20 mg of beta-carotene (which is an insignificant amount). Patients on this regimen saw their adenomas completely disappear after two to four years. Now, there's a cheap, easy way to avoid surgery of the rectum.

If you are at risk for colorectal cancer, you should, in addition to taking fiber, be getting 200 mcg of selenium daily, taking plenty of antioxidants, and eating little to no red meat.

Irritable Bowel Syndrome (IBS)/Colitis

Colitis is a catchall word for many disorders of the large intestine. One of the most common of these is irritable bowel syndrome (IBS). People with IBS tend to have sharp pains in the navel area and alternating diarrhea and constipation. Unlike other forms of colitis, IBS does not involve inflammation. Because people with colitis often have a delayed food allergy, you might want to review our earlier discussion of food allergies. People with IBS tend to be allergic to wheat or gluten, so avoid wheat bran if you have IBS unless you're certain you're not sensitive to it.

Insoluble fiber is often irritating to people suffering from a colitis attack, but soluble fiber can be quite beneficial. Insoluble fiber can be gradually introduced when symptoms aren't present, and that will help prevent a recurrence and keep the gastrointestinal tract cleaned up.

Diabetes

Anything that slows the entry of sugar into the blood can be helpful to those with diabetes. Soluble fiber can slow the emptying of the stomach and coat the small intestine, thus slowing the release of sugar into the bloodstream and reducing the need for large amounts of insulin at one time. This is why it's so much more beneficial to eat an apple than drink apple juice.

Varicose Veins and Hemorrhoids

Varicose veins have become twisted and so large that they can no longer efficiently carry blood. While obesity can certainly aggravate varicose veins, one of the major causes is straining during a bowel movement. Good bowel habits at an early age that prevent constipation and straining can prevent unsightly varicose veins later in life. Fiber is good preventive medicine in more ways than one.

Hemorrhoids are enlarged veins in the rectum and anus, usually caused by constipation and straining. Yet another reason to eat plenty of fiber!

Gallstones

The gallbladder produces a substance called bile, which is squirted into the small intestine to emulsify and digest fats. Gallbladder pain can radiate up to behind the shoulder blades and under the right collarbone. One of the surest remedies for this type of pain is to take a fiber such as psyllium for a few days and avoid fatty foods.

Gallstones, which are hardened deposits of calcium salts and other components of bile, can be prevented by eating plenty of fiber. Now, isn't it easier to eat your bran cereal every morning than to have surgery to remove a gallstone?

Obesity

Fiber can help with weight reduction for the simple reason that it is nearly calorie-free yet provides bulk, giving a feeling of being full. Again, an apple is more filling than apple juice, and an orange is more filling than orange juice.

Increasing Your Fiber Intake

The best way to increase your intake of fiber is to eat more whole grains, as well as fresh fruits and vegetables, and cut down on the amount of white flour and other processed foods you eat. This will keep your bowels moving and keep toxins from accumulating. It's always preferable to get your fiber from your food first and from fiber supplements such as psyllium or bran second.

It's important not to introduce too much fiber or "roughage" into your diet too quickly. If you do, you may suffer from bloating, gas, and abdominal cramps. Gradually introduce more whole grains, more fresh fruits and vegetables, and more water into your diet. If you're not getting some exercise every day, add that, too. Give it three weeks. If that doesn't work, try bran or prunes. Start with a heaping tablespoon of bran and then gradually add more if you need to.

Another reason to increase your fiber very gradually is that as you begin to move the accumulated junk out of your intestines, a lot of toxins can be released, sometimes causing tiredness and headaches. If you do it gradually and drink plenty of clean water (at least six to eight glasses daily), you will minimize these effects. You can also take milk thistle (the active ingredient is silymarin) to support your liver as it helps the body clear out the toxins.

I think that the best all-around fiber food is wheat bran, but as always, moderation is the key. Overdo it and you'll lose the benefits and gain new digestive problems. You'll get bran naturally if you eat whole grains. There are many cereals in the supermarket with bran in them, and they usually advertise it in big letters. You can also buy bran in a jar and sprinkle it on your cereal or in your yogurt. Try starting with a heaping tablespoon. Wheat bran is the most common bran in America, but rice and corn bran also work to relieve constipation.

Fiber-rich prunes and figs work wonders for many people with constipation. Have three or four for breakfast and see what happens. If they are too chewy for you, soak them in water overnight.

Popcorn is a good laxative and fiber for some people.

Beans are a particularly beneficial food for many reasons, including their high-fiber content. They range in fiber from 4–7 g per half-cup serving. They are rich in soluble fiber, which lowers blood cholesterol and blood sugar. Beans also contain insoluble fiber, which can help with constipation.

To get the fiber benefit from wheat, you need to look for "whole-grain wheat" on the label, rather than just "whole wheat."

When you're eating fruits and vegetables, include the skin when possible.

When you're looking for a fruit treat, always go for the whole fruit instead of the fruit juice, which has little or no fiber. Mother Nature's packaging is optimal for good health, and that includes fiber content.

Benefits from Fiber
- Better digestion
- Better elimination
- Lowers cholesterol
- Lowers blood pressure
- Prevents colon cancer
- Prevents appendicitis
- Prevents breast cancer
- Reduces PMS symptoms
- Reduces menopausal symptoms
- Weight loss
- Detoxification
- Healthy gallbladder
- Stable blood sugar

Fiber-Full Foods

- Fruits
- Vegetables
- Brown rice
- Dried beans
- Wheat bran
- Barley
- Rye
- Oats
- Seeds
- Nuts
- Popcorn

Supplemental Sources of Fiber

- Wheat bran
- Oat bran
- Rice bran
- Prunes and figs
- Flaxseed
- Apple pectin
- Legumes
- Psyllium
- Guar gum and other gums
- Whole grains

Some of My Favorite Sources of Fiber (in grams)

1 cup chestnuts, 14.5

½ cup oatmeal, 7.7

1 cup lentils, 6.4

Corn on the cob, 5

½ cup brown rice, 5.5

5 halves dried pear, 4.97

1 large artichoke, 4.5

2½ figs, 4.45

1 small potato, 4.2

1 cup raspberries, 3.69

½ cup black cherries, 2.95

1 apple, 2.8

½ avocado, 2.8

1 cup kidney beans, 2.78

1 papaya, 2.3–2.35

1 cup lentil sprouts, 2.3–2.35

1 cup carrot juice, 2.3–2.35

1 pear, 2.3–2.35

½ cup sunflower seeds, 2.25

½ guava, 2.2

½ cup peanuts, 1.94

½ cup sesame seeds, 1.8

6 PREVENTING HEART DISEASE ~

PREVENTING HEART DISEASE IS EASIER THAN YOU THINK

We all know someone who has died from a heart attack. Heart disease is by far the number one killer of Americans, and yet it is one of the simplest diseases to prevent. Even if your parents and grandparents had heart disease, you can still prevent it in yourself by following some simple guidelines.

If heart disease kills more people every year than anything else, why aren't these simple cures being shouted from the rooftops? Why isn't it the biggest topic of discussion on all the talk shows? First of all, it's too simple, too inexpensive, and not nearly dramatic enough for a talk show. At the same time, these simple cures are the hardest thing to do for many people, because they involve a change in lifestyle and daily habits.

The typical physician believes that his or her patients won't make lifestyle changes and so doesn't even recommend them, even though it is well established that they work better than any drug ever has. In truth, your physician doesn't have the time to help you make lifestyle changes; writing out a prescription is quicker and easier. An expensive drug is prescribed that suppresses the symptoms of heart disease, such as high blood pressure or high cholesterol, and causes a whole range of unpleasant side effects. Pretty soon you're taking other drugs to treat the side effects of the first drugs, and you're on what I call the drug treadmill. I'm going to tell you how to change your lifestyle and get off the drug treadmill. But it's important not to get off drugs suddenly. You'll need to work with your physician.

Many physicians resist taking their patients off these drugs because the drugs make the numbers (blood pressure and cholesterol levels) look good. But suppressing these symptoms does not make the heart disease go away! You need to work on the *causes* of heart disease. If you take the initiative to make positive changes in your diet, get some exercise, lose some weight, and take some supplements, your doctor will be able to see the changes and see your determination. If he or she still resists, I suggest that you get yourself another doctor—one who has your best interest in mind. I'll talk in more detail about the dangers of some popular heart disease drugs later in the chapter.

The single biggest factor contributing to heart disease in America is our poor diet. We eat too much fat, too many processed foods, and not enough fresh vegetables. In the 1950s, the Japanese diet was 16 percent fat, and they had almost no incidence of heart disease. Today their diet is 26 percent fat and heart disease is the second leading cause of death in Japan. In the United States, the average diet contains 36 to 40 percent fat.

I believe that cholesterol and high blood pressure are way overrated as risk factors for heart disease. I haven't even included sections on them in this chapter because if you follow the advice I give here, I can virtually guarantee that your blood pressure and cholesterol will automatically fall. Such risk factors as low antioxidant status or high homocysteine are more telling, but the American public hasn't heard about them because they don't sell drugs. Selling drugs to lower high blood pressure and cholesterol is a billion-dollar industry; yet the evidence that these drugs actually lower your chances of dying from heart disease is extremely skimpy.

A major study published in the *Journal of the American Medical Association* proves my point. This huge trial began in 1958 and included more than twelve thousand men in seven different countries, including the United States, Japan, and five European countries. Total cholesterol was measured in men forty through fifty-nine years of age and followed up at five- to ten-year intervals. Blood pressure, diet, deaths from heart disease, and a variety of other lifestyle factors, such as cigarette smoking, were also tracked.

Statistically, there was a weak relationship between high cholesterol levels and heart disease—but a far stronger relationship between diet and heart disease. From country to country, the rate of death from heart disease varied, and cholesterol levels varied, but the variation in death rate was not at all proportional to cholesterol levels. In other words, those with the highest cholesterol levels did not necessarily have the highest rates of heart disease. For example, in Japan, southern Europe, and the Mediterranean, the rate of death from heart disease did not rise significantly, even when blood cholesterol levels went as high as 250 mg/dl. But death rates *did* rise in the United States and northern Europe with cholesterol, especially when cholesterol went over 250 mg/dl.

What was striking was that cultures eating less meat and more fish, fruits, and vegetables and drinking more wine had significantly lower rates of death from heart disease. Furthermore, there was a strong correlation between diets high in polyunsaturated fatty acids (vegetable oils prone to oxidation/rancidity) and a high rate of death from heart disease (more about that later) and correspondingly lower death rates in those cultures that ate more monounsaturated fats, such as olive oil.

Those countries with the highest intake of antioxidants and bioflavonoids had the lowest death rates from heart disease, with Japan having a much higher intake and a much lower rate of death than any of the other countries.

You're probably aware that cigarette smoking is known as the major preventable risk factor for cardiovascular disease. I think that poor nutrition, lack of exercise, too much stress, an overload of environmental toxins, and a long list of prescription drugs should also be known as preventable risk factors. In this chapter, we'll talk about these lesser risk factors, and I'll give you simple, specific, practical methods for lowering your risk of heart disease.

According to the American Heart Association, the estimated cost for cardiovascular disease in 1994 was $128 billion. This includes the cost of physicians and nursing services, hospital and nursing home services, medications, and loss of productivity. But the personal cost of heart disease is the biggest loss of all because the heart is irreplaceable. Let's work together now to ensure your heart health for years to come!

CUT BACK ON THE SWEETS

Kicking the sugar habit is one of the simplest and most effective steps you can take to prevent heart disease. Americans have the highest rate of heart disease in the world, and I believe that our overindulgence in sugar, combined with poor nutrition and lack of exercise, is the single biggest cause of heart disease.

I strongly recommend that you keep your sugar intake low. For some people, that means not eating it at all, because just a little sugar leads to eating a lot of sugar. Others can have something sweet a couple of times a week and leave it at that. If you fall into the first category, you're best off just avoiding sugar altogether unless it comes in a piece of fruit.

A study of rats and life span published in the *Journal of Clinical Nutrition* illustrates just how detrimental sugar is. One group of rats was given access to a diet that was 66 percent sugar, and the other group was fed a normal diet. The rats fed sugar water had a significantly shorter life span.

Here's a partial list of what sugar does to your body:

- Creates drowsiness and mental sluggishness
- Suppresses the immune system
- Generates free radicals
- Contributes to obesity
- Upsets glucose and insulin balance
- Contributes to diabetes
- Causes hypoglycemia with its symptoms of fatigue, irritability, and weakness
- Contributes to candidiasis, an overgrowth of yeast in the body
- Raises triglycerides, a type of blood fat associated with heart disease
- Damages the kidneys

- Causes premature aging
- Upsets the acid balance in the stomach
- Contributes to arthritis
- Increases cholesterol
- Interferes with the utilization of protein
- Makes food allergies worse
- Contributes to gallstones by raising cholesterol content of bile
- Depletes or interferes with the absorption of vitamin C, B-complex vitamins, chromium, copper, calcium, and magnesium—nutrients that are vital to the proper functioning of the heart and circulatory system

Because the average person in America eats 133 pounds of sweeteners a year, and the average American teenager eats 300 pounds of sugar a year, it should come as no surprise that we have an epidemic of heart disease. Some 20 to 25 percent of our daily calories are consumed in sugar.

Why do we love sugar so much? Sugar quickly and temporarily raises our blood sugar, which stimulates the adrenal glands and creates a "high." The body has a built-in sugar regulator, but it isn't designed to handle the intense concentrations of sugar we get when we eat a pastry or drink a soda. To give you an example of just how far from Mother Nature a soft drink is, you would have to eat 30 yards of sugar cane to get the sugar you get in one can of Coca-Cola. This is the equivalent of 9 teaspoons of sugar. As designed by nature, fruit and sugar cane come packed with fiber and nutrients, which you get none of when you eat the refined version.

You're probably familiar with that rush of energy or sense of well-being after you eat sugar. But within half an hour after eating sugar, your blood sugar plummets. This signals the brain to turn on the adrenal glands, which try to get the blood sugar back up, but in the process, adrenaline is released, too. Adrenaline is the substance that, when we lived in caves, gave us the fight-or-flight response. It's our way of coping with a sudden fright or stress. Our heart beats faster, our blood pressure rises, our muscles prepare for action, and our blood leaves our digestive system for other more survival-oriented parts of our body. When this happens regularly, the adrenal glands become exhausted.

As our body works extra hard to pump its heavy sugar load out of the blood, it will overreact and pump too much out, and blood sugar often ends up below what it was before we ate the sugar. This plunge, along with the adrenaline surge, can cause fatigue, weakness, shakiness, dizziness, "spaciness," headaches, and irritability. So we reach for more sugar to get our blood sugar back up, and pretty soon we're looking for our next sugar fix every hour or so. Meanwhile, the precipitous rise and fall of our blood sugar has a chain reaction all over the body, causing imbalances ranging from too much acid in the stomach to too much cholesterol in the bile, not to mention the depletion of essential vitamins and minerals.

Sugar is hard to get away from in our culture. I know many mothers who have very good intentions about not letting their kids get hooked on sugar but who give up because it's so difficult to keep it out of their diet. Children get sugar from day care on through kindergarten and grade school; they get it when they go over to play at another child's house, at birthday parties, and in many types of processed food. Pretty soon the clamoring for sugary foods is constant, and most parents just get worn down. Sugar in and of itself is not a bad food. But in the amounts we give to our children and ourselves, it is destructive.

The best way to kick sugar out of your life is to start reading labels. Many low-fat foods substitute a lot of sugar or salt. Be aware. Sugar goes under lots of names, but it's all still sugar. "Ose" at the end of a word stands for sugar. There's sucrose (common table sugar), dextrose, and fructose (fruit sugar). Watch out for highly refined fructose, or high-fructose corn syrup, which is used in cola drinks and many of the so-called natural soft drinks, such as Snapple. There's nothing natural about them because they're so concentrated. Brown sugar is also not any healthier for you, contrary to popular opinion. It's just white sugar with molasses coloring. If you give up processed foods, which I'll talk about later, it will be much easier to avoid sugar. Sorbitol is a close relative of the sugars and occurs naturally in fruits and berries. It is used in "dietetic" candy and gum because it is slowly absorbed and doesn't cause bacteria to grow on teeth.

Another hidden source of sugar is alcohol. Most alcohol contains sugar, and many people who drink too much are also sugarholics. If you want to kick the sugar habit, you would be wise to give up alcohol, at least for a month or so, to get your body out of the sugar rut. If and when you decide to drink alcohol again, be alert to whether your sugar cravings return.

There are studies showing that sugar does less harm when you get plenty of exercise. Sugar calories are burned off quickly when you exercise, so if you do have a sweet, be sure to burn it off.

If you have a sweet tooth, have some fruit. Grapes are especially sweet. Apples and pears make good afternoon snacks. Although the sugars in fruit are still sugar, they aren't absorbed as quickly as refined white sugar, and unlike white sugar, which has no nutritional value, a piece of fruit has vitamins, minerals, and fiber. (If you have a craving for chocolate, you may be deficient in magnesium. Try munching on some figs or almonds.) When you get an afternoon or evening craving for fat, try a handful of unsalted nuts such as almonds or cashews. But don't overdo it. Nuts are packed with calories!

CUT BACK ON THE FATS

The promotion of margarine and partially hydrogenated vegetable oils as "heart-healthy" oils is one of the biggest lies ever foisted on the American public. I believe that our consumption of these "fake fats," along with sugar, is one of the major reasons America has the highest rate of heart disease in the world.

Contrary to the doctrines of popular diet fads, fat is not inherently bad for you. However, all fat is bad for you in excess. Some fat is essential to good health. Fats aren't there just to add to your waistline; they are an essential part of the makeup of every cell in the body and participate in nearly every bodily function. A balanced diet will include all the types of fats found in nature in varying amounts and will avoid the refined and synthetic fats.

The most important key concerning fats is to keep your fat calories low: no more than 25 percent of your total daily calories (I keep mine around 20 percent). For most Americans, sticking to this rule means cutting fat intake by half. I don't want you to deprive yourself, but I do want you to become aware of the fats in your diet and gradually work to reduce the amount and replace the unhealthy fats with healthy fats.

For example, the amount of fat that the average adult would want to eat in a day would be 30–40 g. (Growing children can eat up to 30 percent of their calories in fat.) A tablespoon of butter contains 12 g of fat. An ounce of sharp cheddar cheese contains 9 g. A 3½-ounce portion of sirloin steak contains 13 g of fat. If you don't have a sense of how much fat your diet contains, buy one of the many books that lists the fat content of nearly every type of food available in North America. Once you have a sense of how much fat you're eating every day, put the book on the shelf and focus on changing how you eat.

Busting the American Fat Myths

It may surprise you when I tell you that saturated fat is not bad for you. It is *too much* saturated fat that is bad for you. You only need small quantities of saturated fat in your diet to be healthy.

Saturated fat is found in the highest concentrations in red meat, butter, coconut oil, and other tropical oils. They are also found in small concentrations (6 to 20 percent) in all oils. Saturated fats are easy to digest, and we burn them up as energy quickly and efficiently. If you exercise a lot, you can afford to eat more saturated fats.

The total amount of saturated fat in your diet can range from as low as 2 percent of your total calories up to about 10 percent, or half your total fat intake.

While it is true that an excess of saturated fat can contribute to heart disease, let's not go overboard in trying to eliminate saturated fat from our diets. The studies cited to back up the prevailing belief that saturated fat is bad for you are very faulty. Those studies done with tropical oil consumption (coconut oil, palm oil) were done with refined oils. Those populations around the world that consume saturated tropical oils are eating unrefined oils in relatively small amounts, and they are quite healthy and free of heart disease.

Another error in these studies is not comparing *total* fat intake to the amount of saturated fat eaten. In other words, no study has been done that I'm aware of on people whose total fat intake is only 20 percent but who eat a high percentage of that 20 percent in saturated fat. Other factors not taken into account in the saturated fat studies are the amount of exercise; amount of refined sugars and flours in the diet; amount of fiber, fresh fruits, and vegetables in the diet; amount of *trans*-fatty acids in the diet; and stress levels. All of these factors weigh heavily in heart disease. My advice on saturated fat is to go ahead and include some in your diet; just don't overdo it.

EAT HEALTHY FATS AND OILS

Now that we've busted some of America's fat myths, let's take a look at how the various oils and fats fare on the heart-healthy scale. Most of our information about how fats and oils react in the body is based on population studies rather than direct biochemical knowledge. In other words, we know that populations eating lots of olive oil have healthier hearts, but we're not sure exactly why. Although we know a lot about the molecular structure of fats and oils, we know surprisingly little about what they do once they're in the body. One thing we do know for sure is that rancid fats and oils are unhealthy.

Olive oil is a monounsaturated fat, which tends to be stable (it doesn't go rancid easily). Many studies have shown that populations consuming high amounts of olive oil tend to have much lower rates of heart disease. Monounsaturated oils are also found in canola oil, peanuts, almonds, pistachios, pecans, hazelnuts, cashews, macadamia nuts, and avocados.

Although peanut oil is fairly stable, peanuts are highly susceptible to a type of fungus containing aflatoxins, which are poisonous, and peanut crops tend to be heavily sprayed with pesticides and fungicides. I don't recommend peanut oil unless it's organic and from a highly reputable source.

Olive and canola oils are the most stable of the monounsaturated oils—and the healthiest. If you buy canola oil not preserved with vitamin E, open a 400 IU capsule of vitamin E and put the contents in the bottle.

Olive oil is the most stable of the monounsaturated oils, and a high consumption of it has been shown to actually lower heart disease. It's very important to remember, however, that the Italians and Greeks consuming this oil at such a high rate are eating *unrefined* olive oil. Refined olive oil will not have the same benefits, because most of the nutrients are taken out of it, including and especially vitamin E. Therefore, buy unrefined virgin olive oil and—if you can get it—organic. In fact, all of the oils you buy should be unrefined. The refining process uses toxic solvents and takes all the goodness out of the oil.

With the exception of canola oil, which is partially refined, I recommend that as a general rule you avoid all unsaturated, polyunsaturated, hydrogenated, and partially hydrogenated oils. This means that for the most part, you need to avoid vegetable oils unless you can find them unrefined and very fresh or preserved with vitamin E and in a lightproof container.

Vegetable oils, also called polyunsaturated and superpolyunsaturated oils, have caused most of the confusion about oils. Unrefined, very freshly pressed vegetable oils are a wonderful food, and our ancestors often had them delivered weekly from the town oil vendor. They were delivered weekly, along with milk and other products that spoil, because, being unsaturated, these oils are very unstable and thus go rancid very easily, especially when exposed to light and air. Rancid oils create chain reactions of oxidation in the body, setting loose free radicals that do damage to cells, causing disease and aging. To avoid rancidity these days, manufacturers heavily refine vegetable oils, which strips away their nutrients and adds the residues of toxic chemical solvents.

The most common manufacturing method for preventing rancidity is hydrogenation. This process adds hydrogen to unsaturated oils, making them more saturated and thus more stable. You might think that this is good, because it prevents rancidity, but these human-made semisaturated fats are not found in nature, so your body doesn't know what to do with them. Total hydrogenation creates a solid fat such as margarine or shortening. These so-called *trans*-fatty acids have been heavily implicated in heart disease. I believe that they may also be responsible for many of our chronic diseases. Please stay away from them!

I realize that highly unstable oils such as flax oil are very popular right now, but I suggest using them in moderation, and only if you believe that you are deficient in essential fatty acids (EFAs), because these oils are so susceptible to rancidity.

Use your daily allotment of fat calories wisely by consuming nutrient-rich, unprocessed, and unrefined fats and oils as we find them in nature. Our bodies need only tiny amounts of EFAs, so if you eat plenty of fresh, unprocessed fruits and vegetables, you will get all your body needs.

Fish oil contains omega-3 fatty acids, unsaturated oils that seem to help prevent heart disease. The body can also make the omega-3s from alpha-linolenic acid (an essential fatty acid found in flax oil and in smaller amounts in canola oil, pumpkin seeds, soybeans, walnuts, and dark green vegetables).

Omega-3 fatty acids reduce blood clotting without the risk of too much bleeding or hemorrhaging. They also lower blood pressure, improve blood flow, and over time can aid in the process of removing cholesterol from the blood and fatty deposits from the arteries. The omega-3s are also a precursor to prostaglandins, important hormonelike substances that regulate many body functions.

Good fish sources of omega-3s include salmon, herring, mackerel, tuna, sardines, and wild trout. Omega-3s are also found in spirulina, an alga grown in fresh water. If you take fish oil supplements, be sure that they come from deep, northern waters, are unrefined, and have been preserved in some way to prevent rancidity.

Omega-3s used to be found in beef, back in the days when cattle grazed on native grasses and plants instead of being stuffed with corn and other fattening grains and estrogen in feed lots. This may be one reason our ancestors could eat plenty of meat in their diet and not suffer from heart disease. (Unprocessed foods, fiber, and exercise no doubt made a difference, too!) It is becoming increasingly common to find range-fed beef in health food stores and even some supermarkets. Ask around for it.

EAT MORE FRESH, WHOLE FOODS AND FEWER PROCESSED FOODS

You are what you eat, but if you eat a lot of refined foods, you won't be a more refined person—you will be a drastically less healthy person! Our national health began a dramatic decline when refined and processed foods were introduced. The rise of chronic degenera-tive diseases, such as heart disease and diabetes, corresponds with the rise in consumption of foods that have all the nutrients stripped out of them and harmful preservatives and additives put back in. If you're eating lots of canned, packaged, preserved, and frozen foods, gradually begin switching to whole foods. As a bonus, when you fill up on fresh vegetables and fruits, you are likely to eat fewer fats and sweets. Fresh foods are also easier on your wallet. Processed and packaged foods cost more while providing you with less nutrition.

Foods packaged by nature come complete with all the nutrients you need. When I talk about whole foods, I mean essentially as nature made them. You get enzymes, vitamins, minerals, amino acids, and hundreds of other nutritional substances you need for a healthy, energetic body capable of handling stress and fighting off disease.

Whole Foods Are Your Ticket to a Healthy Heart

People who eat plenty of fresh vegetables and fruits have a lower cancer risk as well as less heart disease and a lower risk of diabetes. Instead of buying the canned and frozen varieties of vegetables and fruits, head for the produce section. Treat yourself and your family to daily salads, lightly steamed vegetables seasoned with olive oil and lemon, and a delicious dessert of fresh fruit. Not only will you live longer; you'll feel better along the way.

Grains such as wheat, corn, millet, barley, oats, quinoa, amaranth, and rice are not only delicious; they contain a wonderful potpourri of nutrients as well as fiber. Get reacquainted with whole grains. Try oatmeal or a whole-grain cereal or bread for breakfast. For lunch, have a salad on a bed of brown rice or millet. Add barley to soups and stews, and try some corn tortillas with your vegetables. Add whole grains, which are complex carbohydrates, to your diet gradually. If you switch suddenly, your digestive system may protest with gas and bloating.

Fiber Is a Heart Protector

When you eat whole foods, you get lots of fiber. Fiber is a plant substance that is not digested. You've probably heard a lot about how good fiber is for you. Well, it's true. The American Cancer Institute recommends 25–30 g of fiber a day, and yet most people only get half of that. Try to get 30 g (approximately 1 ounce) of fiber every day, and here's why. Fiber speeds up the movement of food through the intestinal tract. The faster the food moves through, the less time there is for your body to absorb fats. Fiber also acts like a whisk broom that sweeps the small intestine clean, keeping it free of infection, and in the large intestine it absorbs the toxins being removed from the body.

The good news is that increasing your fiber is a piece of cake (so to speak). If you're eating whole foods and plenty of fresh vegetables, it's easy to get your fiber every day. If you're over the age of fifty and need a little help, you can add anywhere from 1 teaspoon to 1 tablespoon of psyllium seed or psyllium husk (pronounced "silly-um") to your diet daily. You know this fiber as Metamucil, but unfortunately, Metamucil has a lot of sugar or artificial sweeteners. Pure psyllium is better for you and it's cheaper. You can buy psyllium in health food stores in bulk 1-pound or 2-pound containers.

Psyllium is easy to use. Just stir it into juice or water and drink immediately. Then drink a glass of water immediately afterward. (You can count these toward your six to eight glasses of water per day.) Be sure to drink plenty of water. Start with a teaspoon of psyllium, and if necessary work your way up gradually to a tablespoon.

If you have a bowel disorder, check with a physician first before using psyllium or increasing the fiber in your diet. It's important to add fiber to your diet gradually if you're not used to it, or you could experience gas and bloating.

There's Good Chemistry in Fresh, Whole Foods

Fruits and vegetables are excellent sources of antioxidants, which are your number one defense against the damage done to your blood vessels by free radicals. Cruciferous vegetables such as broccoli, cauliflower, and cabbage contain dithiolthiones, thiocyanates, isothiocyanates, and sulforaphane, which stimulate the production of enzymes such as glutathione, which is also an antioxidant. Other substances found in fruits and vegetables, such as polyphenols, folic acid, minerals, and chlorophyll, also work to keep your heart healthy.

In whole grains you get vitamin E, some of the B vitamins, and compounds called phenols, yet another form of antioxidant. Other compounds in grains, including lignins, flavonoids, and phytic acid, also contribute to a healthy heart.

An extensive survey of studies done in nineteen Western European and five non-European countries relating heart disease and lifestyle showed that men were far less likely to die prematurely of heart disease if their intake of vegetables was high. The strongest association showed up in vegetables that contain vitamin E.

USE ALCOHOL IN MODERATION

Caution and moderation are the watchwords for drinking alcohol. Studies show that a low alcohol intake, particularly of red wine, does protect against heart disease when included as part of a healthy diet. However, even just a bit too much alcohol can bump up blood pressure and help create nutritional deficiencies that increase your risk of heart disease.

It is well documented that alcohol can be associated with high blood pressure. Supporting evidence comes from studies like one from Belgium, which looked at lifestyle and blood pressure and found that increased alcohol intake led to higher diastolic and systolic blood pressure readings in 405 men and 3,790 women. Keep alcohol intake down, and you'll help keep the lid on hypertension and therefore heart disease, too.

Alcoholics have a greatly increased risk of cardiovascular disease. Chronic alcoholics frequently suffer a deficiency of magnesium, which may have a causative link with heart disease. This was the finding of research done at the University of California Medical Center. For details on magnesium's importance to heart health, see the section on magnesium (page 149).

But, if used in moderation, a little alcohol may lower your risk. A study published in the *New England Journal of Medicine* investigated alcohol consumption and mortality in over eighty-five thousand women ranging in age from thirty-four to fifty-nine with no prior history of cancer or heart disease. Heavy drinking was associated with increased risk of death from cancer and cirrhosis of the liver. Light to moderate drinkers (1.5–29.9 g of alcohol per day), however, were found to have a slightly lower death rate than nondrinkers. Furthermore, this low to moderate intake was of most benefit to women over fifty, and women with risk factors for heart disease. The message coming from the scientific evidence is that a little alcohol can be beneficial, but even just a little too much is bad for you.

The French are known to suffer less heart disease despite relatively high consumption of animal fats—a phenonenon called "the French paradox." You may have read media hype about wine as a magical heart elixir. In fact, the real story isn't so simple.

The French paradox was investigated in a review of heart disease rates, alcohol consumption, diet, and death rate in twenty-one relatively affluent countries. While the study did find that wine does seem to protect against heart disease, drinking more did not increase protection. Interestingly, the study also found lower rates of heart disease in geographical areas where larger amounts of fruit were consumed, indicating that the health benefits didn't rest with wine alone. It was also found that whatever the protection provided by drinking wine, people in France did not live longer as a result. In fact, the French have one of the highest rates of liver disease in the world.

More light on the subject came from a Harvard School of Public Health study that looked specifically at alcohol in the Mediterranean diet. The study found that the Mediterranean diet typically includes one or two drinks per day and large amounts of fruit, vegetables, and grains. The researchers concluded that this kind of responsible consumption of alcohol does appear to reduce the risk of cardiovascular disease.

Red wine is your best bet for heart disease prevention. Components of red wine can reduce the activity of clotting agents in the blood. This was a conclusion of an animal study reported in the *Medical Tribune*. This could help to explain the protective effect of low alcohol intake. Red wine, white wine, and ethanol all produced a reduction in blood-clotting tendencies in rats. As soon as the doses were stopped,

though, levels in the rats fed on ethanol or white wine shot up dramatically, especially in those given ethanol. Clotting activity stayed low, however, in the rats given red wine. Researchers believe that either tannins or polyphenols could be the compounds in red wine that produce this effect. Whatever the particular chemistry, red wine is the preferred form of alcohol for heart-protective effects.

EAT MORE GARLIC

Garlic is the herb of legend and myth. It is mentioned in the Bible, in Homer's *Odyssey*, and in ancient Chinese texts, and it has been found in the tombs of ancient Egyptians. Now we have dozens of scientific studies to back up most of the claims for garlic's prowess in keeping us healthy.

While garlic may or may not work to ward off vampires, it does a great job at neutralizing three risk factors for heart disease—high blood fats, high blood pressure, and blood clotting.

Some two thousand studies by the world's top researchers have established that garlic may have a real impact on the most serious modern diseases, heart disease included. A University of Western Oregon study of diet in fifteen countries showed that rates of heart disease were lower in those with higher garlic consumption.

Getting Your Cholesterol Down with Garlic

Although it's known that cutting down on excessive amounts of high-cholesterol food can help lower LDL cholesterol levels in the blood, more than 70 percent of cholesterol is made inside the body. Cholesterol is essential for the production of all your steroid hormones, including your sex hormones. Garlic helps to keep the production of cholesterol in healthy balance. It slows down internal cholesterol production as well as cutting the negative effects of too much dietary cholesterol.

Rats whose diets were supplemented with garlic extract for two months had significantly lower blood cholesterol, less fat in their tissues, and less cholesterol and fat in their livers. In another study, rats on a high-cholesterol diet supplemented with garlic had LDL levels nearly identical to rats on a cholesterol-free diet.

One study of a vegetarian community in India found that the members eating liberal amounts of garlic and onions averaged 25 percent lower cholesterol levels and 50 percent lower blood fats than those who didn't eat garlic and onions. Subsequent studies support these findings. One, reported in the *American Journal of Clinical Nutrition*, showed that out of the sixty-two patients in the study, the thirty-one given a placebo showed little change in their cholesterol levels. But heart disease patients given garlic oil daily for ten months enjoyed a steady decrease in LDL levels together with a progressive increase in levels of HDL cholesterol, which is protective against heart disease.

A study at California's Loma Linda University School of Medicine gave thirty-two people with high cholesterol levels aged garlic extract for six months. The study was nearly abandoned when patients given the extract at first saw their blood fat levels rise! However, after the initial rise, LDL levels steadily dropped, with the benefit, too, that HDL levels rose. These findings led the researchers to conclude that garlic inhibits LDL production. The initial rise in blood fat levels also indicated that garlic helps to move stored fats from tissues into the bloodstream, helping them eventually to be eliminated.

It may be that the sulfur compounds in garlic inhibit the activity of a key enzyme that initiates cholesterol synthesis. This kind of chemistry helps garlic keep heart disease at bay.

Garlic Unblocks Arteries

Studies by Dr. Arun Bordia, a cardiologist at Tagore Medical College, in India, have revealed that regular garlic consumption not only helps arteries stay clear but also reduces the degree of artery blockage. The reversal of atherosclerosis has actually been measured in rabbits fed on a diet supplemented with garlic.

Heart disease patients have seen the benefits, too. Dr. Bordia conducted a study of 432 patients over three years. Half ate garlic daily and half ate none. Those not eating garlic saw no real cardiovascular changes. But blood cholesterol and blood pressure dropped by about 10 percent in the garlic eaters, who also experienced less angina. Most dramatic of all, deaths among the garlic eaters dropped by 50 percent in the second year and 66 percent in the third.

Garlic Stops the Clots

Ancient folklore has long seen garlic used as a blood tonic—even for horses! Now science has proved the old remedies true. Researchers have discovered four powerful anticlotting agents in garlic, at least one of which is a more effective anticoagulant than aspirin.

German studies at Saarland University, in Homburg/Saar, have demonstrated how garlic compounds help blood clots dissolve faster and improve blood fluidity. A report from the University of Wisconsin has shown how aged garlic extract supplementation inhibits the production of a blood clot trigger. And fifty medical students in India recently saw their blood-clotting time and clot-dissolving activity improve by about 20 percent after eating three raw garlic cloves a day. Coronary thrombosis is the condition in which a blood clot forms in an artery leading to the heart. It can result in myocardial infarction or heart attack. Eating garlic to help prevent the thrombosis in the first place makes good sense.

Garlic Lowers Blood Pressure

Experts estimate that as many as 20 percent of Americans suffer from hypertension, or high blood pressure. As a major risk factor for cardiovascular disease, it is widely treated with drugs. However, most blood pressure medication causes moderate to severe side effects. These can be avoided by simply including the drugs naturally available in plants like garlic.

Garlic has been a hypertension treatment for centuries in China and Japan. It's also widely used today in Germany. In fact, tests were recently performed on a German over-the-counter garlic preparation. A dose equivalent to two daily garlic cloves reduced blood pressure in patients with mild hypertension. The garlic produced a blood pressure reduction over the three-month study, showing that garlic may even have a cumulative effect in the body.

A number of studies involving animals and humans, conducted over the past seven decades, show that garlic lowers blood pressure. Studies on people with diagnosed hypertension as far afield as China and Bulgaria have shown that garlic in various forms produces a fall in blood pressure.

Animal studies show that garlic relaxes the smooth muscles of blood vessels. Another blood pressure–lowering mechanism was reported in the German scientific journal *Planta Medica*. It seems that a small garlic peptide inhibits the production of a blood pressure–raising hormone. Whatever the mechanisms, science and history both provide strong evidence that garlic lowers blood pressure.

How to Take Garlic

Raw garlic has been shown to be beneficial, but it's also true that eating it can have side effects like nausea, vomiting, and diarrhea, and very large intake can damage red blood cells. Many beneficial garlic compounds are actually produced when it is cut, crushed, or heated. Although these processes cause the loss of allicin, a powerful germ-killing substance, research found that allicin kills beneficial as well as harmful cells indiscriminately. Supplemental garlic oil often contains only a small fraction of garlic because it is mixed with other vegetable oils and contains only the garlic chemicals distilled at high temperatures.

After raw garlic, the most effective form of garlic appears to be aged extract of organic garlic, but they all have some beneficial effects.

EAT MORE SOY

The death rate from heart disease in Japan is roughly half the rate in the United States. There are many studies showing how diet plays a key role behind the statistics on heart disease. In the famous Ni-Hon-San Study, researchers found that men eating a traditional Japanese diet had the lowest rate of heart disease. Men who moved to Honolulu and ate a more Western-style diet had a higher rate of heart disease. But the highest death rate from heart disease fell to the Japanese men in San Francisco consuming a typical American diet.

Studies show that a diet high in harmful fats is a major risk factor for heart disease. Because soy contains "good" fats and tends to be lower in fat than food from animal sources, it's a good source of protein. In addition, researchers have shown how isolated compounds in soy may directly prevent heart disease by altering blood fat levels. Extensive research reveals that soy produces a range of effects that are highly valuable in the control and prevention of heart disease.

Soy Is a Cholesterol Buster

In Italy, the government is so convinced of the value of soy that soy protein is provided free of charge to doctors treating patients with high cholesterol levels. Research shows that Italian men and women thirty-three to forty-four years of age with serum cholesterol levels below 220 mg/dl have five times less risk of developing coronary artery disease than those with levels of 256 mg/dl or over.

It is believed that soy may have antioxidant properties in the body, which would explain why it decreases the production of "bad" oxidized LDL cholesterol. In one interesting study by Japanese researchers from Hirosaki University School of Medicine, soy milk was added to the diet of rabbits. The results found soy to be even more effective at lowering unhealthy cholesterol levels than Probucol, a commercial antioxidant supplement.

A University of Illinois study looked at twenty-six men with elevated cholesterol levels who were put on a low-fat, low-cholesterol diet. Over a four-month period, the men substituted half their normal protein intake with soy products or nonfat dried milk. Soy protein gave the best results, producing significant cholesterol level reductions with just 50 g per day. Results from studies in Milan tell the same success story, showing that even when cholesterol is deliberately added to a diet including soy products, soy continues to cut cholesterol levels.

The studies make it clear that by cutting "bad" cholesterol levels, soy makes a powerful addition to a heart disease prevention diet.

Some studies show that blood glucagon levels rise after soy protein consumption. Glucagon is a hormone released by the pancreas. Researchers speculate that a shift in glucagon levels may alter the activity of an enzyme needed by the body to manufacture cholesterol. This is the way a drug called Mevacor works in lowering cholesterol. Soy may well do the same thing naturally.

Animal studies show that as well as lowering cholesterol levels, soy produces an increase in blood plasma levels of thyroxine, a hormone produced by the thyroid gland. Interestingly, the rise in thyroxine always precedes the drop in cholesterol. Sure enough, people with underactive thyroid glands tend to have high levels of blood cholesterol. This leads researchers to believe that soy somehow stimulates thyroxine production, which in turn lowers blood cholesterol.

Phytoestrogens Block Cholesterol

After menopause, estrogen levels drop in women, and cholesterol levels typically rise, bringing an increased risk of coronary artery disease. Some researchers theorize that estrogen decreases the amount of LDL circulating in the blood by increasing the number of LDL receptors in cells. Soy is high in phytoestrogens, which occupy estrogen receptor sites, producing a weak but effective estrogen response in the body without the cancer-stimulating effects of estrogen. Researchers theorize that soy's estrogenic activity could well be linked to its cholesterol-lowering ability.

Soy Is a Chemical Powerhouse

Genistein is a substance unique to soy that has been shown to inhibit cell growth and migration, particularly in tumors. Scientists speculate that genistein may work in the same way to prevent the growth of cells that form plaque deposits in arteries.

Phytic acid, also found in soy, binds to iron and increases copper absorption in the body. Copper deficiency, in several studies, has been associated with high cholesterol. Researchers suggest, too, that soy binds with bile, which is then excreted in the feces. This promotes the production of more bile salts, a process that uses up cholesterol and so reduces levels in the bloodstream.

Studies show that another chemical, the amino acid lysine, increases LDL levels when added to a soy diet. Lysine and other amino acids are at lower levels in soy than in animal protein. This leads scientists to believe that soy's particular mix of amino acids may help to prevent the formation of plaque. Indeed, it's clear that soy's overall chemical makeup makes it a frontline food in heart disease prevention.

Including Soy in Your Diet

Soy products are made from soybeans processed in various ways, including soaking, fermenting, grinding, sprouting, and frying. You can choose from soy milk, tofu, tempeh, miso, soy flour, and soy sauce, although soy sauce is high in sodium and contains the fewest nutrients. There are many possible ways to include soy in every meal. I like to make shakes with soy protein powder. Always be sure to include soy as part of a complete low-fat, whole-food, vitamin-rich, high-fiber diet.

DRINK PLENTY OF CLEAN WATER

Water is your top heart-healthy drink, in a class by itself. Nothing else comes close to clean water's lack of toxicity, safety, and ability to keep your biochemistry whirring smoothly along. It has no calories, no caffeine, no sugar, no additives or preservatives, and no fat. Some 60 percent of the human body is water, and you need plenty of it every day to stay healthy and flush out toxins. Water is more necessary for sustaining life than food. You can survive more than a month without food, but no more than a few days without water.

I recommend everyone drink six to eight glasses of clean water daily. The amount you drink will depend on your body weight, height, biochemistry, and lifestyle. If you are exercising heavily, pregnant, or nursing, you will need significantly more water. Running a marathon on a hot day can deplete the body of as much as 6 quarts of water. A bicycle racer climbing hills can lose up to 3 quarts an hour.

Dehydration while doing vigorous exercise can cause the heartbeat to accelerate abnormally. Chronic dehydration can increase your risk of heart attack and stroke. A study done in Denmark showed that post-operative stroke patients who became dehydrated had a much greater risk of having a second stroke. Another study done in Italy on older men who had heart attacks showed that over half of them were dehydrated. Dehydration can also cause abnormal heartbeats, constipation, urinary tract infections, kidney stones, immune deficiencies, electrolyte imbalances, and skin problems and most likely contributes to many chronic diseases, including arthritis and heart disease. It's so simple to drink plenty of clean water that nobody should subject themselves to this heart attack risk.

Clean water is one of your body's primary weapons against free-radical damage caused by toxins.

Blood and lymphatic fluid, which carry nutrients into cells and toxins out, are primarily made up of water. Water is essential for good digestion and elimination of toxins through sweat and urine. Because water is a solvent, it helps rid your bloodstream of excess fat, which can help to reduce your blood serum cholesterol level.

Cleaning Up Your Water Act

Drinking plenty of water can do your heart more harm than good if it's not pure and clean. Chlorine and fluoride have been clearly implicated in a range of illnesses, including heart disease. Chlorine changes the way the body metabolizes fats, raising LDL cholesterol and lowering HDL cholesterol, the opposite of what you need to keep your arteries clean and clear. Communities with high levels of fluoride in their tap water have significantly higher rates of death from heart disease.

I recommend that you buy bottled water or, even better, use a filtration system. You can purchase an inexpensive water filter or a complete household unit, depending on your needs and budget. The least expensive route is a pitcher with a filter attached. All you do is pour the water through. Even better, of course, would be a more sophisticated filtration system in your home that would eliminate heavy metals, chlorine, benzene, and other carcinogens. Prices start around $200, and you can easily install sink-top units yourself.

Water filtration companies can also install water filtration units in your home. Many companies have units large enough to serve a whole house, apartment, or condominium as well as other units small enough to fit under or even above the kitchen sink. Shop around for the best price. Ask for an analysis of what remains in your water after it has been filtered.

There are currently three types of water filtration systems that eliminate most pollutants from your water. One combines reverse osmosis with carbon filters. Another uses a zinc/copper and charcoal filter. And the third uses a ceramic filter. Check your local telephone book under "Water Filtration" to find companies that sell these systems.

These systems enable you to filter your tap water for pennies a gallon. It tastes great, which makes it easy for you to drink the six to eight glasses I recommend. If you like to drink cold water, store some in the refrigerator. That way you'll always have available a cold, delicious, thirst-quenching beverage with no calories.

PASS ON THE SALT

Sodium, or salt, is one of our most important minerals. We're not healthy without it. Sodium is a metallic element that becomes part of our body chemistry when it combines with other elements, such as chloride. Table salt is sodium chloride, or NaCl.

Here is a list of salt's most important functions in the body:

- It aids in keeping calcium and other minerals soluble in the blood.
- It helps regulate muscle contractions.
- It plays a part in nerve stimulation.
- It plays an important role in maintaining fluid balance in the cells.
- It is necessary for the production of hydrochloric acid in the stomach.
- It helps regulate fluid balance when the temperature rises.

Since the average American consumes about 15 pounds of sodium each year—this amounts to a daily intake of about sixty times what is required by the body—we hardly need to worry about getting enough. Our need for salt will vary according to our weight, our diet, the climate we're in, the amount of exercise we get, and our individual biochemistry, but on average we need no more than 500–1,000 mg daily. Most Americans get five or six times this amount every day. This excess can lead to high blood pressure, migraine headaches, abnormal fluid retention or dehydration, and potassium loss. Much of this excess salt comes from eating processed foods, which are loaded with salt and monosodium glutamate (MSG), another form of sodium (here's another reason to eat whole foods).

Eating heavily salted foods is an acquired taste and can be changed. You'll crave salt after exercising and sweating, but under normal circumstances, you can easily break a salt habit. If you start eating whole foods, you'll find that they are so much tastier that you won't need as much salt. Using herbs and spices to make food taste interesting is fun and makes meals creative.

When you do buy processed foods, try to keep the sodium content (listed on all labels) to under 500 mg per serving (even that's really too high). And beware: Products that are low in sodium are often high in fat or sugar. Your total sodium intake should be no more than 3,000 mg per day.

Places Where Salt Is Hidden

- Antacids
- Cough syrups
- Beer
- Baking soda and baking powder
- Laxatives (check the label)
- Home water softeners
- Cured meats, such as ham, bologna, and hot dogs
- Diet sodas
- Club soda
- Condiments, such as pickles, ketchup, and mustard
- Soy sauce
- Preservatives, such as sodium benzoate and sodium propionate

---

About half of all people with hypertension have excessive sodium. The simplest way to treat this problem is to cut down on salt intake. Some of the drugs that doctors prescribe to lower blood pressure are diuretics that cause the body to lose salt, but these have many side effects. It's much healthier to first try lowering blood pressure naturally with diet, exercise, and supplements.

KEEP YOUR FIBRINOGEN LOW

You may not have heard a lot about fibrinogen as a risk factor for heart disease, but its presence is a key factor. Fibrinogen is a protein substance found in blood that plays an important role in blood clotting. In effect, it makes the blood sticky, or gummy, but too much makes the blood too sticky.

Fibrinogen is an important substance in the body, being the precursor of fibrin, a nondissolving protein that plays a major role in the ability of blood to clot. As with so many substances in our body, having enough fibrinogen is essential to good health, but too much is not healthy.

In nearly every study done on heart disease, high levels of fibrinogen in the blood were found to be directly related to coronary artery disease, probably by interfering with blood flow. Excess fibrinogen is also related to atrial fibrillation, strokes, intermittent claudication (pain in the legs when walking), and high blood pressure. Reducing fibrinogen levels may be your single best protection against having a stroke.

All of the factors that contribute to high fibrinogen, and all the solutions for lowering it, are covered in other chapters in more detail. In other words, most of the factors that raise or lower fibrinogen are the same ones that raise or lower other risk factors for heart disease.

Although researchers don't yet know exactly how fibrinogen works, we do have a pretty good idea of what makes it go up. Women tend to have higher fibrinogen levels, probably because they have more estrogen, which raises it.

What Raises Fibrinogen Levels

Psychological and mental stress can increase fibrinogen levels. High blood sugar and very high LDL cholesterol levels will also raise fibrinogen levels.

Estrogen, which is found in birth control pills and hormone replacement therapy, raises fibrinogen levels, which makes it ironic that the pharmaceutical industry is making claims that estrogen prevents heart disease. It may slightly lower your risk of dying from a heart attack, but it raises your risk of dying from a stroke and from cancer. (More about that later in the section on hormone replacement therapy, page 156.)

In addition, smoking has a direct effect on raising fibrinogen levels, and obesity significantly raises fibrinogen levels.

What Lowers Fibrinogen Levels?

Exercise is the single biggest factor in lowering fibrinogen levels. But consider that a glass of wine with dinner may also slightly lower fibrinogen levels, as might fish oil supplementation. What's more, eating plenty of garlic lowers fibrinogen, as do olive oil, vitamin E, and a vegetarian diet.

A double-blind placebo study of fibrinogen levels in women found that those whose diet was supplemented with fish oil or olive oil had significantly lower levels of fibrinogen, while those on a placebo did not achieve this change. Population studies suggest that the risk of having a stroke is two to four times higher in people with high fibrinogen levels.

KEEP YOUR HOMOCYSTEINE LOW WITH B VITAMINS

In the past few years, it has been scientifically documented that high levels of homocysteine, a by-product of metabolism of the amino acid methionine, is an important risk factor in heart disease and strokes associated with narrowed blood vessels. In fact, I believe that high homocysteine levels will turn out to be a much more accurate marker of heart disease risk than cholesterol or blood pressure.

Researchers currently believe that excess homocysteine damages blood vessels, so it may turn out to be a primary cause of heart disease and not just an indicator. The solution to keeping homocysteine levels low is straightforward for most people. To be neutralized in the body, homocysteine needs B vitamins and hydrochloric acid. A deficiency of any of these can raise homocysteine levels, producing hyperhomocysteinemia, a name I predict you'll be hearing a lot in the next decade or so.

Let's hope it won't be ten or twenty years before mainstream medicine begins admitting that high homocysteine levels are an important risk factor for heart disease. But my guess is that most people will never hear about it because the treatment is so simple and inexpensive. No pharmaceutical company will make excessive profits from this natural treatment.

The Hidden Risk Factor

More than twenty studies involving over two thousand patients have shown that homocysteine levels are significantly higher in people who have coronary artery disease and strokes. In fact, some researchers speculate that high levels of homocysteine may account for the 30 to 40 percent of people who have heart disease without exhibiting any of the other known risk factors such as high cholesterol, high blood pressure, and obesity.

Homocysteine is an amino acid meant to exist only temporarily in the body as a by-product of methionine (another amino acid) metabolism. In a healthy body, it's quickly transformed into harmless substances. If you have a deficiency of certain B vitamins or a genetic predisposition that interferes with the metabolism of homocysteine, the levels of it in your blood will rise, and so will your risk of heart disease and stroke. According to a study from Tufts University School of Medicine, in Boston, if your homocysteine levels are just 20 percent above normal, your risk of cardiovascular disease is significantly increased. If your doctor wants to measure your homocysteine levels, a normal homocysteine level is about 12 μmol/L, and cardiovascular risk increases at about 14–16 μmol/L.

Scientists know that homocysteine damages arteries, but they haven't been able to precisely pin down how. The best evidence suggests that it causes certain kinds of arterial cells called endothelial cells to fall apart. This is the type of damage that attracts cholesterol to the artery walls in an attempt to patch things up. But the "bad" cholesterol accumulates and eventually clogs up the arteries. Antioxidants will help significantly in reducing the amount of "bad" cholesterol in the blood, but if homocysteine levels remain high, the damage to arterial walls will continue.

A large Canadian study compared homocysteine levels in 584 healthy people and 150 people with coronary artery disease. Their levels of vitamin B_{12}, B_6, pyridoxal phosphate (a form of vitamin B_6), and folic acid were also evaluated. The results clearly showed that the higher the homocysteine, the lower the levels of folic acid, B_{12}, and pyridoxal phosphate. Those with low levels of these B vitamins and high homocysteine had a higher risk of heart disease.

How to Reduce Homocysteine Levels

Some drugs can cause high homocysteine levels, particularly if they interfere with folic acid. These include methotrexate, an immunosuppressive drug given to cancer, rheumatoid arthritis, and psoriasis patients; the anticonvulsant drugs phenytoin (Dilantin) and carbamazepine (Tegretol, Epitol); and the bile acid sequestrants for lowering cholesterol levels—cholestipol (Colestid) and cholestyramine (Questran). It's ironic that these cholesterol-lowering drugs, given to reduce heart disease, may actually cause it by raising homocysteine levels.

Other research has shown that homocysteine levels rise when daily folic acid intake is 200 mcg per day or less. This is a typical example of how inadequate the official RDA (recommended dietary allowance) amounts are, because the current RDA for folate is 200 mcg.

Fortunately, for nearly everyone, homocysteine can be easily and inexpensively lowered by taking some B vitamins. If you're taking a daily multivitamin that includes 400 mcg of folic acid, 50 mg of vitamin B_6, and 1,000 mcg of vitamin B_{12}, you should be covered. If your homocysteine levels are high, you should be getting an additional 200 mg of vitamin B_6 (pyridoxine) and 1–4 mg of folic acid daily until your homocysteine levels are back to normal.

Because a deficiency of vitamin B_{12} can also indirectly raise homocysteine levels, and because a high intake of folic acid can mask a vitamin B_{12} deficiency, I suggest that you also make sure that your intake of vitamin B_{12} is at least 1,000 mcg per day. Vitamin B_{12}

is best taken sublingually (under the tongue), in a nasal gel or spray, or as an injection.

If you're having trouble with digestion, you may want to take a liquid B complex that's easier for your body to absorb.

Adding betaine to your supplements, in the form of betaine hydrochloride, can also aid in lowering homocysteine levels when combined with the B vitamins. Any brand of betaine hydrochloride will be fine. Check your health food store and follow the directions on the label.

MAGNESIUM—YOUR MOST IMPORTANT HEART MINERAL

Magnesium is a mineral found in our cells and bones, and it is vital to nearly every major biological process in the body. It helps maintain fluid and electrical balance in our cells and is involved with sending messages through the nerves, relaxing smooth muscles, and maintaining the integrity of our blood vessels. Magnesium also regulates how we absorb and use calcium and is critical to more than three hundred enzyme reactions involved in regulating how the body uses nutrients and other substances such as hormones. For example, both vitamin B_6 and vitamin E need magnesium in order to work properly. This important mineral also plays a role in breaking down and absorbing proteins.

A deficiency of magnesium can result in a calcium deficiency, especially in the bones. When the calcium is directed away from the bones and into the soft tissue because of a magnesium deficiency, it can cause arthritis symptoms.

A combination of magnesium and vitamin B_6 (pyridoxine) has been shown to reduce kidney stones. (The dose used in the study was 300 mg magnesium and 30 mg vitamin B_6.) Magnesium is also helpful in preventing preeclampsia and eclampsia (toxemia of pregnancy that can include headaches, high blood pressure, nausea, and water retention), and some studies even indicate that it can help prevent preterm birth. In some women, magnesium supplementation can help reduce the symptoms of PMS. A magnesium deficiency has also been implicated in migraines. In some studies, up to 80 percent of the people with migraines found relief when they took magnesium supplements. Magnesium has also been found useful in treating asthma and anxiety and can significantly help people with chronic lung disease.

Magnesium and the Healthy Heart

On top of all these other functions, magnesium plays a central role in maintaining a healthy cardiovascular system. In 1978, it was discovered that in areas where magnesium levels in drinking water were low, the rate of death from heart disease was higher.

Because of magnesium's important role in muscle contraction and cell integrity, a deficiency can negatively affect heart function. Several recent studies have shown that when people come into an emergency room with a heart attack, if they are given intravenous magnesium right away, their chances of survival go way up, and if they continue to receive it, their survival rate continues to improve.

A Japanese study published in the *American Journal of Cardiology* found that magnesium deficiency may play a role in coronary artery spasms and in ischemic heart disease, where oxygen is not being delivered to the cells owing to a constriction of the blood vessels. Since magnesium is involved in relaxation of the smooth muscles, it can help with almost any kind of spasm, including those of the heart. I believe that a great deal of angina pain could be relieved simply by bringing magnesium levels up to normal.

A magnesium deficiency can lead to irregular heartbeats (arrhythmias). If you're on digitalis for heart disease, the medication can be toxic if you are deficient in potassium or magnesium.

A Japanese study found that patients with low HDL ("good") cholesterol had low magnesium levels and that when they took magnesium supplements, their HDL levels increased. In addition, animal studies have shown that when magnesium is deficient, the amount of oxidized LDL cholesterol increases, with a corresponding increase in arterial damage.

There have been at least twenty-eight independent studies showing that patients with hypertension (high blood pressure) have a magnesium deficiency. On the average, patients with long-term essential high blood pressure have magnesium levels that are at least 15 percent below normal.

How to Keep Your Magnesium Levels High

A large study by the U.S. Department of Agriculture found that only 25 percent of 37,785 individuals had magnesium intakes at or greater than the recommended daily allowance. In fact, dietary magnesium intake is only a fraction of the RDA, which is only a measure of what you need to avoid being ill, not what you need to be healthy and energetic. Magnesium imbalances are common in hospitalized patients, with magnesium deficiency occurring in 20 to 65 percent of critically ill patients.

Magnesium can be depleted by stress, excessive alcohol, sugar, diabetes, kidney disease, chronic diarrhea, not enough protein in the diet, too much protein in the diet, and thyroid disorders. It's well known that alcoholics are at greater risk for cardiovascular disease and osteoporosis, and this is thought to be caused by the depletion effect that excess alcohol has on magnesium.

Good food sources of magnesium include whole grains (especially oats, brown rice, millet, buckwheat, and wheat), legumes (lentils, split peas, and beans), bran, almonds, peanuts, and broccoli. Chocolate contains large amounts of magnesium, and a craving for chocolate may be an indicator of a magnesium deficiency.

Magnesium by itself can cause diarrhea, so be sure to take it in a multivitamin, in combination with calcium, and in the form of magnesium glycinate, magnesium citrate, or magnesium aspartate.

Most Americans are deficient in magnesium, which is why I recommend that you take 300–400 mg daily as a supplement. Vegetarians usually have very good magnesium levels—yet another good reason to eat lots of whole grains, fresh fruits, and vegetables.

If a health professional wants to test your magnesium levels for some reason, be aware that since magnesium is found in the highest quantities inside the cells, a blood serum test is not a good indicator of magnesium levels. Have your red blood cell magnesium measured instead.

KEEP YOUR ANTIOXIDANT STATUS HIGH

Antioxidants come in many forms, from teas and herbal tinctures to foods and vitamins. Their marvelous power gives a shielding, protective effect against heart disease. You will learn more about the best-known antioxidants, vitamins C and E, a little later in this chapter, where we discuss their individual roles against heart disease. But in this section, I want to tell you about some other important antioxidants—and how all antioxidants protect you against heart disease.

Antioxidants score very high as health-promoting factors in population studies reviewing diet, cholesterol levels, and rates of heart disease. For example, the *European Journal of Clinical Nutrition* reported that some Europeans consume more saturated fat than Americans, yet suffer less heart disease. Part of the key is now thought to be the high level of antioxidants in their diet, mainly from plentiful fruits and vegetables. (Although red wine also provides antioxidants, its benefits have been shown only to apply with moderate intake.)

Japan has the second lowest rate of heart disease in the world for women and the lowest rate for men. The Japanese diet, as well as being high in vegetables and fiber and low in fat, is specifically high in antioxidant-rich foods such as soy and green tea. Where high levels of antioxidants are consumed, rates of heart disease are lower.

The Natural Power of Antioxidants

When a squirt of lemon juice helps food stay fresh, it is working as an antioxidant, protecting against the harmful effects of oxygen. Oxygen harmful? Well, we've all seen rust and tasted rancid oil. Although essential for life, oxygen can also work against it. Unstable oxygen molecules do the damage when their basic paired units, electrons, lose their partners. If an oxygen molecule loses an electron, it stabilizes itself by grabbing another from any body substance or tissue nearby, causing that molecule in turn to become unstable. Every molecule robbed of an electron becomes destabilized itself, and if antioxidants aren't present, a chain reaction can take place, creating damage to tissues. This process is called oxidation and is what antioxidants prevent. Unstable oxygen molecules are called free radicals.

Antioxidants work by preventing oxidants from forming or by putting the brakes on free-radical chain reactions. They form part of a well-balanced system that also repairs oxidation damage and neutralizes toxins.

Oxidants are a natural result of the production of energy in our tissues, and they do serve many useful purposes in the body. However, a healthy body is designed to keep free radicals in check or directed only where they are useful, such as attacking invading bacteria. Out-of-control oxidation is a causative factor in much illness, including heart disease and strokes. In today's polluted world, our bodies have to cope with far higher levels of free radicals than ever before. Free-radical culprits include smog, cigarette smoke, pesticides, and food additives. The average American doesn't eat nearly enough antioxidant-rich fresh fruits and vegetables to counteract these environmental toxins. Our bodies are in double oxidant jeopardy, which makes taking antioxidant supplements an important part of preventing heart disease.

Antioxidants and the Cholesterol Connection

Cholesterol is essential for the formation of many important substances in the body, including steroid hormones. High levels of "good" HDL cholesterol actually help to prevent heart disease. It is elevated levels of "bad" LDL cholesterol that are known to contribute to heart disease. The trouble comes from oxidized LDL cholesterol. Destabilized, it damages blood vessel walls, beginning the buildup of artery-blocking plaque.

Unlike drugs, which may lower "bad" cholesterol levels but do not tackle the underlying cause, antioxidants work directly against the oxidation of LDL cholesterol. In fact, low levels of antioxidants in the body could be said to be one of the causes of heart disease, since low antioxidants mean high oxidized LDL cholesterol, which in turn can lead to cardiovascular problems, stroke, and heart attack.

One of the many studies showing that antioxidants reduce LDL cholesterol was performed by the NIH (National Institutes of Health). An antioxidant combination of 30 mg of beta-carotene, 800 IU of vitamin E, and 1,000 mg of vitamin C was taken by nineteen middle-aged people with high LDL levels. After one month, the rate of oxidation was decreased by 26 percent and the onset of oxidation had been delayed significantly.

Beta-Carotene

In 1993, researchers reviewing the diets of 87,000 nurses reported an interesting connection between eating carrots or spinach and the risk of stroke. A 68 percent lower risk of stroke was found in nurses eating five or more servings of carrots a week than in those eating one or less a month. Eating spinach each day produced a 43 percent lower risk than for women consuming less. Both vegetables are rich in beta-carotene.

In the Physicians' Health Study, monitoring a group of 333 doctors with angina pectoris and coronary revascularization, beta-carotene supplementation at 50 mg on alternate days was shown to produce a remarkable 44 percent drop in all major coronary events, including death, and a 49 percent fall in cardiovascular problems, including stroke and death.

A report from the Netherlands described how a study of 674 heart attack patients supported the theory that beta-carotene may protect against heart attacks by protecting polyunsaturated fatty acids from oxidation.

Taking a multivitamin and eating a lot of fresh fruits and vegetables may provide enough beta-carotene. But if there's any doubt, a 10,000–25,000 IU daily supplement is recommended. Beta-carotene is best taken with meals, giving most benefit when it is consumed with fatty foods.

Ginkgo Biloba

Ginkgo biloba extract is made from the tree of the same name. It is particularly rich in antioxidant substances that act synergistically. One of its properties leads to improvement in circulation to the heart. As

might be expected, it also reduces oxidized LDL cholesterol levels and lowers LDL cholesterol generally. In addition, it raises "good" HDL cholesterol and lowers blood fat levels.

Ginkgo biloba takes time to produce its effects and should be taken in repeated doses for a fairly long period of time. Ginkgo biloba extract (GBE) with at least 24 percent ginkgo flavoglycosides is the best form to take. Standardized, semipurified, and concentrated, GBE provides consistent levels of its most active compounds. Take the recommended dosage on the package up to three or four times a day.

Glutathione

Glutathione is one of the most universal and important antioxidants, particularly renowned for its detoxification properties. As a protein made up of three amino acids, cysteine, glycine, and glutamic acid, glutathione is called a tripeptide. It is found in the cells of almost all living organisms and represents the front line of your body's antioxidant defenses. In fact, you could not survive without it.

Glutathione catches free radicals before they start chain reactions. Then it neutralizes them and hands them on to compounds such as vitamin E before starting the cycle again. Glutathione also binds to toxic substances in the liver, aiding in their excretion, and neutralizes free radicals threatening red blood cells. As a partner with selenium, glutathione protects the blood, the heart, and other organs as a coenzyme, changing toxic oxidants into more manageable forms.

Higher cholesterol, higher body weight, and a 24 percent higher rate of illness and death were all linked to low levels of glutathione in one study of elderly people in England.

When you have a good supply of glutathione's three amino acid components, glutathione is constantly renewable, extremely abundant, and highly active in your body. If you have high LDL cholesterol levels or are otherwise at risk of heart disease, it is worth trying to raise your glutathione levels. Of the three amino acids, cysteine is the one you are most liable to run short of, and it can be taken as the supplement NAC (*N*-acetylcysteine). Be sure to follow label recommendations and do not overdose, as the body chemistry in this area is in delicate balance. Foods high in cysteine include wheat germ, red meat, yogurt, onions, and garlic.

Overexposure to drugs that are hard on the liver, such as aspirin and Tylenol, and an overload of rancid oils can deplete glutathione levels. Aging also causes glutathione levels to fall. Keep up your levels of selenium and vitamins C and E to ensure that glutathione works efficiently in the body with these nutrient partners.

Green Tea

Green tea is a polyphenol, an aromatic, organic compound that acts as a potent antioxidant in the body. Like others in this family, it prevents the oxidation of LDL cholesterol, lowers cholesterol, raises "good" HDL levels, and lowers triglyceride levels. It also reduces blood coagulation and prevents the clumping of red blood cells, both good steps for the prevention of heart disease.

Studies in Japan have shown that green tea even outperforms synthetic vitamin E, vitamin C, a synthetic antioxidant called BHT, and glutathione when it comes to the prevention of oxidation in fatty substances.

PCOs

PCOs are procyanidolic oligomers, which are bioflavonoids found in grapeseed, lemon tree bark, peanuts, cranberries, and citrus peels. Known to improve circulation, PCOs strengthen blood vessel walls and prevent the clumping of blood-clotting substances, providing protection against stroke. These properties come on top of PCOs' very strong antioxidant powers that preempt LDL oxidation.

To address high cholesterol with PCOs, 150–300 mg per day is recommended. Otherwise, 50 mg of PCOs daily make a good supplement if you're over fifty. Many studies have shown that PCO extract from grapeseed is one of the most powerful antioxidants known. It also increases the performance of other antioxidants.

The best grapeseed extract is packaged with phytosomes, by a process in which the molecules are combined with a natural component of lecithin. This combination increases the absorption and effectiveness of the PCO extract in your body.

Making Your Diet Antioxidant Rich

Your main food sources of antioxidants are fresh fruits and vegetables. Top scorers are cabbage, cauliflower, and broccoli; spinach and kale and other green leafy vegetables; carrots, sweet potatoes, and other "yellow" vegetables; and garlic and onions.

Remember, some antioxidants such as vitamin C are lost when you boil vegetables. Eat vegetables steamed or raw if you don't want to see your heart protection go down the drain.

VITAMIN E—YOUR MOST IMPORTANT HEART VITAMIN

Vitamin E is your greatest ally and protector when it comes to vitamins and heart health, and yet most people are deficient in vitamin E. In one study, the vitamin E intake of elderly, affluent Americans was less than three-quarters of the RDA.

A World Health Organization (WHO) review of European populations, nutrient levels, and health showed that those with higher levels of vitamin E had a lower rate of coronary artery disease. The same result held, even where saturated fat intakes were high, in non-European and European countries.

Impressive results were shown in two major Harvard University studies of health professionals. A survey of over 39,000 male professionals showed that they enjoyed a 37 percent lower risk of coronary artery disease when they took 100 IU or more of vitamin E daily. The Nurses' Health Study of 87,000 women showed a 40 percent lower risk of heart disease for women on the same dose of vitamin E.

A European population study looked at one hundred apparently healthy men aged forty to forty-nine. Blood levels of vitamin E were found to be the most important risk factor for heart disease, even beyond smoking. Levels of vitamins E and A in the blood were so significant that researchers could use them with 73 percent accuracy to predict which of the men studied would die from a heart attack.

Vitamin E Keeps Blood Vessels Free and Flowing

Vitamin E is the oldest recognized biological antioxidant. Animal and human studies done at the University of Texas Southwestern Medical Center have shown that supplementation with vitamin E reduces the extent of "bad" LDL cholesterol oxidation. Studies by Japanese scientists have also shown that vitamin E reduces levels of oxidized fats in the bloodstream. Vitamin E also works closely with glutathione, an antioxidant enzyme that is particularly important to the layer of cells that line the heart, blood, and lymph vessels. And Swedish researchers working with rabbits concluded that vitamin E supplementation halted and in some cases even reversed arterial damage caused by oxidation.

Several studies show that vitamin E inhibits the release of clotting agents in the bloodstream that cause blood to clump and clot, increasing the risk of stroke. A report in the *American Journal of Clinical Nutrition* on vascular diseases of the legs, which often occurs with heart disease, described how patients treated with vitamin E enjoyed increased blood flow, less painful walking, and far fewer amputations. Another study looked at 1,476 patients with general atherosclerosis who had taken supplemental vitamin E for ten years. The patients' ten-year survival rate was higher than for any patient in similar studies who had not been treated with vitamin E.

There is evidence, too, that vitamin E dissolves clots, helps the heart pump more efficiently, naturally makes arteries widen, and increases the oxygen available in the blood.

How to Get the Vitamin E You Need

Vitamin E is a fat-soluble oil found in many foods, including unrefined vegetable oils, whole grains, butter, organ meats, eggs, a variety of nuts, sunflower seeds, fruit, soybeans, and dark green leafy vegetables.

I recommend that you take vitamin E either mixed as tocopherols or *d*-alpha-tocopherol. I do not recommend the synthetic form of vitamin E, called *dl*-alpha-tocopherol.

Although vitamin E is very safe, even at high doses, 400–800 IU (dry form) daily should be an adequate dose for adults. The dry form is recom-

mended for anyone sensitive to oils or with problems absorbing nutrients. (If you're over the age of sixty-five, you probably fall into the latter category.) Vitamin E works well taken with its partners in the body, the nutrients vitamin C, beta-carotene and other flavonoids, and selenium.

VITAMIN C MAKES EVERYTHING WORK BETTER

It's now well established that vitamin C, which is ascorbic acid, has a preventive and therapeutic effect against infectious diseases like the common cold. It is, in fact, important for a wide range of bodily functions from the production of antistress hormones to the healing of wounds. An increasing number of studies show that vitamin C is also highly valuable as protection against heart disease.

Several population studies single out vitamin C intake as a major factor protecting against heart disease. Over forty years ago, a California study concluded that vitamin C was the most important of twenty-five factors in preventing death—the most usual cause of which was heart disease. Another study of a large population in England found vitamin C to give the greatest protection against ischemic heart disease caused by a narrowing and constriction of the blood vessels.

"C" for Cholesterol Control

Vitamin C is useful against that known heart disease villain, "bad" LDL cholesterol. It's important to remember that most of our cholesterol is made within our bodies, and studies show that high-cholesterol foods do not cause significant changes in blood cholesterol. LDL cholesterol becomes harmful when it is oxidized by free radicals. Vitamin C works directly against internally generated oxidized LDL. As early as 1947, a Russian study showed that vitamin C could bring down high cholesterol levels. Many studies since then have confirmed this result.

One of the ways the body regulates cholesterol is by converting it into bile acids, which are excreted into the intestines. When the body needs more cholesterol, it will reabsorb some of the bile acids and pull out the cholesterol. Two good studies have shown that the rate at which cholesterol is removed from the blood by being converted into bile acids is increased by a high intake of vitamin C. In addition, vitamin C can act as a laxative, speeding up the removal of bile acids from the bowel. This, of course, means less bile acids get converted back into cholesterol.

A German study gave patients with high cholesterol levels 1 g of vitamin C per day for three months. The patients saw their cholesterol levels drop by an average of 10 percent. Another German study looked at patients with extremely high cholesterol levels and found an even greater average drop of 18 percent in cholesterol levels when the patients were given 3 g of vitamin C for just three weeks.

Vitamin C produces little change in people with normal cholesterol levels. One researcher studied 280 men and women with a range of low to high cholesterol levels. Given 300–1,000 mg of vitamin C, average cholesterol levels stayed the same in people with normal cholesterol and decreased by 10 to 20 percent for those with high cholesterol.

Additional evidence of vitamin C's beneficial role in cholesterol regulation comes from recent studies showing that vitamin C not only lowers levels of "bad" LDL cholesterol but also raises "good" HDL levels.

Vitamin C for Cardiovascular Health

Vitamin C is indirectly beneficial to the heart through its partnership with vitamin E. Vitamin E is an antioxidant that helps prevent the oxidation of unsaturated fatty acids and LDL cholesterol. Vitamin C is also an antioxidant but has a special role in restoring "spent" vitamin E.

Thrombosis, or blood clotting, in the coronary arteries is a major cause of heart attacks. The root cause is the body's blood-clotting system going seriously awry. Studies show that a deficiency of vitamin C often lies behind this.

It is known that people with coronary artery disease have lower levels of vitamin C than healthy people. In one study of postsurgical patients, the number of blood clots developed in patients given 1 g of vitamin C daily was significantly lower than in patients who did not receive the supplement. The research shows that the chemistry of vitamin C both boosts clot-dissolving activity and inhibits the clumping of

cells that leads to clots. These actions make it a valuable heart disease preventive.

As well as helping to prevent blood clotting, studies show that a diet high in vitamin C helps keep blood pressure down. Research on elderly people performed at the U.S. Department of Agriculture's Human Nutrition Research Center on Aging showed that taking the amount of vitamin C in four oranges a day kept blood pressure four times lower than did eating the vitamin C in one orange.

Research shows that low levels of vitamin C raise both systolic and diastolic blood pressure readings. It's clear that a diet rich in vitamin C is a simple way to help treat high blood pressure, a condition that plagues over sixty million Americans and is intimately linked to heart attacks and strokes.

How to Boost Your Vitamin C

Statistics show that vitamin C is the most widely taken dietary supplement. It cannot be made in the body and must come from food or supplements. There is evidence that taking flavonoids with vitamin C raises its concentrations in some tissues and helps to trigger some of its effects.

Because some vitamin C is lost through excretion, it's best taken in a dose divided throughout the day. Recommended levels vary, but 500 mg twice daily should be sufficient for adults and children over ten. Illness, stress, smoking, and injury all increase the need for vitamin C. Megadoses of vitamin C can wash out B_{12} and folic acid, so increase your B vitamins if you're taking a lot of vitamin C.

Of course, supplementation is no substitute for a diet naturally rich in vitamin C. Fresh fruits (especially citrus) and vegetables are the best source. Raw is best, as cooking destroys vitamin C. Include vitamin C in a low-fat, low-sugar, high-fiber diet with lots of fish and little meat, and your heart will be well protected.

TWO REMARKABLE HEART STRENGTHENERS: CoQ10 AND HAWTHORN BERRIES

One of the best-kept secrets is the well-proven ability of two remarkable heart strengtheners—coenzyme Q10 (CoQ10) and hawthorn berries.

The Benefits of CoQ10

CoQ10 has been shown to protect and strengthen the heart, to lower blood pressure, to strengthen the immune system, and, as an added bonus, to cure gum disease. It also happens to be extremely safe and nontoxic.

CoQ10 is a vital enzyme, or catalyst, to the production of energy in our cells. Without it, our cells simply won't work. Its chemical name is *ubiquinone*— it is ubiquitous, or everywhere, where there is life. Its levels in the human body are highest in the heart and liver. When we are ill or stressed, and also as we age, our bodies are less able to produce CoQ10.

According to a study done by CoQ10 expert Karl Folkers, published in the *International Journal of Vitamin and Nutrition Research*, patients with a variety of cardiac disorders consistently demonstrate a blood deficiency of CoQ10. A double-blind Japanese study with one hundred patients who had cardiac failure showed that as little as 30 mg per day of CoQ10 for two to four weeks produced a measurable improvement in symptoms. Many older people whose heart function has degenerated and who try CoQ10 report an almost immediate boost in their energy levels.

People who suffer from angina report that with CoQ10 their pain disappears and they can do some exercise. In a double-blind placebo study using CoQ10 and other drugs traditionally used to treat angina, it was found that CoQ10 was far more effective in reducing or eliminating angina pain than any of the other medications. Other studies have shown that people on heart medications can greatly reduce their dosage of medicine if it is combined with CoQ10.

I know you're asking the question, "If this stuff is so good, why isn't it being prescribed for everyone who has heart disease?" Like so many of the heart helpers in this book, CoQ10 is a natural substance, so it can't be patented. Therefore, the drug companies can't have exclusive use of it or charge high prices for it, so they have no interest in selling it, have no reason to promote it, and in fact have every reason to wish it would go away. There are literally volumes of good research done on CoQ10, much of it sponsored by the government.

CoQ10 should come as a powder in a capsule and be a deep yellow color. If it's not, or if it's cut with fillers, find a brand that's pure and the right color. Also, be sure that the product says "coenzyme Q10" or "CoQ10." Variations of it will not be as effective. The purity and quality of CoQ10 do vary, and since it's not a cheap supplement, it pays to get a high-quality brand. Most CoQ10 comes in 30 mg capsules and costs about $16 for one hundred capsules. You can take one 30 mg capsule up to three times a day with meals.

If you want to know more about CoQ10, a good book to read is *The Miracle Nutrient: Coenzyme Q10* by Emile G. Bliznakov, MD, and Gerald L. Hunt (Bantam, 1987).

Hawthorn Berries

Hawthorn berries (*Crataegus oxyacantha*) have been used as a heart tonic for centuries and are widely used in Europe as a heart medicine for angina and for lowering blood pressure. They are rich in bioflavonoids, which help strengthen the blood vessels. Hawthorn is also a vasodilator, which increases the flow of blood and oxygen to the heart, lowers blood pressure, and strengthens the heart muscle.

Hawthorn berries work gradually, and you may not notice a difference for a month or so. You can find hawthorn berries in capsule or tincture form. Because the amounts vary widely, follow directions on the bottle. Some of the tinctures can be very powerful, so it is very important, if you're already on heart medicine, that you work with your physician. However, in and of themselves, hawthorn berries are very nontoxic and safe.

IF YOU NEED HORMONES, TAKE THE NATURAL ONES

That estrogen protects against heart disease has become an accepted "fact" in mainstream medicine, but in reality, there is little evidence to support this claim. The supposed benefits of estrogen are much less established than drug company advertising would have you believe, but the increased risk of cancer and stroke are very well established.

We do know that estrogen can improve lipid profiles slightly (raise HDL cholesterol and lower LDL cholesterol), but it's a big leap to say that it must also protect against death from heart disease, especially considering that estrogen raises fibringen levels, a significant risk factor for heart disease.

The mainstay of the claim that estrogen will prevent heart disease is the famous Harvard Nurses' Study. But the information regarding estrogen in this study is seriously flawed. First of all, two very unequal groups of women were compared. Doctors do not (or should not) prescribe estrogen to women who are obese, diabetic, have kidney or liver disease, are at risk for cancer or stroke, or smoke cigarettes. Therefore, the women who took estrogen were, by elimination, a healthier group to begin with and less likely to have heart disease with or without the hormone replacement therapy. (Other studies also show that women who use hormone replacement therapy are more likely to be better educated and healthier.) To the best of my knowledge, there are no other studies showing that estrogen or hormone replacement therapy of any kind truly reduces the risk of dying from heart disease. Despite the fact that they were healthier to begin with, the women who took estrogen in this study had a much higher risk of stroke than those who did not take it.

The *New England Journal of Medicine* published a study by the highly respected Harvard researcher Dr. Graham Colditz, showing that women who use estrogen for more than a few years have a 46 percent higher risk of breast cancer. Colditz is one of the primary authorities on the link between estrogen and breast cancer, and his results came from more than 121,700 women tracked for twenty-four years in the Harvard Nurses' Study. It is also well established that estrogen causes ovarian cancer.

In addition to an increased risk of stroke, breast cancer, and ovarian cancer, estrogen causes weight gain, bloating, headaches, irritability, depression, tender breasts, fatigue, thinning of scalp hair, foggy thinking, and decreased libido. Why would anyone want to subject themselves to that?

Getting What You Really Need at Menopause

Somehow, mainstream medicine has forgotten about the important role that the hormone progesterone

plays in a woman's hormonal cycles. A woman's level of progesterone actually drops much more dramatically at menopause than estrogen levels do, and this accounts for more of the menopausal symptoms than a drop in estrogen does.

Even competent doctors seem to confuse progesterone with the synthetic progestins found in birth control pills and hormone replacement therapy (Provera, for example), but one is a safe, natural hormone and the other is a dangerous synthetic drug. They are most emphatically not the same.

Progesterone has no known side effects other than some sleepiness at very high doses, but the progestins have a long list of negative side effects. For example, the progestins can cause miscarriage and fetal malformation, but progesterone is essential for a successful pregnancy. This alone should be a major clue to physicians and their patients that these two substances are very different. The progestins also cause bloating, headaches, weight gain, breast tenderness, depression, migraines, asthma, breakthrough bleeding, liver damage, decreased glucose tolerance, excess hair growth, and an increased risk of stroke. Makes you wonder why it's allowed on the market, doesn't it?

All the maladies for which doctors are prescribing estrogen can be prevented and reversed with diet and lifestyle changes and, when necessary, some natural progesterone cream. (Please do not confuse natural progesterone cream, which is often identified on the label as wild yam extract, with another wild yam extract substance called diosgenin. Some manufacturers are claiming that diosgenin becomes progesterone in the body and are selling it as progesterone. Diosgenin is not progesterone, and there is no evidence whatsoever that it becomes progesterone in the body. Diosgenin is used to make natural progesterone in the laboratory but not in the body.)

Progesterone does not raise fibrinogen levels, and high levels of progesterone in the body are actually associated with a reduced risk of breast cancer. It will also raise HDL levels and lower LDL levels as well as or better than estrogen.

It is very well known now that heart disease is one of the most preventable of all chronic diseases with diet and lifestyle changes. Why should a woman increase her risk of breast cancer and stroke and suffer from all the estrogen and progestin side effects when she can accomplish the same heart benefits naturally and increase her quality of life in every way?

Women who keep their weight within reasonable limits, who keep their fat intake low and their vegetable intake high, and who get regular exercise rarely suffer from distressing menopause symptoms. Those who add soy products such as soy milk and tofu to their daily diet are even less likely to complain about menopause symptoms. High soy consumption and low fat consumption are almost certainly the primary reasons that hot flashes and breast cancer are virtually unknown in Japan.

Estrogen's benefits for osteoporosis have also been greatly exaggerated. It will slow bone loss for a few years around the time of menopause, but after that it has no benefit. Women who are at risk for osteoporosis can prevent it with a combination of diet (not too much protein, a minimum of carbonated beverages, and plenty of fresh vegetables), weight-bearing exercise, and some progesterone cream, which has been convincingly shown by Dr. John Lee to stimulate bone growth and reverse osteoporosis.

For a very small percentage of women, diet, exercise, and natural progesterone do not relieve menopause symptoms such as severe hot flashes and vaginal dryness. If you fall into this category, find a doctor who will give you a small amount of natural estrogen, rather than something like Premarin, which is made from pregnant mares' urine. If you decide to use natural progesterone, do so with an experienced health care practitioner, and use a brand known to contain actual progesterone.

GET MOVING AND SHED THE EXTRA POUNDS

Our bodies are designed to move. Movement is essential for health, and exercise is simply a way of making sure your body gets the movement it needs. Scientific research has shown that the internal benefits of exercise include improved circulation, increased oxygen uptake, better lymph circulation and therefore better immune functions, and elimination of toxins. Digestion and absorption improve, and muscles, joints, tendons, and ligaments are all strengthened. Exercise is especially good for the heart, but really, every part of the body benefits.

If you've been a couch potato, once you begin exercising, you'll soon experience many worthwhile "side effects" of exercise. People who exercise regularly find that they have more energy, can relax and unwind more easily, and sleep better. Many say that their mood brightens, stress tolerance increases, and even their sex life improves. Exercise for a healthy heart and you'll gain much more besides—except weight, of course—unless it's muscle weight you're building.

Exercise Lowers Risk Factors

You can show the power of a really good laundry detergent by using it on very dirty clothes. Well, the power of exercise is demonstrated when it improves the health of smokers. This was the case in a study from the University of California. A group of twenty-eight healthy female cigarette smokers (averaging seventeen cigarettes a day for an average of twenty years) was studied. After exercise, it was found that they enjoyed a reduction in risk factors for coronary artery disease and stroke. Levels of harmful agents in the blood came down, and oxygen uptake improved. And they didn't have to become fanatics to get these benefits. Any exercise program over 2 hours per week for longer than six months produced a decreased risk of coronary artery disease.

Further evidence comes from a French study that showed that if physical exercise is sustained, it can reduce fibrinogen in the blood and therefore reduce the risk of having a stroke.

Running 7 to 14 miles a week can increase your levels of HDL cholesterol. This was shown in a study of 2,906 healthy, nonsmoking males by the Veterans Affairs Medical Center. What's more, ratios of "good" HDL to "bad" LDL cholesterol also improved. Don't overdo it, however. No more heart protection advantage seems to come from running further, and the risk of joint injury goes up.

A New Zealand study found that individuals with hypertension who walked briskly for 40 minutes three times a week showed significant reductions in systolic blood pressure. Along similar lines, a Belgian lifestyle research study showed a connection between blood pressure and exercise. As calories were burned up in sports, so blood pressure, and therefore risk of heart disease, went down.

Men who were thinnest at the beginning of a twenty-seven-year study were more than twice as likely to be alive at the end of it. This was the result of a study of 19,297 men by the Harvard School of Public Health. Keep that heart ticking—especially to lose that excess weight!

Get on the Move—Starting Now!

Research shows that most Americans have as much trouble sticking to exercise as they do sticking to a diet. Part of the solution lies in making your life itself a workout that you don't have to think about. Walk the dog. Join your children playing. Walk or bike to work and during your lunch hour. Get busy with chores and kill two birds with one stone. Raking, digging, and weeding are all good aerobic movement. Weather bad? Dusting, mopping, sweeping—add them all to your exercise list. Park a few blocks away. Use the stairs instead of elevators. Even standing instead of sitting to watch TV is helpful. Add a few on-the-spot stretches, too. Get moving!

Make exercise as much a priority as eating or sleeping and make it enjoyable. Plan an exercise schedule and, at least for the first six months, build in support like classes, videos, exercise partners, and weekend recreation.

Walk Your Heart to Health

Simple and easy, one of the best physical workouts is a brisk, daily 30-minute walk. Starting from scratch, three days a week is fine, building up gradually to about 2 miles in a half hour. Remember, always consult your doctor first if you have a medical condition that might make brisk walking hazardous to your health.

Equipment is minimal and inexpensive: a good pair of walking shoes (rather than tennis or running shoes) with energy-absorbing soles to lessen the strain on your ankles, knees, hips, and back, and cotton and Lycra walking socks with reinforced heels and toes, as toes and heels are stressed when you walk quickly.

As you walk, move your arms in time with your pace. You'll find that your whole body perspires a little by the end of your walk. Using weights gives the upper body more of a workout, and, of course, your heart is an upper body muscle. Start with 1-pound hand weights and build up gradually to 4 or 5 pounds each over about a year. Aim at a pace of around 3 or 4 miles per hour, which is a mile every 15 to 20 minutes. An inexpensive pedometer can help you figure out the mileage. As much as possible, gear your walk to a time of day when your energy levels are high, remembering that urban pollution levels are lowest in the morning before rush hour. Get outdoors with local walking or hiking groups or take designated walking routes in your local shopping malls. Find friends to join you in this very simple way to protect your heart.

Move the Eastern Way

Instead of fast, sweaty aerobics, you might prefer to give your heart a workout with the gentler mind-body-spirit approach of the Eastern movement arts of yoga and chi gong (also called chi kung or qi gong). Begin by taking a class. Follow up with books and videotapes if you enjoy them. A number of videos on chi gong, tai chi (a form of chi gong), and yoga are available from the Sounds True Catalog (1-800-333-9185).

"LIFE'S TOO MYSTERIOUS, DON'T TAKE IT SERIOUS"

Stress is a major contributor to heart disease, and the title of this section, which I first saw on a greeting card, sums up a heart-healthy approach to life. I don't mean to suggest that we should shirk personal responsibility, only that we could all benefit from approaching life with a sense of humor, a sense of detached compassion for ourselves and others when we can't change the things we don't like, and a sense of possibility for the wonders that each day can bring us. As any healthy ninety-year-old will tell you, life's true value is found in time spent with loved ones, helping others, laughter, fun, and, for many, a spiritual focus.

How the Heart Responds to Stress

Mental and emotional stress cause the body to react as if it's in danger, increasing heart rate and blood pressure, releasing adrenaline that makes us jittery and tense, increasing muscle tension, and shunting blood away from digestion and other organ functions. Constant stress causes wear and tear that sooner or later will show up as illness: heart disease, stroke, headaches, chronic pain, back problems, indigestion, and psychological disorders such as anxiety and compulsive behavior.

Recent research has given us even more detail on how stress causes heart disease. When blood pressure rises due to stress, the heart responds by narrowing arteries, which can cause them to spasm and increase blood-clotting factors. When stress occurs over a long enough period of time, the heart muscle simply begins to wear out, and if nutritional deficiencies are present, such as low B vitamins, antioxidants, or magnesium, that will accelerate the chances of having a heart attack or stroke.

Some prominent researchers who have studied stress and cholesterol levels believe that stress plays a much greater role than diet in raising cholesterol levels. (Actually, there is very little evidence that high-cholesterol foods raise cholesterol levels in the body, but that's another story.)

The evidence that stress plays a major role in heart disease is so overwhelming that some insurance companies are now paying for their high-risk policyholders to participate in lifestyle programs designed by Dr. Dean Ornish to reverse heart disease. These programs include a low-fat vegetarian diet, participation in a support group, an exercise program, and meditation.

The Relaxation Response

When Dr. Herbert Benson published *The Relaxation Response* more than twenty years ago, it was part of a revolutionary new concept: By de-stressing our lives, we could be healthier, happier people. This espe-cially applies to heart disease. Since then, we've also discovered that having frequent feelings of anger, hostility, powerlessness, or loneliness can also contribute significantly to heart disease.

A number of studies have found that people who feel isolated and alone and without a sense of community are as much as twice as likely as the "averagely" sociable to have a heart attack. Even having a pet can alleviate some of these feelings, but volunteering at a local soup kitchen will help even more.

It's also very helpful to learn a relaxation response, such as a form of meditation or a breathing exercise, that you can use when you feel tension rising. Yoga and chi gong, mentioned earlier, are Eastern disciplines that incorporate a relaxation response into their practice. In fact, many hospitals now routinely teach yoga or chi gong to their heart attack patients. One study showed that people with high blood pressure who participated in support groups, learned a relaxation response, and got some exercise were able to lower their blood pressure significantly enough to reduce their blood pressure medication by 80 percent, and 20 percent of them were able to stop using it altogether.

Try These Nutritional De-stressors

Certain nutritional deficiencies can increase your mental and emotional stress levels. These include the B vitamins, which help regulate brain function, and the minerals calcium and magnesium, which play a part in relaxing muscles. For some people, a sublingual B vitamin is just the ticket to an energy boost that can be calming at the same time. If you know you're going to be under a lot of stress, be sure to increase your intake of these supplements.

If you're under stress, avoid stimulants. Especially avoid drinking too much coffee. More than two or three cups will make you jittery, deplete your adrenal glands, and rob you of needed vitamins and minerals. Also avoid sugar. It can pick up your energy for a short time, but you're likely to feel even lower as little as a half hour later. If you're craving something sweet, try fruit, which contains a lot of sugar but in a form better tolerated by the body. A banana contains potassium, which will calm you down, natural sugars, which will give you a bit of life, and carbohydrates, which will give you long-term energy.

Ginseng tea gives a lift without stressing out the adrenal glands and without a letdown. It actually supports and balances the body. A brisk walk can get your circulatory and lymphatic systems moving, making you more alert.

The bottom line is that it's not healthy to be stressed out all the time, and there are many ways to alleviate and eliminate stress. Start today, and your heart will thank you for the rest of your life.

IS YOUR HEART DRUG DOING MORE HARM THAN GOOD?

As a pharmacist, I'm well versed in just how much damage prescription drugs, and particularly drugs to treat heart disease, can do to people. Over the past few decades, it's become clear that prescription drugs are not the magic bullets we thought they would be. It's true that these drugs have saved many lives, but it's also increasingly true that they are taking a great many lives and ruining even more with debilitating side effects.

One quarter of the elderly population, or 6.6 million people, are taking a drug they should never take. Many people are prescribed a drug, then prescribed another one to counter the side effects of the first, and then a third to counter the side effects of the first two. I call this getting on the drug treadmill. People typically get put on the drug treadmill by their doctor in their sixties, and never get off it. The average senior citizen is taking eight different drugs every day!

According to government figures, some 140,000 people die every year from pharmaceutical drugs, and many more are hospitalized. This is absolutely unnecessary. I don't want you to be part of those statistics. I believe that the side effects of prescription drugs cause most symptoms of aging, such as fatigue, forgetfulness, and impotence. Take as few prescription drugs as possible, and learn to treat risk factors for heart disease, such as high blood pressure and high cholesterol, naturally. That simply means following the steps outlined in this chapter.

It's important to make the distinction between a drug that effectively treats a symptom and a drug that actually reduces the chance that you'll die from a heart attack. Most heart disease drugs treat the symptom effectively, such as lowering blood pressure or cholesterol, but not the underlying problem, and your risk of dying of heart disease remains the same. If these drugs were working such wonders, the United States wouldn't continue to have the highest rate of death from heart disease in the world.

You can avoid the vast majority of pharmaceutical drugs simply by using the information given in this chapter. When you do need to treat a cold, allergy, illness, or symptoms of aging, you can nearly always use simple, effective, natural remedies and herbs.

If you're not taking any prescription drugs, congratulate yourself. And if your doctor wants to put you on one, go on the defensive. Ask some important questions, such as: Exactly what will this drug do? How long will I need to take it? Are there any safe, effective ways to treat this problem without drugs? Is this the lowest dose I can take? What are the side effects?

If you are on a prescription drug, don't go off it without consulting your doctor. At the same time, I encourage you to consider how much your quality of life will improve if you treat heart disease symptoms with the suggestions given in this chapter rather than with drugs that reduce your quality of life with their unpleasant side effects. I realize it's more difficult to change old habits than to pop a pill, but the benefit you will receive in a better quality of life and increased energy will make it well worth the effort.

Treating High Blood Pressure and Cholesterol

Taking medication to lower blood pressure or cholesterol should not have to be a fact of life for so many Americans. The truth is that these drugs don't work very well to lower your risk of dying from heart disease, and most of them will make you feel awful. Diuretics used to lower blood pressure can starve your body of minerals important to your heart function, such as magnesium, and actually raise your risk of disease. Drugs that lower cholesterol can make you feel tired and impotent and can increase your risk of dying in an accident or committing suicide.

It's important to always begin treating mild to moderate high blood pressure and high LDL cholesterol with nondrug methods. The biggest risk factors for both high blood pressure and high cholesterol are obesity, alcohol, smoking, a high-fat diet, stress, and lack of exercise.

If you reduce your fat calories to 20 to 25 percent of your caloric intake, eat a diet that's mostly whole grains, fresh fruits, and vegetables, take a brisk 20-minute walk every day, and cut way down on sugar and refined carbohydrates, I guarantee you'll lose weight. If you make these diet and lifestyle changes, quit smoking, and keep your alcohol consumption low, it is a near certainty that your blood pressure and cholesterol will drop. If you do all of these things and your blood pressure and cholesterol are still high, take a good look at the stress in your life, and take steps to reduce it.

BAN PESTICIDES FROM YOUR LIFE

Chronic exposure to pesticides is a known heart disease risk, but one that most people never think of when they douse their lawn with chemicals, spray their garden, go after bugs in the house with a can of spray, or have their house fumigated. If you're pouring poisons down gopher or mole holes, and dousing your aphids with pesticides and your dog with flea dip, you're exposing yourself, and your heart, to unacceptable levels of poison.

These poisons may not kill you on the spot, but they will create free-radical damage in your tissues and accumulate in the body. A study done in the Ukraine of agricultural workers showed that those frequently exposed to pesticides had a higher rate of heart disease as well as a higher rate of spontaneous abortions and birth defects. There is also evidence that fetal exposure to pesticides can cause congenital heart disease.

Other Toxins Promote Heart Disease

Pesticides aren't the only toxins that can cause heart disease. Others, usually found in the workplace, but also in the garage, include solvents, glues and other binding materials, dyes, lacquers, paints, PCBs, met-als, and vinyl chloride. In many cases, workers only need to be exposed to fumes or dust from these materials to increase their risk of heart disease.

Don't take it for granted that just because you buy a pesticide, herbicide, fungicide, cleaning solvent, paint, or other chemical from the hardware store that it's safe. The industries that make these substances are largely unregulated. There are literally thousands of these products on the shelves that have never been tested for safety. In fact, I recommend that you assume that they are harmful unless you find out otherwise, and avoid contact with skin and avoid breathing the fumes. Even simple household chemicals, such as ammonia and chlorine, can be harmful.

Another source of chronic exposure to heart-harming substances is air pollution. A number of studies have shown that many thousands of people die each year of heart attacks caused by poor air quality. Granted, their hearts may have been in bad shape to begin with, but a good dose of carbon monoxide can push people over the edge. Avoid sitting in traffic and breathing car exhaust, and avoid exercising outside around heavy traffic. Neither your lungs nor your heart will thank you for it!

Reduce Your Exposure

Here are some tips for reducing your exposure to pesticides and other environmental toxins:

- Control fleas on your pets and in your home with substances such as boric acid compounds (now found in most pet stores, or call Flea Busters) and aromatic oils such as pennyroyal rather than flea powders.
- If you're a gardener, learn how to do it the organic way. There are plenty of books and magazines on the subject, and local classes are easy to find. You *can* create a beautiful lawn and garden without chemicals, and in the long run, you'll have far fewer pest problems.
- Don't drink tap water. (See the section on drinking clean water on page 145.)
- If you are exposed to pesticides, take a cool shower and drink plenty of clean water to help flush out the poisons.

- Wash, peel, or even scrub fruits and vegetables well, and eat organic produce whenever possible.
- If you think something at work is making you sick, pursue it. It could be mold or fungus in the heating or cooling system, fumes from wall paneling or carpets, or a coworker's cigarette smoke.
- Stop using fungicides, herbicides, and pesticides. Get out of the habit of blasting indoor and outdoor pests with a can of spray. Learn how to control pests naturally. There's a wealth of information at your library and in your bookstore.
- Don't move next door to an agricultural field or orchard unless you know it's organic and likely to stay that way.

QUIT SMOKING

If you're not convinced that smoking is dangerous to your heart, you haven't read the studies. A major scientific review of disease prevention in health care reform found that the major preventable risk factor for cardiovascular disease—which costs $128 billion a year in treatment and in lost productivity—is cigarette smoking.

Regular or low tar—it makes no difference. Your risk of a heart attack is still a hefty four times greater than that of nonsmokers. This was the finding of a study published in the *British Medical Journal*. When it comes to heart disease, the choice is not about tar levels, it's about stopping now!

Smoking Raises Fibrinogen Levels and Lowers Your Vitamin C

At least ten large studies have shown how a high-fibrinogen level is a major risk factor for cardiovascular disease, including atherosclerosis (clogged arteries) and thrombosis (stroke). Fibrinogen is a blood-clotting agent. It is at least as important as other well-known factors like cholesterol levels. Fibrinogen levels can be used to assess the severity of coronary artery disease and stroke and the risk of arteries becoming blocked again after surgery. And you guessed it: Smoking increases fibrinogen levels.

Studies continue to reveal the ways in which smoking is a threat to your health. One study of forty-four smokers and forty-four nonsmokers between twenty-two and twenty-eight years of age showed that smokers had lower levels of vitamin C than nonsmokers. Furthermore, when smokers took vitamin C, there was no corresponding rise in their blood levels of vitamin C. As reported in the *British Journal of Nutrition*, this finding indicates that smoking lowers the body's antioxidant status as well as bombarding it with very high levels of the harmful substances that antioxidants help to neutralize.

Making Quitting Easier

Did you know that your senses of taste and smell improve greatly if you give up smoking? That's just one more incentive to quit. Fortunately, there are several strategies to try, although statistics show that

---

Passive Smoking Creates Active Risk

An article in the *Journal of the American Medical Association* reviewed the research on passive smoking and heart disease. Predictably, it concluded that nonsmokers exposed to secondhand smoke on a daily basis have an increased risk of heart disease, nonfatal and fatal. The danger lies in the cocktail of chemicals in cigarette smoke, which includes carbon monoxide, nicotine, and hydrocarbons. The result of breathing in these noxious chemicals is decreased oxygen supply to the heart and compromised heart function. In addition, secondhand smoke increases blood-clotting activity and artery lesions and promotes tissue damage following heart attacks. Secondhand smoke? You don't want even a whiff of it!

essful method is actually to go cold

...ods include nicotine patches, which
...bed by your doctor. These give a gradually reduced dose of nicotine over the course of a few months. This is designed to wean you off the nicotine, which is highly addictive.

It makes sense to support your body while you reduce its dependency. Funnily enough, raw, shelled, unsalted sunflower seeds can help. Keep them with you to munch on whenever you feel a craving for a cigarette. Sunflower seeds are rich in B-complex vitamins and zinc. These nutrients help to lower blood acidity and lessen the stress of withdrawal on your body.

It's a good idea to use supplements as an anti-stress measure while you are quitting smoking. Recommended daily are 50 mg of B complex; 2,000 mg of vitamin C; 15 mg of zinc, taken at night to avoid interference with copper absorption; and 800 mg of magnesium per day, with 400 mg taken just before bedtime to help you relax.

Making the decision to quit smoking is a major move toward a healthier heart and a healthier life in general.

7 NATURAL HEALTH FOR WOMEN ~

TAKING CONTROL OF YOUR OWN HEALTH CARE

It is a misconception that the United States has the world's greatest health care system. Here are a few statistics about women's health care in particular:

- Our rate of death from heart disease is the highest in the world. It is the number one cause of death in women over age seventy. But this fact was only recently discovered because heart disease studies focused on men, so women weren't being diagnosed and treated for heart disease.
- Women are often prescribed medications that have only been tested on men. Women's bodies are more complicated to study—they have menstrual cycles, they get pregnant, and they go through menopause. Women of childbearing age aren't asked to participate in many studies because experimental drugs may carry the risk of pregnancy complications and birth defects.
- U.S. doctors perform some 500,000 unnecessary hysterectomies each year, condemning those women to a lifetime of hormone replacement.
- According to the Centers for Disease Control and Prevention, U.S. doctors performed 349,000 unnecessary cesarean deliveries in 1991, at a cost of $1 billion, not to mention the cost to mothers—severe pain and scarring, the risks of major surgery, higher rates of infection, and longer hospital stays. (Only Brazil and Puerto Rico have higher rates!) Cesarean deliveries don't necessarily make for better infant mortality rates, either. The U.S. infant death rate is still worse than that of twenty-two other countries.

Women's health care in North America is no safe, healing haven. If you are a woman and you want the best health care, it's up to you to become your own best advocate. Educate yourself about your choices, and, if necessary, educate your doctor. Once you've made your way through this chapter, you'll learn some facts about the female body that most mainstream physicians don't know.

HORMONES AND HOW THEY AFFECT YOU

Your body's biochemistry is a beautiful, complex, and intricately balanced system that is largely still beyond the comprehension of science and medicine. One of the most important and finely tuned chemical systems in your body—and one that profoundly affects every other system in your body—is the steroid hormones. The steroid hormones include pregnenolone, progesterone, DHEA (dehydroepiandrosterone), the estrogens, the androgens, the cortisols, and testosterone. You probably recognize that these are the hormones secreted by your ovaries and adrenal glands.

The building block for all these hormones is cholesterol, which in turn is made from the breakdown products of the foods you eat. The steroid hormones regulate and play a part in a seemingly endless list of functions in the body, including sex characteristics, sex drive, thyroid metabolism, insulin regulation, blood pressure, behavior and moods, inflammation, and allergies.

These hormones work together, and when one is out of balance, the others tend to follow, so you can imagine how important it is to help your body maintain hormone balance. Let's take a brief look at some of these hormones.

Estrogen: The Hormone of Femininity and Cell Division

Estrogen is actually the name of a class of hormones. Some of its better-known members are estradiol, estriol, and estrone. To confuse matters, the drug companies refer to their weird not-found-in-nature estrogenlike drugs as estrogens. But don't be fooled. Premarin, for example, is made from a plant-derived human estrogen and a pregnant mare–derived estrogen. The plant-derived estrogen is chemically identical to human estrogen until it is altered in drug company labs and combined with equine estrogens. This is called a conjugated estrogen, but it certainly doesn't resemble anything found in the human body.

When girls reach puberty and begin to experience bodily changes such as growing breasts, underarm hair, and pubic hair, as well as the unseen changes of development of the uterus, vagina, and fallopian tubes, estrogen is the hormone driving these changes. It is also responsible for a woman's curves, those extra deposits of fat that aren't particularly popular in our culture at this time. (At one time they were considered the epitome of beauty and femininity.) When a young woman's estrogen levels, along with the levels of other hormones, rise high enough, she will begin ovulating and having menstrual periods.

Like her other hormones, a woman's estrogen will ebb and flow during the course of her menstrual cycle. Estrogen is highest at the beginning and middle of the cycle, when it is stimulating the uterine tissue to grow, providing a rich, blood-filled womb for embryo growth. This property of stimulating cell growth is both what makes estrogen a feminine hormone and what makes it dangerous when it is found in the body in excess or unbalanced by progesterone. Estrogen doesn't just stimulate cell growth in the uterus; it can also stimulate the growth of cells in breast tissue, ovarian tissue, and cervical tissue.

Estrogen also causes the body to retain water. This accounts for its ability, when it is the dominant hormone, to cause weight gain, bloating, irritability, headaches, and other brain symptoms, such as foggy thinking, memory loss, and depression.

Estrogen Dominance

Dr. John R. Lee, the leading authority on the use of natural progesterone to balance hormones and author of *What Your Doctor May Not Tell You About Menopause* (Warner Books, 1996), has coined the term *estrogen dominance* to describe what happens when a woman has an imbalance of hormones characterized by estrogen unbalanced by the hormone progesterone. Even if a woman's estrogen levels have dropped, as happens at menopause, if her progesterones have dropped even further, her hormones will be unbalanced and she will suffer from estrogen dominance. In other words, it's not an estrogen excess per se that causes estrogen dominance; it's too much estrogen relative to not enough progesterone.

Both women who have suffered from premenstrual syndrome (PMS) and women who have suffered from menopausal symptoms will recognize the hallmark symptoms of estrogen dominance: weight gain, bloating, mood swings, irritability, oversensitivity, tender breasts, headaches, fatigue, depression, hypoglycemia, clumsiness, uterine fibroids, endometriosis, and fibrocystic breasts, just to name the more common symptoms.

Because progesterone is supposed to be the dominant hormone during the premenstrual phase of a woman's cycle, for years PMS was blamed on progesterone. Ironically, it is precisely a *deficiency* of progesterone that is causing the problem at a time in the cycle when it is supposed to be dominant.

Dr. Lee believes that many illnesses that afflict women in the United States are caused by estrogen dominance, including uterine fibroids, fibrocystic breasts, hypoglycemia, low thyroid, gallbladder disease, autoimmune diseases such as lupus, miscarriages, and breast, ovarian, and uterine cancer.

With progesterone playing such an important role in hormone balance, let's examine it more closely.

Progesterone: The Hormone of Pregnancy and Balance

Progesterone is the building block of all the other steroid hormones. In contrast, estrogen is an end-product hormone, meaning that no other hormones are made from it. Progesterone's primary role as a hormone precursor means that a deficiency of progesterone can result in a deficiency or imbalance of other steroid hormones, throwing the entire body out of balance. This is why symptoms of PMS and menopause can be so severe for some women.

In the female body, progesterone is made in the ovaries, the adrenal glands, the placenta during pregnancy, and even, some researchers speculate, in the brain. The ovaries produce the vast majority of a woman's progesterone on a monthly cycle. But the production of progesterone is dependent on ovulation. Without ovulation, there is no ovarian progesterone. How does ovulation work?

Each month, a follicle, which is a sac inside the ovary containing an egg, migrates outside the ovary and ruptures, releasing the egg. The egg then begins its journey down the fallopian tube to the uterus, while the ruptured sac, now called the corpus luteum, produces progesterone. If for some reason ovulation doesn't occur that month, there is no progesterone made by the corpus luteum, which sets the stage for estrogen dominance.

Rising progesterone levels at mid-cycle have the effect of maturing the cells of the uterine lining that estrogen has stimulated to grow, preparing them either for an embryo or to be shed in menstruation. When pregnancy doesn't occur, the brain sends out signals to the ovaries, and both progesterone and estrogen levels fall, creating the end of a menstrual cycle with the shedding of the uterine lining.

Dr. Lee theorizes that the ability of progesterone to mature cells may partly account for its potential to prevent and even reverse reproductive cancers in women (and, I might add, in men). And remember, I am not talking about the synthetic progestins here, which seem to stimulate cancerous growth.

Progesterone is also the primary hormone of pregnancy. After about the third month, the placenta begins producing progesterone, and by the third trimester, the placenta is producing 300–400 mg of progesterone every day! This is a whopping dose for a hormone!

Moreover, progesterone plays a large part in sex drive, or libido, which is logical, since it is the hormone present in the greatest amount at ovulation, when a woman is fertile.

Why Isn't Natural Progesterone Used In Hormone Replacement Therapy?

Many doctors would answer this question by saying, "Of course progesterone is used in hormone replacement therapy! What do you think Provera is? What do you think the progestins are?" And herein lies a misconception that has caused harm to millions of women. The progestins such as Provera (medroxyprogesterone acetate) are most emphatically *not* the same as progesterone. They are synthetic versions of progesterone, molecules not found in nature, and the body does not respond to them in the same way it does to the natural progesterone found in your body. They're close, but close doesn't count in hormones. The molecular difference between testosterone and estrogen is less radical than the difference between progesterone and the progestins, and yet the difference between testosterone and estrogen is the difference between a man and a woman!

If your doctor argues with you about this, point out that the placenta produces 300–400 mg of progesterone during the last few months of pregnancy, so we know that it's the ultimately safe hormone to have in the body during pregnancy. But the progestins can cause birth defects with a fraction of that amount! I'd hardly call that the same hormone! The progestins also cause many other side effects, including partial loss of vision, breast cancer in test dogs, an increased risk of strokes, fluid retention, migraine headaches, asthma, cardiac irregularities, depression, and a whole list of other side effects caused by combining the progestins with the synthetic estrogens. Natural progesterone, on the other hand, has never been shown to have any side effects except sleepiness at very high doses.

You may wonder why the drug companies would produce a drug with so many side effects when the real thing is easily available and cheaper, with no known side effects, and even more appalling, why the FDA would ever approve it! The answer is money. Natural progesterone can't be patented because it's a natural substance; therefore, the drug companies can't charge outrageous prices for it. So they create a synthetic, patentable drug, pretend it's the same thing, and drop millions and millions of advertising dollars into perpetuating the illusion that the two are the same. Even most doctors believe it. Now you see why I keep telling you that neither the drug companies nor the FDA is looking out for your best interests. You must take the initiative to educate yourself and protect your own health.

Where Does Natural Progesterone Come From?

There is an enormous amount of confusion about exactly what a natural progesterone is. My definition is the same as Dr. Lee's: To be called progesterone, it must be the same molecule as the progesterone made in a woman's body.

But the progesterone used for natural hormone replacement doesn't come from people—or from animals; it comes from either diosgenin, extracted from a very specific type of wild yam (*Dioscorea* spp.) that grows in Mexico, from a substance extracted from soybeans called stigmasterol, or from cholesterol derived from wool fat.

In the laboratory, diosgenin, stigmasterol, and cholesterol can relatively easily and cheaply be converted to the exact molecular structure of all the human steroid hormones, including estrogen, testosterone, progesterone, and the cortisones. And in fact, this is where nearly all pharmaceutical hormones originate.

Is Wild Yam Extract the Same as Progesterone?

Some companies are trying to sell diosgenin, which they label "wild yam extract," as a medicine or supplement, claiming that the body will then convert it into hormones as needed. This is a very neat and logical-sounding theory, and I wish it were true, but unfortunately there is no evidence that this is what happens. There are piles of papers proving that this can be done in the laboratory, but nothing showing that it's the way it happens in the human body. I keep hearing promises that research is under way that is going to prove it, but it never surfaces.

Diosgenin, or wild yam, has been used by herbalists to relieve menstrual cramps and abdominal pain, and it has been shown in studies to lower cholesterol a little bit, so it may very well be a useful medicinal plant. Just be aware that it will not have the same effect as progesterone cream and that by taking it you are not taking progesterone—or any other steroid hormone, for that matter. In addition, wild yam is used in Mexico as a fish poison, so I would avoid taking it in high doses if you should decide to try it.

Unfortunately, the consequences of this type of "theoretical marketing" can be tragic. I recently got a call from the owner of a health food store, telling me that a woman in a wheelchair was in his store, demanding to know why the progesterone she was taking hadn't helped her osteoporosis. She had taken a bone density measurement, faithfully used progesterone cream as instructed, and here she was six months later with a hip fracture caused by a minor fall and lower bone density than when she started.

My friend was puzzled, having seen many good results with progesterone and osteoporosis. I told him to ask her what brand of progesterone cream she was using. Well, it turns out she wasn't using a progesterone cream at all; she was using a diosgenin cream labeled "wild yam extract" and advertised as giving all the benefits of progesterone. Please don't make this mistake—the consequences are too serious. And by the way, to confuse matters even more, real progesterone cream is often labeled "wild yam extract," so the best thing to do is know your sources. I will give you a list of reliable sources of natural progesterone cream at the end of the book.

Why Some Women Stop Ovulating

There are many reasons why women don't ovulate. Perhaps the most common reason is stress. Our bodies are intimately and intricately connected to the brain, and the brain's response to stress is to signal the body not to reproduce. Another common reason for nonovulatory cycles, also called *anovulatory* cycles, is strenuous exercise. Many female athletes don't ovulate, and some don't even menstruate. Is it possible not to ovulate and still have a menstrual period? Absolutely! That just means that there is enough estrogen to stimulate the uterine lining to build and then shed its blood-rich tissue. A lack of menstruation means that there isn't enough estrogen in the body to stimulate tissue growth in the uterus, so there's nothing to shed at the end of the cycle.

The consequences of anovulatory cycles are serious: All of the estrogen dominance symptoms can come into play, including uterine fibroids and fibrocystic breasts, as well as endometriosis. Weight gain, fatigue, depression, sleep disturbances, and foggy thinking can dog the heels of a woman who's not ovulating. And she may not even be aware that she's not ovulating because she's continuing to have menstrual periods.

The Threat of Xenoestrogens

According to Dr. Lee, one cause of anovulatory cycles is follicle burnout caused by *xenoestrogens*, which are environmental estrogens that come from pesticides, herbicides, fungicides, some types of soap, air pollution, plastics, and the meat of animals fattened for slaughter with estrogenlike drugs, an almost universal practice in the United States. These xenoestrogens are not identical to estrogen but are enough alike so that they behave somewhat like estrogen in the body. They are usually very potent and are especially dangerous to a growing fetus because they can cause reproductive abnormalities that show up later in life.

Remember, in addition to creating female characteristics, one of estrogen's primary jobs in the body is to stimulate cell growth. Xenoestrogens may very well be a cause of the rising rates of reproductive organ cancer (for both women and men), including breast cancer, testicular cancer, ovarian cancer, and cervical cancer, as well as the rapidly dropping sperm count in men and the epidemic of infertility among couples in their thirties.

I strongly encourage you to avoid xenoestrogens as much as possible. Here's how:

- Eat organic fruits and vegetables whenever possible.
- Never spray your garden or lawn with pesticides, herbicides, or fungicides (there are plenty of effective ways to control pests without pesticides).
- Never spray or "bomb" your home with insecticides.
- Minimize your consumption of meat unless you know it's hormone free.

- Use environmentally friendly soaps that do not contain nonylphenols, a type of surfactant.
- Do not cook in plastic, which sheds when heated.

Hormones and Menopause

Estrogen is not the hormone most women need to be taking for menopausal symptoms. Estrogen will do most women more harm than good, making them feel great for a few months and then dropping them into a kind of permanent postmenopausal PMS.

Estrogen levels only drop 40 to 60 percent at menopause, which is just enough to stop the menstrual cycle. But progesterone levels may drop to near zero in some women. In a healthy woman, hormone levels will fall off very gradually over time, with a gradual lessening of menstrual cycles and with very little in the way of menopausal symptoms.

Menopause is relatively uneventful in most Third World countries, and in Japan there's not even a name for hot flashes! According to Dr. Lee, this is because the high-stress, high-calorie, and low-exercise lifestyle of most American women creates higher-than-normal hormone levels, which drop more abruptly at menopause, creating the unpleasant symptoms of hot flashes and night sweats, along with all the estrogen dominance symptoms.

Later in this chapter, I'll talk in more detail about a lifestyle for a healthy menopause.

The Male Hormones

Although testosterone is the hormone that confers "maleness," women also have some testosterone in small amounts. Testosterone, along with progesterone, plays an important role in sex drive. It also builds bone, helps define muscle, and speeds up metabolism. DHEA (dehydroepiandrosterone), an important hormone mainly made by the adrenals, also tends to be an androgen, or male hormone. It is clear that some men can benefit from DHEA supplementation as they age, as high as 150 mg a day, but very little research has been done with women. However, there is some indication that older women may benefit from 20 mg a day of DHEA. Please don't take high doses of DHEA. The research we do have indicates that it may increase insulin resistance and the risk of heart disease in women at high doses. And again, do not take diosgenin, or "wild yam extract," thinking you are getting DHEA. As far as we know, that doesn't happen reliably.

NATURALLY HEALTHY BREASTS

Women's breasts are very sensitive to hormones, especially to estrogen and progesterone. Women who experience breast tenderness premenstrually will attest to this.

Virtually every risk for breast cancer is associated with excessive estrogen in some way. This makes sense, because estrogen stimulates tissue growth, particularly tissue in the breasts and reproductive organs.

According to the American Cancer Society, more cancers are detected by women examining themselves than by mammogram. This is a simple, effective routine that should be done by every woman, every month, for her entire life. It's best to do a breast exam just after a menstrual period, so that premenstrual breast lumps can be distinguished from lumps that are independent of monthly cycles.

Fibrocystic Breasts

Some estimates are that 60 percent of women in their premenopausal years experience fibrocystic breast changes. The symptoms include lumps and tenderness. Some women have many lumps, some women have only one. Fibrocystic breasts generally worsen premenstrually. When menopause begins, fibrocystic breasts end for most women.

The breasts are composed of fatty tissue interwoven with ducts and glands for milk. Breast ducts and glands are the parts of the breasts influenced by hormones, particularly estrogen, which stimulates duct growth and branching. If they are overstimulated, they can become swollen and blocked, leading to the formation of cysts. Fibrocystic breasts are probably caused by estrogen dominance and can nearly always be relieved with the use of some progesterone cream.

If you have fibrocystic or tender breasts and you're premenopausal, you can use the recom-

mended dose of progesterone cream, usually ¼ to ½ teaspoon daily, from day 12 of your cycle (day 1 is the first day of menstruation) to two days before your period is due, usually twenty-six to twenty-eight days for most women. *Do not* use progesterone cream if you are trying to become pregnant, because starting the cream before you ovulate can block ovulation, and stopping it at day 26 or 28 brings on menstruation because an abrupt drop in hormones triggers menstruation.

If you are under the age of thirty-five, I recommend that you try dietary and lifestyle changes and some herbs before resorting to progesterone. (Women over thirty-five should try these remedies first, too, but they are more likely to have a progesterone deficiency leading to estrogen dominance.)

Exercise is one of the best things you can do to relieve tender or fibrocystic breasts. Moving your body moves your lymphatic system, which is composed of millions of tiny channels, glands, and ducts that transport toxins out of the body. One of the primary lymph gland sites is under the armpit, near the breast.

The lymphatic system moves when you do. Stretching is one of the best types of exercise you can do for your lymphatic system. Many yoga, tai chi, and chi gong movements are specifically designed to move the lymphatic system.

Diet for Healthy Breasts

There are a few basic changes that have helped many women reduce or eliminate fibrocystic breasts. Perhaps the most important is cutting out coffee. For some reason, coffee seems to aggravate fibrocystic breasts, probably because it's so hard on the liver. Many women have eliminated their problem simply by eliminating coffee.

It may seem contradictory to tell you to drink plenty of water when water retention can aggravate breast tenderness, but water is your body's favorite cleanser. Drink at least six to eight glasses of clean water daily when you are premenstrual.

Another important step is eliminating hydrogenated oils such as those found in margarine and nearly all processed baked goods and chips. These synthetic oils block important biochemical pathways of essential fatty acids, promoting inflammation. It's also important to avoid processed, unsaturated vegetable oils, which are usually rancid by the time they get onto your dinner table. Stick to the monounsaturated oils, such as olive oil and canola oil, and small amounts of saturated oils, such as butter and coconut oil. Yes, contrary to popular opinion, saturated fats are perfectly fine as long as you eat them in moderation. They shouldn't comprise more than 10 percent of your fat and oil consumption. I would much rather have you eat butter than margarine or other hydrogenated oils.

Meat is a good food to go easy on when you are premenstrual. It takes a lot of energy to digest meat, and you'll avoid those estrogenlike drugs that are used to fatten cattle, as well as the pesticides (xeno-estrogens) that become concentrated in fatty tissues.

Eating fish a couple of times a week, as well as plenty of nuts, fresh fruits and vegetables, and whole grains, will give you the essential fatty acids you need. You can take an essential fatty acid supplement, too. These are usually derived from evening primrose oil or borage oil and fish oils.

Herbs for Healthy Breasts

Although fibrocystic breasts are most likely caused by hormonal imbalances, once you have them, you're dealing with inflammation and tissues that have in effect become clogged or toxic. Some of the herbs I'm going to recommend are for hormonal balance, and some are for detoxification. The liver is the organ most responsible for excreting excess estrogen, so it's very important to specifically support your liver. Because the liver has to expend a lot of energy to get rid of excess fat, you can also support your liver by strictly avoiding fried foods and keeping your fat intake moderate.

Check your health food store for formulas and teas made from these herbs. They can be very effective in relieving symptoms and helping your body restore itself to normalcy. All of these herbs can be taken as a tincture, tea, or capsule, following the directions on the container.

Black Cohosh (Cimicifuga racemosa)

This is one of the ultimate women's herbs, used extensively by the American Indians for menstrual-related problems. It contains phytoestrogens (plant estrogens that occupy estrogen receptor sites, lessening the effect of the body's estrogen) and many other nutrients that strengthen and balance the female reproductive system. Black cohosh nourishes the adrenals and kidneys, improves circulation, is calming, helps relieve the swelling caused by water retention, and improves digestion.

This is not an herb to use if there is a possibility that you are or may become pregnant.

Dandelion (Taraxacum officinale)

Sore, tender breasts can often be caused or aggravated by water retention. In this case, a diuretic, which helps the body eliminate excess water, can be very helpful. Dandelion is a wonderful medicinal herb that is a gentle diuretic and contains helpful minerals, including potassium. It is also high in lecithin, a substance that supports liver function, your most important route of detoxification.

Sage (Salvia officinalis)

Named from the Latin for "to save," sage has been associated for centuries with longevity. It has a long-standing reputation as an aid for painful periods and tender breasts, and it will aid in the digestion of fat. Other cooking herbs, such as rosemary and thyme, also have a beneficial effect on fat digestion.

Besides its powerful oils, sage contains estrogenic compounds, which can soften the effect of excessive estrogen by taking up estrogen receptor sites on cells. It also contains antibacterial agents and antioxidants.

Sage should only be taken as a remedy for a week or two at a time, since it has another substance, thujone, that can have potentially toxic effects. Don't mistake "garden sage" for desert sage (Artemisia tridentata).

Vitex/Chasteberry (Vitex agnus-castus)

Traditionally, chasteberry was very popular in Europe as a woman's remedy for regulating the reproductive system, treating PMS, and treating unpleasant symptoms associated with menopause, such as hot flashes.

Research has revealed the presence of a volatile oil in chasteberry that tends to balance the production of women's hormones. This oil is believed to contain a progesteronelike substance, which could explain the herb's therapeutic effect in relation to PMS symptoms such as anxiety, nervous tension, insomnia, and mood changes, as well as tender breasts and cramping. Chasteberry has also been used to treat irregular menstruation, heavy bleeding, and fibroid cysts. Vitex needs to be taken regularly over a period of at least a month or two to have its effect.

White Willow Bark (Salix alba)

For pain relief, white willow bark tea, capsules, or tincture can provide the same analgesic effect as aspirin without the stomach distress caused by aspirin. Willows have been used since antiquity for pain relief and reduction of fever. Ancient manuscripts of Egypt, Greece, and Assyria refer to willow bark, and even Hippocrates recommended willow to counter pain.

Yellow Dock (Rumex crispus) and Milk Thistle (Silybum marianum)

These are both wonderful herbs for supporting and tonifying the liver. When you support your liver, your body rids itself of toxins more quickly.

Supplements for Healthy Breasts

It is important to maintain a good daily vitamin regimen for optimal nutritional support (see chapter 1). In addition, the following supplements will help prevent tender and fibrocystic breasts.

Vitamin B_6

This vitamin will help balance hormones because it is an important part of the body's process of transforming one hormone into another. Without adequate B_6, your body may be unable to make the hormones it needs to keep everything in balance. Vitamin B_6 will also help relieve water retention. Take 50 mg two times a day between meals.

Calcium and Magnesium

These minerals are important for maintaining proper fluid balance in the cells and for muscle relaxation. Be sure you're getting 1,200 mg of calcium and 400–500 mg of magnesium daily.

NATURALLY HEALTHY MENSTRUAL CYCLES

A woman's monthly cycles are perfectly designed by nature to prepare the body for impregnation. We call them monthly cycles, but they more accurately reflect the lunar cycle (the cycle of the moon).

At the beginning of a cycle, prior to ovulation, the brain releases hormones that instruct the uterus to build a thick, blood-rich lining that will act as a temporary incubator for an embryo should the monthly egg be released and fertilized. This process is stimulated by estrogen. By the end of the third trimester, the placenta will be fully surrounding and protecting the fetus and producing progesterone in copious amounts.

Around the middle of the cycle, called the luteal phase, the brain again signals the ovaries, this time to release a follicle, which is a sac inside the ovary containing an egg. One follicle makes it to the surface of the ovary and releases an egg. While the egg is making its way down the fallopian tube, where it may meet up with sperm, the empty follicle sac, now called the corpus luteum, is releasing progesterone. At this point in the cycle, both progesterone and estrogen levels are fairly high.

When impregnation doesn't happen, progesterone levels and estrogen levels begin to drop, falling abruptly at the end of the cycle, around day 26, and stimulating the uterine muscles to contract and release their bloody lining.

What I've just outlined is a very simplified version of a woman's monthly cycle, and while the body is adept at adjusting for all kinds of variations, from diet to stress, there are many ways this cycle can be thrown out of balance.

Menstrual Cramps

Nearly all women have experienced menstrual cramps—what doctors call dysmenorrhea—at some time in their life, but for some women, an estimated 10 percent, their monthly cycles are a source of pain and misery that will cause them to miss work and school. Until recently, the medical mind-set toward menstrual cramps was that they were psychologically caused and that women should just endure them or take a painkiller. Of course, this is not true. Cramps can be made worse by stress, but they are caused by very real biochemical imbalances in the body.

Menstrual cramps may have more than one cause, but the primary one is an excess of "bad" prostaglandins called PGF2, which are normally released to stimulate gentle muscle contractions of the uterus, allowing the shedding of the uterine lining, or endometrium. In excess, the muscle contractions become cramps.

An excess of "bad" prostaglandins is primarily caused by doing things that block the "good" prostaglandin pathways. The prostaglandin pathways are largely regulated by our intake of essential fatty acids (EFAs). Eating hydrogenated oils (found in margarine and most baked goods and chips) and rancid oils can block the EFAs, starting a chain reaction down the bad pathways. Many women can avoid cramps simply by avoiding hydrogenated oils and limiting their oils to olive oil, canola oil, and butter. But to balance your prostaglandins, you need a balanced intake of EFAs. This means eating fish two or three times a week and including a variety of nuts (except peanuts), seeds, whole grains, and fresh vegetables in your diet. You also need to minimize your intake of coffee, dairy products, red meat, and alcohol, all of which will stimulate the bad prostaglandins.

A diet high in refined carbohydrates and sugar will also drive oils down the bad pathways. Viral illnesses and excessive adrenal hormones secreted in response to stress can also create more bad prostaglandins and a deficiency of good ones. This is why we can accurately say that stress does contribute to menstrual cramps.

Some doctors will prescribe birth control pills to relieve menstrual cramping. If they help, this is an indication that the cramps may be caused by estrogen dominance—an imbalance of estrogen caused by a progesterone deficiency. In this case, it would be far safer to use the natural hormones found in proges-

terone cream. To use progesterone cream, follow the directions given in the section on naturally healthy breasts. However, if you are under the age of thirty-five, it is far preferable to try the lifestyle and dietary changes recommended first. You might use progesterone cream for a few months while you are getting your system back in balance, but always try the simplest solutions first.

Painkillers such as aspirin and ibuprofen help relieve the symptoms of menstrual cramps by blocking both prostaglandin pathways. This will provide symptomatic relief for some women, but suppressing the good prostaglandins has the effect of suppressing the immune system. These types of drugs are also very hard on the stomach. I suggest you try to correct the underlying cause of your cramps and bring your body back into balance.

I recommend the book *Women's Bodies, Women's Wisdom* by Christiane Northrup, MD (Bantam, 1998), for an in-depth look at how the emotional and stress-related causes of menstrual cramps can be healed.

If you use tampons, be sure they aren't the cause of your cramps. Try a couple of cycles without them and see if that helps. Gas and constipation can aggravate cramps, so when you are premenstrual, try to avoid foods that cause those symptoms.

Herbs for Menstrual Cramps

Herbs can be very useful for gently and safely relieving the pain and muscle spasms of menstrual cramps. But do not use them if you are trying to get pregnant, as some of them can encourage menstruation. Some women can experience cramping as an early sign of pregnancy.

As always, use herbs in moderation, follow the directions on the container, and be cautious about mixing them with other drugs. Herbs are generally much safer than prescription drugs, but it always pays to be cautious. All the herbs listed here can be taken as teas, as tinctures, or in capsule form. You can also check your health food store for formulas made specifically for menstrual cramps that contain some or all of these plants.

In this section and elsewhere later in the book, you will notice that some information is repeated.

This is because certain herbs and nutrients operate on several conditions, and the full information should be available in each place where it will be called for, even if it also appears elsewhere.

Anise (Pimpinella anisum)

This common plant is mainly an antispasmodic, used for relieving the muscle spasms associated with menstrual cramps. You can chew on anise seeds, drink it as a tea, or take it in capsules.

Chamomile (Matricaria chamomilla)

Chamomile makes a mild, relaxing, and soothing tea that can help promote menstruation when it is delayed.

Cramp Bark (Viburnum opulus)

This aptly named bush will help relieve cramps anywhere in the body. It relaxes muscles and nerves.

Dong Quai (Angelica sinensis)

This is one of the most popular Chinese herbs for balancing women's hormones. It works specifically on the uterine muscles and appears to contract or relax them, as needed, to bring balance. This type of herb is known as an *adaptogen*, because it tends to bring the body into balance. Contrary to popular opinion, dong quai does not contain estrogenlike substances or have an estrogenic effect on the body. It has a mild sedative effect, a mild diuretic effect, and enhances liver function.

Sage (Salvia officinalis)

Sage has a long-standing reputation as an aid for painful periods. See page 171 for more information on this herb.

White Willow Bark (Salix alba)

White willow bark tea, capsules, or tincture can provide the same pain relief as aspirin. See page 172 for more information on this herb.

Supplements for Menstrual Cramps

Taking an essential fatty acid (EFA) supplement normally in the form of EPA (eicosapentaenoic acid) and GLA (gamma-linolenic acid) supplements can significantly help prevent and relieve menstrual cramps. The EPA usually comes from fish, and the GLA from borage oil. Take them starting at least a week before your period is due. Take them in a 2-to-1 ratio, so that you get twice as much EPA as GLA. It is also important to maintain a good daily vitamin regimen (see chapter 1) for optimal nutritional support. In addition, the following supplements will help prevent menstrual cramps.

Vitamin B_6

Take 50 mg two times a day between meals. (See page 172.

Calcium and Magnesium

Magnesium is one of the most effective remedies for muscle spasms. Be sure you're getting 1,200 mg of calcium and 400–500 mg of magnesium daily. You can double your magnesium intake the week before your period. Be sure to take it in a buffered form or it can cause diarrhea.

Vitamin E

This vitamin has been shown to help prevent and relieve menstrual cramps. You should be taking 400 IU daily as part of your daily vitamin regimen. You can add another 400 IU during the week before your period.

Bioflavonoids

Bioflavonoids can help reduce the inflammation associated with some menstrual cramping. There are many bioflavonoid formulas available. Three of my favorite bioflavonoids are quercetin, grapeseed extract, and hesperidin.

PMS

PMS, or premenstrual syndrome, has achieved wide recognition in the past few decades. Like menstrual cramps, PMS was first thought to be a product of a woman's unbalanced psyche. Now we know that it can be caused by a complex interplay of factors that include genetics, nutrition, hormones, and stress.

It is estimated that 50 percent of all women experience mild PMS, but my guess is that nearly all women experience some form of PMS between the time menstruation begins and menopause. An estimated 30 percent of women experience moderate PMS symptoms, and some 5 percent experience symptoms that are severe enough to interfere with their daily lives.

PMS symptoms occur a week or ten days before menstruation begins and go away shortly after. They include a lot of mental/emotional symptoms such as depression, weeping, anxiety, irritability, foggy thinking, memory loss, confusion, inability to focus, and anger. Other symptoms include clumsiness, dizziness, fatigue, headaches, muscle aches and pains, water retention and the resulting weight gain, nausea, low back pain, acne, breast tenderness, and food cravings, particularly for chocolate, sugar, and refined carbohydrates such as cakes and cookies.

Women who suffer from PMS dread those times of the month, and so do their families and friends. If you look at Dr. John Lee's list of estrogen dominance symptoms and then look at a list of PMS symptoms, you'll find that they are very similar. Katharina Dalton, a British medical doctor, pioneered the use of progesterone for PMS decades ago. She had great success in relieving symptoms, but the vaginal or rectal suppositories she used to deliver the hormone were not popular. Meanwhile, back in the United States, many doctors were blaming progesterone for causing PMS because that was the dominant hormone present at the end of the menstrual cycle. Somehow, it never occurred to them that a progesterone *deficiency* could be causing the symptoms.

Many women can relieve their PMS symptoms by using some natural progesterone cream, but it should not be treated like a magic bullet. Severe PMS symptoms are the body's way of letting you know that something is very much out of balance, and if you fail to address those imbalances, they will reappear somewhere else in the body.

There are a variety of factors that can contribute to PMS. A thyroid deficiency can imitate many PMS symptoms, including headaches, fatigue, and mental fogginess. Women who have allergies, who abuse alcohol, or who have chronic gastrointestinal problems are more prone to PMS. Lack of exercise will contribute to PMS. And pervasive petrochemical pollution and the resulting prevalence of xenoestrogens (potent environmental estrogens) are also no doubt contributing to PMS.

Reduce Stress Levels

Stress can certainly push a woman over the edge into PMS. Chronic stress stimulates the release of adrenal hormones that in excess can throw the rest of the body's hormones out of balance and block the good prostaglandin pathways. Women whose PMS symptoms include cramping and abdominal pain may be especially susceptible to stress.

To uncover the source of your stress, it may help to talk to a sympathetic friend or relative, or even a therapist—someone who will listen and help you sort things out. Good nutrition, exercise, plenty of sleep, and a life that is balanced with work and play will go a long way toward reducing stress. Meditation or the Eastern disciplines of yoga, tai chi, or chi gong can also greatly help relieve stress. Again, I recommend Dr. Christiane Northrup's book, *Women's Bodies, Women's Wisdom* (Bantam, 1998), for good advice on handling stress.

Diet for a PMS-Free Month

Poor nutrition is a primary factor aggravating PMS. The PMS-free diet is similar to the diet for healthy breasts and a healthy menstrual cycle. These few basic dietary changes have helped many women reduce or eliminate their PMS symptoms.

The most important step you can take is eliminating hydrogenated oils such as are found in margarine and nearly all processed baked goods and chips. These synthetic oils block important biochemical pathways of essential fatty acids, promoting inflammation. It's also important to avoid processed vegetable oils, which are usually rancid by the time they get to your dinner table. Stick to the monoun-saturated oils, such as olive oil and canola oil, and small amounts of saturated oils such as butter and coconut oil. Coconut oil is perfectly good for you when eaten in moderation. It is high in medium-chain triglycerides, beneficial oils that can help balance prostaglandins.

The next important step you can take is to eliminate the very foods many women crave—namely, sugary, highly refined carbohydrate foods such as cakes, cookies, and candy. These foods only aggravate the insulin and blood sugar imbalances caused by excess estrogen. Taking the supplements recommended here will greatly help reduce your sugar cravings. Try eating some fresh fruit or raw carrot sticks when a sugar craving comes on.

Meat is a good food to go easy on when you are premenstrual. It takes a lot of energy to digest meat, and you'll avoid those estrogenlike drugs that are used to fatten cattle, as well as the pesticides (xeno-estrogens) that concentrate in fatty tissue. Protein in general seems to aggravate PMS symptoms. It may help to eat primarily vegetarian foods and fish when you are premenstrual.

Eating fish a couple of times a week, as well as plenty of fresh fruits and vegetables and whole grains, will give you the nutrients and fiber you need. Fiber is an important part of a PMS-free diet, because it helps the body eliminate toxins, including excessive estrogen.

It's very important to drink plenty of water to assist your body in detoxifying itself and staying hydrated. Dehydration in itself can cause cramping, headaches, and irritability. Drink at least six to eight glasses of clean water daily when you are premenstrual.

Herbs for a PMS-Free Month

Herbs can play a major role in preventing and treating PMS symptoms. But do not use them if you are trying to get pregnant, as some of them can encourage menstruation. Some women can experience cramping as an early sign of pregnancy.

As always, use herbs in moderation, follow the directions on the container, and be cautious about mixing them with other drugs. Herbs are generally much safer than prescription drugs, but it always pays to be cautious. All the herbs listed here can be taken as teas, as tinctures, or in capsule form. You can also check your health food store for formulas made specifically for PMS that contain some or all of these plants.

Black Cohosh (Cimicifuga racemosa)

See page 171.

Dandelion (Taraxacum officinale)

PMS can often be aggravated by water retention. In this case, a diuretic, which helps the body eliminate excess water, can be very helpful. Dandelion is a wonderful medicinal herb that is a gentle diuretic and contains helpful minerals, including potassium. It is also high in lecithin, a substance that supports liver function, your most important route of detoxification. (See page 171 for more information.)

Dong Quai (Angelica sinensis)

See page 174.

Ginger (Zingiber officinale)

Ginger is one of the most versatile plants on earth, being widely used both as a medicinal plant and as a spice. Its major action is to stop cramping, especially in the digestive system and in the uterus.

Ginger is best known for its effectiveness in relieving indigestion and most types of nausea. Researchers believe that it is ginger's mild suppressing effect on the central nervous system that prevents nausea, and this would also account for its ability to relieve PMS symptoms. Ginger can relieve some migraine headaches, which often occur premenstrually in women. Ginger also contains antioxidants and anti-inflammatory and antibacterial substances. It has been used to help regulate heartbeat, and like aspirin, but without its side effects, it reduces the tendency of blood to clump, thus reducing the risk of heart attacks and strokes. As well as using fresh gingerroot in food or taking it as a tea, you can also take it in a powdered form in capsules.

Vitex/Chasteberry (Vitex agnus-castus)

See pages 171–172.

Yellow Dock (Rumex crispus) and Milk Thistle (Silybum marianum)

These are both wonderful herbs for supporting and tonifying the liver, an important part of maintaining hormone balance and preventing PMS. When you support your liver, your body rids itself of toxins more quickly.

Supplements for a PMS-Free Month

It is important to maintain a good daily vitamin regimen for optimal nutritional support (see chapter 1). In addition, the following supplements will help prevent PMS symptoms.

Essential Fatty Acids (EFAs)

EFAs can significantly help relieve PMS. Take a supplement with a 2-to-1 ratio of EPA oils to GLA oils. Flaxseed oil can be taken for a week or so premenstrually to relieve symptoms, but I don't recommend that you take it every day long-term because it can suppress both good and bad prostaglandin pathways. Also, always make sure that flaxseed oil comes in a lightproof container and that it is refrigerated and dated, and don't use the same bottle for more than two weeks. Flaxseed oil is one of the most unstable of all the unsaturated oils, and if it becomes rancid, it will certainly do you more harm than good. To avoid the problem of rancidity, you can also buy the seeds and grind them just before you eat them.

Vitamin B$_6$

Take 50 mg two times a day between meals. (See page 172.)

B Complex

B-complex vitamins can help with the mental and emotional symptoms of PMS. Take a B-50 complex the week before your period, in addition to your regular vitamins. The B-50 complex contains 50 mg of most of the B vitamins.

Calcium and Magnesium

Magnesium is one of the most effective remedies for muscle spasms. Be sure you're getting 1,200 mg of calcium and 400–500 mg of magnesium daily. You can double your magnesium intake the week before your period. Be sure to take it in a buffered form or it can cause diarrhea.

Vitamin E

This vitamin has been shown to help PMS symptoms to some degree. You should be taking 400 IU daily as part of your daily vitamin regimen. You can add another 400 IU during the week before your period.

Bioflavonoids

The bioflavonoids quercetin, grapeseed extract, and hesperidin are all good choices.

Copper, Zinc, Manganese, Selenium, and Chromium

These minerals should either be present in your multivitamin supplement or taken as an additional supplement premenstrually. Chromium can help reduce sugar cravings. For those symptoms, take 200 mcg twice daily for the premenstrual week.

A NATURALLY HEALTHY URINARY TRACT

Urinary tract infections (UTIs) are one of the most common and painful infections that can plague women. Chronic UTIs are poorly handled by mainstream medicine. Most women get at least one UTI during the course of their lifetime, and it is estimated that as many as 20 percent of all women suffer from chronic UTIs.

A UTI can be caused by trouble in the kidneys, the bladder, or the urethra, the tube leading from the bladder through which urine is excreted. Most often the symptoms are caused by a bacterial infection in the urethra or bladder.

One of the first symptoms of a UTI can be a burning or cramping sensation in the lower abdomen or behind the pelvic bone. Other symptoms of a UTI are a burning pain on urination; urgency, or the feeling of a strong need to urinate frequently (but only a small amount of urine is voided); foul-smelling urine; or blood and/or pus in the urine. Symptoms such as vomiting, chills, and low back pain may be a sign that the kidneys are involved. It is important to see a doctor if you have blood in your urine, vomiting, a high fever, or chills.

The vast majority of UTIs are caused by bacteria that find their way up the urethra from the genital area, resulting in bladder infection, but this is only part of the story. For an infection to take hold, the urinary tract has to be out of balance.

One of the primary functions of the kidneys and bladder is to eliminate bacteria from the body, so bacteria usually are washed out of the urethra when you urinate. In fact, urine itself will usually kill bacteria. A bladder infection usually involves some type of blockage or pooling of urine in the bladder. Thus, it's clear that an imbalance must be present to create a UTI.

One such imbalance may be in the pH of the urine, or the acid/alkaline balance. Stress, poor diet, and some medications, such as antibiotics, can throw off the pH of the urinary tract, creating a susceptibility to infection.

Too much protein is one of the biggest dietary offenders when it comes to UTIs. A high-protein diet produces an acidic condition in the body, which creates a high stress load on the kidneys. If the kidneys can't keep up, a UTI often results. Sugar will also aggravate a UTI, so it's important to avoid sweets while you're healing an infection or if you're susceptible to chronic UTIs.

Pregnancy, diabetes, and a sudden increase in sexual activity can also trigger UTIs. Other contributing factors can be chronic dehydration; resisting the urge to urinate and delaying urination; diaphragms used for birth control; a yeast infection; tight pants; or sports such as horseback riding and bicycling, which may force bacteria up the urethra, irritate the urethra,

or block the flow of urine. It is also important to urinate soon after having sexual intercourse.

If your immune system is compromised by stress, poor nutrition, alcohol or drug abuse, excessive caffeine, and excessive sugar, it makes it much easier for a UTI to find a hold in your body.

Some UTIs occur primarily in menopausal women. They are caused not by a bacterial infection but by an estrogen deficiency that thins the tissue of the vagina and urethra and shrinks the genitalia. The thinning of tissue can cause easy bruising and tissue damage, creating the symptoms typical of a UTI. These symptoms can often be cured with a *natural* estrogen cream applied topically in the genital area.

Mainstream medicine tends to treat urinary tract infections with antibiotics, but in chronic cases with underlying imbalances, antibiotics only cause rebound infections and compromise the immune system as well as upsetting the digestive system. Antibiotics also encourage yeast infections, which can precipitate a UTI! So don't resort to antibiotics unless the kidneys are involved or the infection is serious.

Your best treatment for a UTI is prevention, but if you do get a UTI, there are some safe, natural remedies you can try. But sure to see a health care professional if the symptoms are severe for more than a few days, if there is blood in your urine, or if you have a high fever, chills, and pain in your kidneys or lower back.

One of the simplest and most important remedies is to drink plenty of clean water, up to six to eight glasses a day. This may seem like the last thing you'd want to do when it hurts to urinate, but you need the cleansing action of water.

Herbal Diuretics

Diuretics help encourage the flow of fluids through the kidneys, which cleanses the urinary tract. Diuretics should be used in moderation, since you don't want to overstress the urinary tract.

Uva-Ursi (Arctostaphylos uva-ursi)

This herb is an honored old folk remedy for UTIs. It acts as a diuretic, antibacterial agent, and astringent.

A tea is the most recommended way to take it, but tinctures and capsules are also available. Do not take more than the recommended dose of bearberry (uva-ursi), as it can be toxic at high doses.

Parsley (Petroselinum sativum)

This herb is also a diuretic and it contains nourishing chlorophyll and minerals that are healing to the urinary tract. It also happens to be good for digestion and is a wonderful breath freshener. Do not drink parsley tea if you are pregnant or trying to become pregnant.

Herbs That Fight Infection

Echinacea (Echinacea angustifolia) and Goldenseal (Hydrastis canadensis)

These herbs are powerful immunostimulants. Goldenseal is soothing to mucous membranes and has antibacterial properties, so it is well worth trying in place of antibiotics if the infection is not serious.

Garlic (Allium sativum)

Garlic is a potent antibacterial agent, especially against one of the most common UTI invaders, *Escherichia coli*. Put raw garlic in your salad, use it in cooking, or—if you don't like the odor—take the odorless capsules.

Cranberry Juice

For decades, the medical profession pooh-poohed the use of cranberry juice for fighting UTIs, but women never stopped using it because it's such an effective remedy. Finally, some studies were done showing that indeed, cranberry juice was effective in clearing up UTIs. The original theory was that cranberry juice acidified the urine, but scientists have since discovered that a substance in the cranberry prevents bacteria from clinging to the wall of the urethra, allowing them to be washed out during urination. Please don't buy cranberry juice heavily sweetened with sugars, including corn syrup or fructose, which will negate any good the cranberry is doing. Either mix it with the smallest possible amount of a sweeter juice, such as grape juice, or water it down enough so that you can drink it unsweetened. Drink at least two 8-ounce glasses a day.

Warm Baths and Compresses

A warm bath with aromatic oils or soothing minerals can work wonders to speed the healing process of a urinary tract infection. A hot water bottle or warm compress on the lower abdomen can also help relieve pain and soothe inflammation.

A NATURALLY HEALTHY PREMENOPAUSE

Many women nearing menopausal age continue to menstruate but stop ovulating. This is a setup for what Dr. John Lee has coined "premenopause syndrome," caused by progesterone lack and estrogen excess. (See the section on hormones, page 165, for details). Anovulatory cycles may begin as early as a woman's early thirties and can be a setup for years of seemingly undiagnosable symptoms.

A woman who is not ovulating can still be menstruating—she is still producing enough estrogen to cause the buildup of tissue in the uterus—but if she doesn't ovulate, she won't be producing any progesterone.

Premenopause syndrome is particularly apt to occur in highly stressed women who are trying to maintain a career, a family, and a marriage. Weight gain, bloating, depression, mood swings, cold hands and feet, irritability, blood sugar imbalances, and fatigue are among the symptoms of premenopause syndrome. Infertility, endometriosis, uterine fibroids, and fibrocystic breasts may also appear in women who have stopped ovulating. Premenopause syndrome is also a setup for osteoporosis, as the lack of progesterone, a hormone that stimulates bone growth, will result in loss of bone and decreased bone density. (The fact that osteoporosis begins at least a decade short of menopause is well documented.)

If premenopause symptoms are being caused by anovulatory cycles, then the straightforward solution is to supplement the body with natural progesterone in the form of a cream. Because progesterone is fat soluble, it is easily absorbed through the skin. The cream can be rubbed anywhere on the body, but areas where the skin is thin, such as the palms, inner arms, sides of the torso, and upper inner thighs, are probably best.

A progesterone cream delivers a fairly reliable dose. Oral progesterone is more problematic because most of it is promptly excreted by the liver before having any effect on the body. Therefore, to get a proper dose of 30–40 mg of progesterone daily, you have to take 100–200 mg of oral progesterone in the hope that the liver will miss a small percentage of it. However, depending on diet, liver function, the toxin load on the liver, and many other factors, the dose you actually get is unpredictable, and it is very easy to get too much progesterone, resulting in sleepiness. In addition, oral progesterone puts the liver to a lot of unnecessary work.

The progesterone cream should be used from day 12 to day 26 or 28 of the menstrual cycle (the first day of menstruation is day 1). When you stop using it, menstruation should begin within forty-eight hours. But do not use progesterone cream without professional guidance if you are trying to get pregnant, since progesterone can influence ovulation, and the abrupt cessation of daily progesterone cream usually brings on menstruation.

It is vital that you follow the dietary and lifestyle advice given earlier in this chapter. The use of progesterone cream is addressing a symptom underlying a deeper problem that is blocking ovulation. Premenopause syndrome is a signal from the body that it is out of balance, and you need to address that imbalance on many levels.

For a detailed explanation of premenopause syndrome and other women's hormone balance issues, as well as detailed descriptions of how to use natural progesterone, I highly recommend the books *What Your Doctor May Not Tell You About Menopause: The Breakthrough Book on Natural Progesterone* (Warner Books, 1996) and *What Your Doctor May Not Tell You About Premenopause* (Warner Books, 1999) by John R. Lee, MD.

Herbs for Premenopause

Black Cohosh (Cimicifuga racemosa)

See page 171.

Dong Quai (Angelica sinensis)

See page 174.

Vitex/Chasteberry (Vitex agnus-castus)

See pages 171–172.

Yellow Dock (Rumex crispus) and Milk Thistle (Silybum marianum)

See pages 172 and 177.

Supplements for Premenopause

Essential Fatty Acids (EFAs)

EFAs can significantly help relieve premenopause symptoms. Take a supplement with a 2-to-1 ratio of EPA oils to GLA oils.

Vitamin B$_6$

Take 50 mg two times a day between meals. (See page 172.)

B Complex

B-complex vitamins can help with the mental and emotional symptoms of premenopause syndrome. Take a B-50 complex in addition to your regular vitamins.

Calcium and Magnesium

These minerals counteract the fatigue and weakness that can accompany premenopause. Be sure you're getting 1,200 mg of calcium and 400–500 mg of magnesium daily. You can double your magnesium intake the week before your period. Be sure to take it in a buffered form or it can cause diarrhea.

Vitamin E

This vitamin has been shown to help balance women's hormones to some degree. You should be taking 400 IU as part of your daily vitamin regimen, and you can add 400 IU when you have symptoms.

Bioflavonoids

Bioflavonoids can help reduce inflammation and relieve fatigue and weakness. Try quercetin, grape-seed extract, or hesperidin.

Copper, Zinc, Manganese, Selenium, and Chromium

These minerals should either be present in your multivitamin supplement or taken as an additional supplement premenstrually. Take 200 mcg of chromium twice daily in the week before your period to fight off sugar cravings.

A NATURALLY HEALTHY MENOPAUSE

Nothing gets commercialized faster or cashed in on faster in medicine than women's health problems. Pregnancy has been treated like a disease for nearly a century, and as a result, the United States has one of the highest infant mortality rates in the industrialized world. Menopause, too, has been regarded as a disease to be treated. The result? Nearly half a million unnecessary hysterectomies are performed every year in the United States, condemning those women to a lifetime of hormone replacement therapy. This all adds up to a steady source of cash flow for drug companies and doctors but a source of side effects and greater susceptibility to disease for the women.

Since the 1960s, the drug companies have been trying to convince doctors and women that menopause is, as Dr. John Lee has coined it, "an estrogen deficiency disease" that needs to be treated with synthetic, not-found-in-nature hormones. Menopausal women are at higher risk of heart disease and osteoporosis, but I promise you, estrogen is not the solution. After an initial period of feeling better, estrogen and the synthetic progestins cause most women to feel as if they have permanent PMS. The synthetic hormones prescribed by most doctors do vastly more harm than good, and their ability to protect against heart disease and osteoporosis is grossly exaggerated by drug companies.

The problems associated with menopause are also grossly exaggerated by the drug companies and the media. In truth, it is women who have had a hysterectomy (instant menopause) who have the most problems. The vast majority of other women pass through menopause relatively uneventfully.

The Real Story on Estrogen

Estrogen has been touted by the drug companies and the media as an elixir of youth, but in fact, estrogen is more like the grim reaper. Progesterone levels actually drop much more dramatically at menopause than estrogen levels do, and this accounts for more of the menopausal symptoms than a drop in estrogen does.

Most articles on hormone replacement therapy do not distinguish between estrogen therapy alone and estrogen combined with the synthetic progestins. Most of the beneficial side effects attributed to estrogen are, in reality, more likely attributable to the progestins. Estrogen causes weight gain, bloating, headaches, irritability, depression, tender breasts, fatigue, thinning of scalp hair, foggy thinking, decreased libido, and (most life threatening) an increased risk of strokes. Adding the progestins to the mix gives some benefits, but once again you get bloating, headaches, weight gain, breast tenderness, and depression. You also get migraines, asthma, breakthrough bleeding, liver damage, decreased glucose tolerance, excess hair growth, and an increased risk of stroke. Furthermore, *every* risk factor for breast cancer is directly or indirectly related to estrogen.

As I mentioned earlier in this chapter there is a vast difference between the synthetic progestins and natural progesterone as made by the ovaries. The progestins have a long list of negative side effects, including possible miscarriage and fetal malformation, while progesterone is essential for a successful pregnancy. This alone should be a major clue to physicians and their patients that these two drugs are very, very different.

Sadly, very few studies have been done with progesterone, as it is a natural substance and therefore not patentable and profitable. Those that have been done show no side effects (aside from some sleepiness at very high doses), and many benefits, especially for menopausal women.

Does Estrogen Really Protect Against Heart Disease?

That estrogen protects against heart disease has become an accepted "fact" in mainstream medicine, but in reality there is little evidence to support this claim. We do know that estrogen can improve lipid profiles (raise HDL cholesterol and lower LDL cholesterol), but it's a big leap to say that it must therefore also protect against heart disease. Doctors do not (or should not) prescribe estrogen to women who are obese, are diabetic, have kidney or liver disease, are at a risk for cancer or stroke, or smoke cigarettes. Therefore, the women who took estrogen in the largest study purporting to show that estrogen reduces heart disease were, by elimination, a healthier group to begin with and less likely to have heart disease with or without the hormone replacement therapy. (Other studies also show that women who use hormone replacement therapy are more likely to be better educated and healthier.)

Furthermore, the women who took estrogen had a much higher risk of stroke, even though they were a healthier group. To the best of my knowledge, there are no other studies showing that estrogen or hormone replacement therapy of any kind truly reduces the risk of heart disease. Somehow, the fact that estrogen can increase the risk of stroke never makes it into the mainstream media.

It is very well known now that heart disease is one of the most preventable of all chronic diseases with diet and lifestyle changes. So why should a woman increase her risk of breast cancer by 46 percent and stroke by up to 75 percent and suffer from all the estrogen and progestin side effects when she can accomplish the same thing naturally and increase her quality of life in every way?

Natural Remedies for a Healthy Menopause

Now that you know the truth about estrogen and progesterone, it's easy to see why progesterone cream (not the synthetic progestins) is a far better choice for menopause symptoms. Sticking to a vegetable-rich, soy-rich diet without much added fat is also important for a smooth transition into menopause.

Women who keep their weight within reasonable limits, who keep their fat intake low and their vegetable intake high, and who get some regular exercise rarely suffer from distressing menopause symptoms. Those who add soy products such as soy milk and tofu to their daily diet are even less likely to complain about menopause symptoms. High soy consumption and low fat consumption are almost certainly the primary reasons that hot flashes and breast cancer are virtually unknown in Japan. For more on the amazing benefits of soy, refer to chapter 2.

Your best bet for preventing and relieving menopause symptoms such as hot flashes and vaginal dryness is plenty of exercise, clean water, and a nutrition-rich, low-fat diet emphasizing vegetables and soy products. Menopause symptoms are virtually nonexistent in Japan, where fat consumption is low and soy consumption is high.

Any woman with menopause symptoms such as hot flashes, night sweats, vaginal dryness, hair loss, dry skin, and decreased libido not relieved by the recommended lifestyle guidelines plus the supplements named here should try natural progesterone cream. Any woman at risk for heart disease or osteoporosis should also be using natural progesterone cream. Recent research indicates that natural progesterone may also be protective against breast cancer.

A menopausal woman can use progesterone cream as directed three weeks out of the month, with a week off to resensitize cell receptor sites. According to Dr. John Lee, a very small percentage of women may need a small amount of natural estrogen cream applied topically to relieve the symptoms of vaginal dryness and hot flashes. Only a small amount is needed, and after six months to a year, it can be *gradually* discontinued.

The herbs for menopausal symptoms are the same as those listed in the premenopause syndrome section on page 180.

NATURAL REMEDIES FOR OSTEOPOROSIS

Although cardiovascular disease is the leading cause of death among American women, osteoporosis is the disease they are most likely to develop as they age. Four out of ten white women in the United States will fracture a hip, spine, or forearm as a result of osteoporosis. As many as five out of ten will develop small fractures in their spine, causing great pain and a shrinking in height. This amounts to fifteen to twenty million people affected by a crippling and painful disease that is almost entirely preventable and reversible.

Osteoporosis is a gradual decrease in bone mass and density that can begin as early as the teen years. Bone mass should be at its peak in our late twenties or early thirties, but thanks to a poor diet and lack of exercise, many women are already losing bone in their twenties. Bone loss occurs more rapidly in women than in men, especially right around the time of menopause, when an abrupt drop in estrogen and progesterone accelerates bone loss.

When you think of your bones, you may imagine a dead skeleton, but your bones are living tissue, just like the rest of your body, and they need a good supply of nutrients and regular exercise. New bone is constantly being made, while old bone is being reabsorbed and excreted by the body. Our larger long bones, such as our arm bones and leg bones, are very dense, and they are completely replaced about every

ten to twelve years. Our less dense bones, such as our spine and the ends of our long bones, turn over every two to three years. Thus, as you can see, we always have the opportunity to be creating better bones for ourselves.

In osteoporosis, the old bone is being reabsorbed faster than new bone is being made, causing the bones to lose density and become thinner and more porous. The integrity and strength of our bones is related to bone mass and density. The bones of a woman with osteoporosis gradually become thinner and more fragile.

A progressive loss of bone mass may continue until the skeleton is no longer strong enough to support itself. When that happens, bones can spontaneously fracture. As bones become more fragile, falls or bumps that would not have hurt us before can cause a fracture. Bone loss seems to be most severe in the spine, wrists, and hips. Unfortunately, there are usually no signs or symptoms of osteoporosis until a fracture occurs.

We all hear about how having enough calcium in the diet and taking estrogen can help prevent osteoporosis, but there is a much bigger nutritional and lifestyle picture to look at when we are talking about preventing this bone-robbing disease. You'll be happy to know that for the vast majority of women, there is no need to take estrogen to prevent osteoporosis.

The most important element of bones is minerals. Without minerals, we don't have bones. The most important bone minerals are calcium, magnesium, potassium, phosphorus, and fluoride. Equally important is the balance between the minerals. Too much phosphorus or fluoride will create poor bone structure. (Nearly all of us already ingest too much fluoride.) Without enough magnesium, the calcium can't be absorbed into the bone. Vitamins are also involved. For example, vitamin B$_6$ works with magnesium to get calcium into your bones.

Some of the things that cause you to lose bone are coffee, alcohol, cigarette smoking, aluminum, diuretics, fluoride, and high-dose synthetic cortisones such as prednisone. The hormones testosterone, estrogen, and progesterone are also actively involved in the making and unmaking of bone.

Early Signs of Osteoporosis

- Sudden insomnia and restlessness
- Nightly leg and foot cramps
- Persistent low back pain
- Gum disease, loose teeth
- Gradual loss of height

How Aware of Osteoporosis Are You?

A Gallup poll sponsored by the National Osteoporosis Foundation found that:

- 75 percent of women believed that they were knowledgeable about osteoporosis, *but*:
- 80 percent were not aware that it was responsible for disabling fractures,
- 90 percent were surprised to learn that osteoporosis frequently causes death, and
- 60 percent could not identify the risk factors of osteoporosis.

Your Risk of Osteoporosis Is Higher If You:

- Are a woman
- Have a family history of osteoporosis
- Are white
- Are thin
- Are short
- Went into menopause early
- Have a low calcium intake
- Don't exercise
- Smoke cigarettes
- Drink more than two alcohol drinks daily
- Are on chronic steroid therapy (for example, prednisone)
- Are on chronic anticonvulsant therapy
- Are taking drugs that can cause dizziness
- Are hyperthyroid
- Eat too much animal protein
- Use antacids regularly
- Drink more than two cups of coffee daily

Testosterone and progesterone build bone, while estrogen appears to indirectly slow bone loss.

Will Hormone Replacement Therapy Prevent Osteoporosis?

There is a misconception that osteoporosis begins at menopause. According to Dr. John Lee, bone mass begins declining in most women in their mid-thirties, accelerates for three to five years around the time of menopause, and then continues to decline at the rate of about 1 to 1.5 percent per year.

Because bone loss accelerates at menopause, and because estrogen levels decline at menopause, conventional medicine has adopted the belief that osteoporosis is an estrogen deficiency disease that can be cured with estrogen replacement therapy. This is only partly true. Once again, thanks to the courageous and pioneering work of Dr. John Lee, we have found that the missing piece of this puzzle is diet and lifestyle, plus the bone-building hor-

mone progesterone, which drops much more precipitously at menopause than estrogen does. (When I refer to progesterone, I mean the natural hormone, not the synthetic progestins.) There is no question that estrogen can slow bone loss around the time of menopause, but the scientific evidence is very clear that after five to six years, bone loss continues at the same rate, with or without estrogen.

A very large study published in the *New England Journal of Medicine* in 1995 analyzed the risk factors for hip fractures in white women. The study, which followed over 9,500 women for eight years, found no benefit in estrogen supplementation in women over the age of sixty-five. As Dr. Lee has pointed out, if estrogen was the only known treatment for osteoporosis, it might be worth taking it to get the small saving in bone density, despite all the risks and side effects. But since it's clear that progesterone, combined with proper diet and exercise, steadily increases bone density regardless of age, there are *very* few women who should ever need to take estrogen for osteoporosis.

Dr. Lee has suggested that the most important factor in osteoporosis is a lack of progesterone, which causes a decrease in new bone formation. He and others have extensive clinical experience showing that using a natural progesterone cream will actively increase bone mass and density and can *reverse* osteoporosis. After treating hundreds of patients with osteoporosis over a period of fifteen years, Dr. Lee found that those women with the lowest bone densities experienced the greatest relative improvement, and those who had good bone density to begin with maintained their strong bones.

Postmenopausal women using a transdermal (on the skin) progesterone cream or oil should use the equivalent of 20–40 mg daily for three weeks out of the month, with a week off each month to maintain the sensitivity of the progesterone receptors.

Dietary Guidelines to Prevent Osteoporosis

Getting adequate calcium is only a small part of the dietary prevention picture for osteoporosis. Slowing the excretion of calcium is much more important than getting enough calcium in the diet. The primary factors in calcium depletion in American women are high-protein diets, soda pop, and antacids. Advertising that antacids can be taken for their calcium is false advertising, because antacids actually deplete calcium, so at best you're replacing what you lose when you take the antacid.

It is important for women to make sure they're getting adequate calcium. Some good food sources of calcium are snow peas; broccoli; green leafy vegetables, such as spinach, kale, and beet and turnip greens; almonds; figs; beans (soybeans are best); and nonfat milk, yogurt, and cottage cheese. Don't depend on milk to get your calcium, because milk has a poor calcium-to-magnesium ratio. Your body needs a certain amount of magnesium to get the calcium into your bones. Without magnesium, calcium can't build strong bones.

In fact, magnesium deficiency may be more common in women with osteoporosis than calcium deficiency. Although many fruits and vegetables contain some magnesium, especially good sources of magnesium are whole grains, wheat bran, leafy green vegetables, nuts (almonds are a very rich source of magnesium and calcium), beans, bananas, and apricots.

Trace minerals are also important in helping your body absorb calcium. Eating plenty of green leafy vegetables gives you calcium along with these helpful trace minerals. Boron and manganese are especially important. Foods that contain boron include apples, legumes, almonds, pears, and green leafy vegetables. Foods that include manganese include ginger, buckwheat, and oats.

Collagen is the tissue that makes up your bone. To build collagen, you need vitamin A (beta-carotene), zinc, and vitamin C. Vitamin C is especially important, as it is the primary ingredient in the collagen matrix. I recommend that you take 1,000–2,000 mg daily of vitamin C in an esterified form to prevent stomach problems.

Use 'Em or Lose 'Em

Lack of exercise is one of the primary causes of osteoporosis. Using your bones keeps them strong and healthy. Weight-bearing exercise is the only thing besides progesterone found to actually *increase* bone density in older women. By weight-bearing, I mean exercise that uses your bones. Brisk walking counts as weight-bearing exercise, but add some light hand-held weights and it's even better. Pushing a vacuum cleaner or lawn mower, gardening, dancing, and aerobic dance also qualify.

Your exercise plan should include a minimum of twenty minutes of weight-bearing exercise three to four times a week. An hour is even better. In contrast to women who exercise, those who don't continue to lose bone, regardless of what else they are doing. Studies of elderly people who fall and break a bone show that these people had poor flexibility, poor leg strength, instability when first standing, and difficulty getting up from and sitting down in a chair.

Exercise can help increase flexibility, strength, and coordination. A weight-lifting program of just half an hour three or four times a week can significantly improve bone density. You don't need to go to the gym to do a weight-lifting program. You can lift a can of peas or a small carton of milk.

Women with advanced osteoporosis should work with a physical therapist to create a safe, effective program to reduce the risk of fracture. The Asian movement exercises such as yoga, tai chi, and chi gong are also excellent for improving strength, flexibility, and coordination.

Sunshine Is the Best Medicine

Vitamin D is another important ingredient in the recipe for strong bones because it stimulates the absorption of calcium. A deficiency of vitamin D can cause calcium loss. The best way to get vitamin D is from direct sunlight on the skin. Sunlight stimulates a chain of events in the skin leading to the production of vitamin D in the liver and kidneys. (This is why liver and kidney disease can produce a vitamin D deficiency.) Going outside for just a few minutes a day can give us all the vitamin D we need, and yet many people don't even do that. They go from their home, to their car, to their office, and back home, without spending more than a few seconds outdoors. Many elderly people are unable to get outside without assistance, but this should be a priority for their caregivers.

Supplements for Bone Building

Women concerned about osteoporosis should take the following supplements:

- Calcium, 1,200–1,500 mg daily with meals
- Magnesium glycinate, 600–900 mg daily with meals
- Folic acid, 200 mcg daily
- Vitamin C, 1,000–2,000 mg twice daily
- Vitamin B_6, 50–100 mg daily between meals
- Zinc, 15 mg daily with meals
- Beta-carotene, 15,000 IU daily
- Trace minerals, including 1–3 mg of boron and manganese daily

In addition, the herbs oat straw (*Avena sativa*) and horsetail (*Equisetum arvense*) are high in silica, which enhances calcium absorption.

8 NATURAL HEALTH FOR MEN ~

GETTING REACQUAINTED WITH THE MALE ANATOMY

With his best-selling book *Men Are from Mars, Women Are from Venus*, author John Gray created a new vocabulary of male-female relationships based on the differences between the sexes. While some of these differences stem from cultural values, most are based on the biological facts of anatomy and hormones. Although as human beings the sexes are more alike than different, men do have unique physical attributes, challenges, and concerns.

Testosterone: The Male Hormone

Testosterone is the hormone that transforms a boy into a man. Men produce ten times more testosterone in their bodies than women do. Most of it is produced in the testes, but some is also produced in the adrenal glands.

Testosterone levels in a male during fetal development in the womb are higher than they are from shortly after birth until puberty. When the fetus is only four weeks old, testosterone begins to stimulate the growth of the penis, testes, scrotum, and prostate gland and suppress the growth of female characteristics. Testosterone also causes the testes to descend into the scrotum.

When a boy reaches puberty, increased levels of testosterone cause his penis and scrotum to enlarge by eight to ten times. At the same time, his voice becomes deeper, his skin becomes thicker, the amount of hair on his body increases, and his muscles become better defined. Testosterone is also responsible for male pattern baldness and men's tendency to be more aggressive than

women. For more information on men and hormones, I recommend the book *A Woman's Guide to Male Menopause* by Marc Rose, MD (Keats Publishing, 2000).

The Testes: The Male Reproductive Organ

The testes in the man are essentially the same organs as the ovaries in the woman. In fact, if you look at an anatomical drawing, they appear nearly identical in outer shape, except that the ovaries sit up in the abdomen, whereas testes hang down between the legs in a sac called the scrotum. However, a key difference is that the ovaries produce relatively large amounts of estrogen and progesterone, while the testes produce relatively large amounts of testosterone.

The testes have two jobs to do in the male body: to participate in the production of sperm and to secrete hormones into the bloodstream. If there is a deficiency of testosterone or an excess of estrogen, the testes may not descend. Some 10 percent of boys are born with an undescended testicle, but 97 percent of them descend within a few weeks of birth. Of those that don't descend in infancy, the vast majority descend under the influence of increased testosterone at puberty. An undescended testicle will produce hormones, but it won't produce viable sperm. A testicle that doesn't descend by about the age of five usually won't be able to produce live sperm.

The testes rest in a loose sac of skin called the scrotal sac. There is a good biological reason for the testes to be located outside the body: Sperm develop better in temperatures that are lower than body temperature. If the temperature drops too much, special muscles pull the testes back up into the body. If the temperature goes too high, the testes drop more.

Men who are concerned about their fertility should wear all-cotton boxer shorts and avoid hot baths to keep from overheating the testes.

Xenoestrogens and Their Effect on Men

Because boys produce minimal amounts of testosterone, the presence of an undescended testicle after infancy would suggest the presence of excess estrogen.

Some herbalists recommend saw palmetto for boys with an undescended testicle to enhance the activity of the small amount of testosterone present in a young boy. I strongly recommend that boys with an undescended testicle avoid environmental estrogens, known as xenoestrogens, as much as possible. Pervasive petrochemical pollution has dropped us all into a sea of xenoestrogens, and the long-term consequences for men are devastating. The rate of undescended testicles in boys has doubled since the end of World War II, when petrochemical products and by-products, including pesticides, plastics, and air pollution, were introduced into our environment. During that same period, men's sperm count has dropped by half, with a corresponding rise in infertility. Some studies indicate that an undescended testicle has a much higher risk of becoming cancerous in adulthood.

Testicular cancer, which tends to strike men between the ages of thirty-five and fifty and is the most common type of cancer among men aged fifteen to thirty-five, has quadrupled since the 1940s. Biopsies done on testicular tumors in children show the presence of abnormal fetal-like cells, suggesting that whatever went awry had its source in the womb. Studies of reproductive abnormalities in animals such as seagulls demonstrate that exposure to excessive estrogen in the womb causes reproductive abnormalities in the offspring. While the predisposition to testicular cancer may be genetic, or begin in the womb, living a healthy lifestyle and avoiding xenoestrogens are the best preventive strategies men can employ.

How to Avoid Xenoestrogens

While no one source of normal exposure to xenoestrogens is likely to cause estrogen excess, it has a cumulative effect, as we are exposed to it in many small doses. Avoiding xenoestrogens involves avoiding all meat and fowl unless you know for sure that it is organic, meaning raised without hormones. Nearly all livestock raised for eating in the United States is given estrogenlike substances to increase fat content.

Pesticides, herbicides, and fungicides, which can act as potent xenoestrogens in the body in very small amounts, must also be avoided. This means no lawn or garden sprays, no bug sprays or flea bombs of any kind, and organically grown—without the customary application of pesticides or artificial fertilizers—fruits and vegetables.

Many soaps, including laundry soaps and dish soaps, contain substances called nonylphenols, which are surfactants that also act as potent xenoestrogens. I recommend that you look in your health food store for environmentally friendly "green" products without nonylphenols.

Many types of plastic shed xenoestrogens, so avoid heating or cooking in plastic.

At the same time, it is important to eat vegetables, which contain phytoestrogens. This type of plant estrogen will take up estrogen receptors in the body, effectively blocking the action of xenoestrogens.

Sperm and Semen

Sperm are manufactured in the testes, but they don't leave the body directly from there. First they make their way to the epididymis, a long tube attached to the back of each testicle, where each sperm picks up a tail, enabling it to swim. Then the sperm move on to another tube called the vas deferens, where they travel up into the groin, behind the bladder, and into the prostate. The sperm are stored in the end of the vas deferens until they enter the urethra at the time of ejaculation. On their journey from the vas deferens to the penis, sperm are mixed with various fluids from the prostate and the seminal vesicles. This fluid protects the sperm, makes them swim faster and harder, and makes the vagina more receptive. This mixture is called semen, or ejaculate. Semen is made up of fructose, glucose, citric acid, zinc, selenium, vitamin E, proteins, and enzymes.

Although sperm make up an extremely tiny percentage of ejaculate, just 3 percent, there are an average of four hundred million sperm in one batch of semen. Only a few will make it all the way to the waiting egg, which is gigantic in size compared to the sperm, and only one sperm will actually penetrate the egg and cause conception.

The Urethra and Penis

The tube descending from the bladder and out to the end of the penis and which carries both urine and semen is called the urethra. On its way to the penis, the urethra passes through the prostate gland, where it picks up fluids for semen during ejaculation. During ejaculation, a muscle in the urethra clamps down, blocking urine from the passageway. This also keeps semen headed down into the penis instead of back toward the bladder. You will hear a lot more about the urethra when we discuss the prostate.

The penis is made up of three cylindrical spongelike bodies that contain blood, the urethra, and the head, or glans, at the end. When the penis is erect, the spongelike bodies are engorged with blood, and the veins that carry blood out of the penis are constricted. The process of erection is under the involuntary control of the autonomic nervous system and can be brought about by psychological or physical stimuli. Interestingly, the penis can become erect through psychological stimulation alone, such as a daydream, or physical stimulation alone, such as masturbation. The glans is the part of the penis most sensitive to stimulation.

The average penis is about 3.5 inches long flaccid and 5 inches long erect, representing a 300 percent increase in volume! Men get an average of five erections a night. Contrary to popular notion, penis size doesn't vary much and has little to do with how large or tall a man is. Penis length *is* affected by obesity. Fat around the waist can, in effect, absorb the base of the penis, making it shorter.

HOW TO PREVENT IMPOTENCE

Impotence, or the inability to attain or maintain an erection, can be caused by either psychological or physical factors. Researchers estimate that some 25 percent of men over the age of fifty suffer from some form of impotence, also called erectile dysfunction. In older men, the cause of impotence is nearly always of physical origin.

There is something to be said for the axiom "Use it or lose it" when it comes to sexual function. Having regular sex may be one of the best deterrents to impotence. It stimulates circulation, hormones, and seminal secretions and brings energy to the genital area, not to mention the fact that it's fun, feels good, can be good exercise, and is an opportunity for closeness and intimacy with a loved one—always an important factor in good health. Masturbation certainly doesn't have all the benefits of having sex with another person, but it can be an important outlet when a sexual partner isn't available.

The four major physical causes of impotence are alcohol, cigarette smoking, prescription drugs, and the types of heart disease that produce clogged blood vessels. Other causes include poor diet—especially too much sugar—diabetes, hypothyroidism (low thyroid), excess estrogen, stress, and depression. According to research done at the Boston University School of Medicine, men who have heart disease, diabetes, or high blood pressure have four times the risk of becoming impotent as they age as do men who are free of these chronic diseases.

Avoid Alcohol

Alcohol interferes with many parts of the body related to sexual performance, and excessive alcohol use will actually shrink the testicles and lower your production of testosterone. Men who are under the influence of alcohol often think they are better lovers because their inhibitions are lowered, but their erections tend to be significantly softer, their coordination compromised, and their reflexes slower. Shakespeare probably said it best in *Macbeth* when he described alcohol as that which "provokes the desire, but . . . takes away the performance." Alcohol is also a vitamin robber, which can interfere with sexual performance over the long term.

Don't Smoke

Cigarettes interfere with sex drive and with erections via many mechanisms, including clogged blood vessels, poor physical condition, and poisoning from the wide array of toxins present in tobacco (most of these toxins are added by the tobacco companies, by the way). The nicotine in tobacco acts to constrict your blood vessels. Every cigarette smoked means less blood will reach the penis when it is stimulated. The Boston University research on impotence showed that even after being treated for heart disease, men who continued smoking had a 56 percent higher risk of becoming impotent, while those who didn't smoke only had a 21 percent risk. Men who quit smoking generally notice that they have firmer erections after just a few weeks.

Avoid Prescription Drugs

Many prescription drugs, particularly those prescribed for older men, can cause impotence. The vast majority of men should be able to remain sexually vigorous well into their eighties. My guess is that the myth that sex drive drops around the age of fifty has more to do with the drugs that doctors start handing out to men of that age rather than to any real physical incapability. This is one of the best reasons I can think of to live healthily and avoid prescription drugs if at all possible. Chronic problems such as high blood pressure and high cholesterol can almost always be solved with a healthy lifestyle and some nutritional and herbal supplements. Nearly every heart disease drug has a natural counterpart that doesn't cause side effects. Only a tiny percentage of men ever need to suffer from impotence due to prescription drugs.

If you're suffering from impotence and are taking a prescription drug, call your pharmacist or doctor and ask if one of the side effects of the drug is impotence. Combining one or more drugs can also cause unreported side effects, including impotence. If you're taking more than one drug, including over-the-counter drugs, it could be causing your impotence, even if that is not listed as a side effect.

Unclog Those Arteries

Clogged arteries are the leading cause of death in the United States, and they may also be the leading cause

---

Some Common Types of Drugs That Cause Impotence

- Antibiotics
- Antihistamines (for allergies and sinus congestion)
- Anticholinergics (used for ulcers and other gastrointestinal disorders, for nausea, for tremors caused by Parkinson's disease and psychiatric drugs, and sometimes for asthma)
- Anticonvulsants
- Antihypertensives (drugs that lower blood pressure)
- Antipsychotics
- H2 blockers such as Tagamet, Pepcid, and Zantac
- Sedatives and tranquilizers
- Many of the drugs used to treat heart disease, including beta-blockers, calcium channel blockers, ace inhibitors, and antiangina drugs
- Painkillers such as indomethacin, naproxen, and naltrexone

---

of impotence. Think about it. The physical mechanism of erection depends on blood flow. The arteries around your heart aren't the only ones that become clogged when you have heart disease. The arteries in your penis are suffering the same fate. In fact, impotence can be one of the first outward signs of clogged arteries.

Contrary to what mainstream medical doctors would have you believe, clogged arteries (and most types of heart disease for that matter) *are* reversible through good nutrition and a healthy lifestyle. This has been conclusively proven by Dr. Dean Ornish, who put his heart disease patients on an intensive heart-healthy lifestyle program and got excellent results.

America's poor diet contributes heavily to its rate of heart disease. We eat too much fat, too many processed foods, and not enough fresh vegetables. In the 1950s, the Japanese diet was 16 percent fat, and they had almost no incidence of heart disease.

Today, their diet is 26 percent fat, and heart disease is the second leading cause of death in Japan. In the United States, the average diet contains 36 to 40 percent fat.

Worldwide, cultures eating less meat and more fish, fruits, and vegetables and also drinking more wine have significantly lower rates of death from heart disease. Furthermore, there is a strong correlation between diets high in polyunsaturated fatty acids (vegetable oils prone to oxidation/rancidity) and a high rate of death from heart disease and correspondingly lower death rates in those cultures that consume more monounsaturated fats, such as olive oil.

Those countries with the highest intake of antioxidants and bioflavonoids have the lowest death rates from heart disease, with Japan having a much higher intake and a much lower rate of death than any other country.

Eat Right

A poor diet doesn't just clog your arteries; it also robs you of important vitamins, depletes cells of oxygen and energy, and creates blood sugar imbalances. One of your keys to a physically healthy sex life is good circulation, and a good diet and exercise are your keys to good circulation. In addition, men who have low HDL ("good") cholesterol have a much greater risk of being impotent than those who have normal or high HDL cholesterol. I'll talk about how to maximize your sex life by maximizing your diet a little later in this chapter.

Control Diabetes

Diabetes afflicts millions of Americans, and impotence is one of the most distressing side effects of this disease. The most tragic part of this scenario is that nearly all adult-onset diabetes can be prevented and even reversed, if caught early enough, with diet and lifestyle.

Because diabetes medication theoretically has to be taken every day for the rest of your life, it's a huge business that generates big bucks. That's why you don't hear much about people who beat diabetes by changing their lifestyle. And it's much easier for a doctor to prescribe a daily shot or pill to control your diabetes than it is for him or her to encourage you to lose weight, exercise, and start eating a nutritious diet. More than 90 percent of the diabetes in the United States is caused by obesity, poor diet, and lack of exercise. All of these causes are under your control, and it's a lot easier to prevent diabetes than it is to treat it once you have it.

In countries where people eat a diet low in fat and sugar and high in whole foods such as unrefined grains and fresh fruits and vegetables, diabetes is almost nonexistent.

Most mainstream doctors are unable to help their patients control their diabetes naturally because they don't understand the basics of nutrition. They recommend a high-carbohydrate diet that avoids sugars, but they fail to distinguish between refined carbohydrates and complex carbohydrates! If you eat pancakes, bread, or baked goods made from white flour, your blood sugar will rise almost as fast as it would if you just ate white sugar. It's important for diabetics to eat unrefined carbohydrates such as whole-grain bread, brown rice, and beans. If you have a hard time digesting whole grains, introduce them to your diet gradually, and eat them in small amounts. You don't need a lot of carbohydrates to stay healthy. What's more important is the *quality* of your carbohydrates.

I find it fascinating that the very nutrients that are stripped out of refined carbohydrates—chromium, zinc, manganese, and vanadium—are the same ones that are critical to maintaining stable blood sugar and are also the very ones that diabetics have been found to be deficient in. If you are at risk for diabetes or have adult-onset diabetes, the major focus of your diet should be fresh vegetables, legumes (such as beans and soy products) and nuts, followed by lean protein, unrefined carbohydrates, and small amounts of fresh fruits. Refined carbohydrates and sugar should never be consumed if you are at risk for diabetes or have it. Foods that raise blood sugar include refined sugar, refined grains, carrots, potatoes, processed cereals, raisins, pasta, yams, and oranges. Another key to maintaining a stable blood sugar and beating diabetes is keeping your weight down and getting plenty of exercise. That may sound tough, but isn't it tougher to suffer from the effects of diabetes, which include heart disease, blindness, and numbness in the extremities?

Herbs and Supplements That Help Control Diabetes

While it may not be possible for many diabetics to get off insulin completely, you can dramatically reduce your need for insulin by taking the following supplements. Your need for insulin can drop quickly if you follow my advice, and the less insulin you need, the less chance you'll suffer from the effects of diabetes. I can't stress enough that if you have diabetes, it is important to work with a health care professional who can help you monitor your blood sugar carefully as you take these steps. This program does work!

Chromium picolinate. Chromium picolinate works hand in hand with insulin to stabilize blood sugar. Take 200–600 mcg daily.

Vanadyl sulfate. This is a form of vanadium. Start at 6 mg and increase the dose until you get results, up to 100 mg daily. You can use this trace mineral, with chromium, to stabilize your blood sugar. At high doses, vanadyl can cause cramping and diarrhea; lower the dose if that happens, and don't use high doses for more than three weeks. Also, don't use vanadyl sulfate if you are hypoglycemic.

Zinc. This mineral will help your body use insulin more efficiently. Be sure you're getting 15 mg daily. Most multivitamins contain this amount.

Manganese. This mineral plays an important role in regulating blood sugar. You should be getting 2–5 mg daily. Check your multivitamin.

Onions and garlic. These foods can also help lower blood sugar naturally and should be a regular part of a diabetic's diet. Other herbs and foods that can help lower blood sugar include fenugreek seeds, ginseng, fresh berries, fish, soybeans, fresh vegetables, and cinnamon.

Control Hypothyroidism

The thyroid gland is one of your body's central command posts for regulating metabolism, the rate at which you generate energy in your body. Hypothyroidism is a deficiency in the production of thyroid hormones by the thyroid gland. It is more common in women than men, but when it afflicts men, one of its side effects can be a decrease in sex drive. Other symptoms of hypothyroidism are weakness, slow speech, cold hands and feet, unexplained gain in weight and difficulty losing it, fatigue, dry skin, and headaches.

Blood tests that check your thyroid levels may not accurately diagnose mild hypothyroidism. One of the best ways to find out whether your thyroid gland is up to par is to take your basal body temperature. This is your body temperature upon waking, before doing anything else, even sitting up. You take your basal body temperature by putting the thermometer under your armpit. Your basal body temperature should be between 97.8 and 98.2 degrees Fahrenheit.

If your temperature is low and you suspect that you may have hypothyroidism, the first thing to do is find out whether you're getting enough iodine in your diet. You only need very small amounts of iodine, 1 mg daily, but not getting it can seriously impact the functioning of your thyroid gland. Table salt that you buy in the supermarket has iodine in it, and if your salt consumption is normal, you should be getting plenty of iodine in your daily diet. If you're on a salt-restricted diet, you may not be getting enough iodine. Seafood is the best source of iodine.

Another way to boost your thyroid gland is to buy a desiccated thyroid supplement, which you can find at most health food stores. This may be enough to boost you out of a mild thyroid deficiency. If that doesn't help and you still suspect a thyroid deficiency, see a doctor for a prescription thyroid supplement.

Avoid Xenoestrogens

As mentioned earlier, petrochemical pollution has dropped us all into a sea of synthetic chemicals that behave like estrogen. These are the xenoestrogens. No one source of xenoestrogen is going to cause a man to grow breasts or show other signs of feminization, but the effects are cumulative and have an especially potent effect on a fetus.

I believe that the steadily rising rate of prostate enlargement, prostate cancer, testicular cancer, and infertility among men is due to chronic long-term exposure to xenoestrogens through meat, pesticides, plastic residues, and surfactants in soaps. One group of researchers in England even found that the estrogens excreted in the urine of women taking birth control pills were making their way intact through sewage treatment plants and into the food chain. Remember, estrogen is the female hormone, and its presence will actually oppose testosterone, in effect reducing testosterone levels.

Let's review the steps you can take to reduce your exposure to xenoestrogens:

- *Avoid all meat and fowl unless you know for sure it's organic*, meaning raised without hormones. Nearly all livestock raised for eating in the United States are given estrogenlike substances to increase fat content.
- *Avoid pesticides, herbicides, and fungicides*, which can act as potent xenoestrogens in the body in very small amounts. This means no lawn or garden sprays, no bug sprays or flea bombs of any kind, and only organic fruits and vegetables.
- *Avoid exposure to laundry soaps and dish soaps that contain substances called nonylphenols*, which are surfactants that also act as potent xenoestrogens. Instead use environmentally friendly, nonylphenol-free "green" products. Even though you do not eat or drink these substances, they are fat-soluble and will enter directly through your skin.
- *Avoid heating food or cooking in plastic, as many plastics shed.*
- *Eat plenty of fresh, organic vegetables and soy products*, which contain phytoestrogens. This type of plant estrogen will take up estrogen receptors in the body, effectively blocking or reducing the action of xenoestrogens. Soy is my favorite phytoestrogen.

These steps are especially important if you are trying to father a child, and they are also important for a woman who is trying to become pregnant or is pregnant. The most significant harm by xenoestrogens is caused by exposure in the womb, where it can cause reproductive abnormalities, particularly in males.

PRESCRIPTION FOR A LONG AND ACTIVE SEX LIFE

Why is it so difficult to change our unhealthy habits? By now you would have to live in a cave or on a mountaintop not to know that a high-fat diet of junk food is going to take you straight down the road to heart disease. Mainstream medicine considers it so difficult to change an unhealthy lifestyle that most doctors will write you a prescription for a drug they know has unpleasant side effects before they will even consider suggesting you lose weight and get some exercise. We could save billions of dollars every year in health care costs if we just changed our eating habits and our sedentary lifestyles a little bit.

Food is an emotionally charged subject. Our "comfort foods," which we eat when we're upset or stressed, are usually fat laden, sweet and soft, or salty and crunchy. In other words, what Americans reach for when they want a snack or when they're stressed, which is most of the time, is sugar, white flour, salt, and hydrogenated oils. When we eat a meal it often comes out of a can or a box and is stripped of its nutritional value, with a few token vitamins thrown back in. To add insult to injury, processed foods contain a veritable chemistry lab of additives, preservatives, and dyes, many of which cause allergic reactions.

Combine fatty, sugary, salty snacks and processed nutrition-free foods with little to no exercise, and you have a recipe for chronic illnesses such as arthritis, diabetes, and heart disease. Headaches, back pain, fatigue, depression, foggy thinking, memory loss, and high blood pressure are some other common effects of this type of diet. Lack of sex drive and impotence by the age of sixty are frequently the long-term consequences of the typical American lifestyle.

If you begin feeling the debilitating effects of the standard American diet when you're in your fifties, and your life expectancy is seventy-five, that gives you about twenty-five years of a less-than-optimal life, complete with drugs, surgeries, and chronic pain. But there is no reason to suffer that fate! You will be amazed at how dramatically your energy will pick up and how much better you'll feel emotionally and mentally when you start eating whole foods and getting some exercise. I call this a "high-potency" lifestyle!

When you change your lifestyle and start giving up the pastries and potato chips, it's important to do it gradually and give yourself substitute treats. You can't just yank away your favorite comfort foods and expect to experience success. For example, if you're working to give up sugary desserts after dinner, substitute your favorite sweet fruits, even if they're out of season and expensive. You're worth it, and it will help ease you out of the habit. (Please don't use the sugar substitute aspartame; it's a brain excitotoxin that is likely to cause more problems than it will solve.) If you're working to give up potato chips, substitute roasted nuts or seeds (fresh, not rancid), which may be equally high in fat but will spare you the hydrogenated oils found in snack foods and will add all kinds of good nutrition.

Can Water Improve Your Sex Life?

Water may be the cheapest, easiest way to improve your sex life. Americans are so chronically dehydrated that you'd think we lived in a desert and that water was a scarce commodity. In truth, clean water *is* scarce, and we often drink coffee, tea, and soft drinks instead of water. Drinking plenty of clean water is essential to good health. I recommend that everyone drink six to eight glasses a day.

And guess what, guys—I know this sounds too simple to be true, but drinking a tall glass of clean water half an hour or so before having sex can make all the difference in your ability to get and maintain an erection. It makes sense, doesn't it? Blood, which is what an erection is made of, is made primarily of water. If your body is dehydrated, it's not likely to give up some of its precious water for an erection. It's amazing what staying hydrated can do for your sex life.

Sugar Is a Sex Buster

I can't say enough bad things about sugar. It will do more to diminish your sex life than almost any other food (alcohol and drugs can do more harm, but they aren't foods). While glucose, a form of sugar, is essential to life, what Americans stuff into their bodies by the dozens of pounds every year in the form of white, refined sugar is not only *not* essential to life, it is detrimental to life and to good health.

Your body can make all the sugar it needs from carbohydrates, and we all get plenty of those when we eat grains, legumes, potatoes, rice, corn, and other starchy vegetables. The sugar we get from cakes, candies, ice cream, pastries, soft drinks, and dozens of other sources will contribute to heart disease, diabetes, and arthritis. It will make your capillaries "baggy" and less able to deliver oxygen and other nutrients to your cells. It will run your life because you'll always be looking for your next sugar fix to boost your flagging energy caused by your last sugar fix.

Do not fall for the advertising gimmick that refined fructose is not as bad a sugar as the others. It may even be worse, because there is evidence that it suppresses the immune system when eaten regularly. Sucrose and malt are also sugars. Regardless of how quickly or slowly your body processes a sugar, it's still a sugar. If you don't burn it off, it will add to your fat.

You can get away with occasional sugar snacks if you're athletic and burning off calories intensively. But if you're not burning off those sugar calories right away, they're not doing you any good. They are devoid of nutrition beyond supplying glucose to your brain and muscles (most of us have a more than adequate supply), and any energy benefit they give you will result in lower energy within half an hour to an hour.

I'm not against having a sweet now and then. But most Americans are addicted to sugar. If you're eating foods high in refined sugars more than a few times a week, kicking the sugar habit may be the single best thing you can do for your health.

Hydrogenated Oils Damage Arteries

I'm really down on the hydrogenated oils found in nearly every processed snack food in America. I'm convinced that they've contributed heavily to our astronomical rate of death from heart disease. These vegetable oils are chemically processed so that they're partially saturated to keep them from going rancid. They damage your arteries and take up receptor sites for the essential fatty acids so important to good health. These extremely harmful oils have been pushed on the public for years by the very powerful vegetable oil industry, to the great detriment of our national health.

Eating unprocessed vegetable oils isn't the answer, either, unless you're pressing them by hand in your home and using them immediately. Vegetable and nut oils (corn, safflower, peanut, soy) are very unstable polyunsaturated oils and go rancid easily. In fact, most vegetable oils are rancid before you even open the bottle, and they are certainly well on their way within a few days of exposure to air. Rancid oils smell bad, but even worse, they wreak havoc on your arteries by setting loose more free radicals than any amount of antioxidants can handle. And these free radicals proceed to damage your arteries. The body attempts to repair this damage with cholesterol, but if you have too much LDL, or "bad," cholesterol, the repair job will just act like a magnet for more LDL cholesterol.

Cholesterol in and of itself is not bad for you. In fact, it is necessary to good health. All of your steroid hormones (including testosterone) are made from cholesterol. Cut out too much cholesterol from your diet and you're likely to suffer from a low sex drive, fatigue, and depression. Your body manufactures about 75 percent of its own cholesterol, and the remaining 25 percent comes from diet. Any excess cholesterol is simply excreted in a healthy person and does not clog the arteries. What *is* bad for you is oxidized cholesterol, the kind that is created when it meets up with rancid oils and hydrogenated oils or when you're low on antioxidants.

Your best sources of healthy oil for everyday use are olive oil and canola oil. Olive oil is a stable monounsaturated fat that doesn't go rancid easily and in its unrefined form is packed with nutrition. It can improve "good" HDL cholesterol levels and doesn't break down when used in cooking at low heats. Canola oil is also a monounsaturated oil. Although it is processed to remove some harmful ingredients and is not packed with nutrition like olive oil is, it is a good choice for baking because it doesn't have much flavor and is a light oil.

Don't be scared of saturated fats, either. Saturated fat has been unjustly maligned by the vegetable oil industry. In truth, it's an *excess* of saturated fat that will contribute to heart disease. Moderate amounts of saturated fat are fine, as long as they're combined with plenty of fresh fruits and vegetables and exercise. Moderate means a maximum of one or two small portions (4 ounces) of red meat per week. Don't worry about eating coconut oil or meat; just eat them in small amounts. I like to keep my fat calories to about 25 percent of my calories, and my saturated fat intake is about 10 to 12 percent of that.

Too much fat will beef you up, but it won't beef up your sex life. In a study measuring fat consumption and testosterone levels, men who drank a fatty shake watched their testosterone levels drop by 30 percent within four hours.

Essential fatty acids (EFAs), on the other hand, are vital to good health. It's important to get your essential fatty acids by eating fish once or twice a week and by eating a variety of whole grains, fruits, vegetables, and legumes. Most Americans are badly deficient in EFAs, raising the risk of heart disease and arthritis because they're eating nutrition-free hydrogenated oils.

As I mentioned earlier, soy is one of my favorite phytoestrogen sources. I recommend that you incorporate it into your daily diet in place of red meat for many reasons. It is an excellent protein, it is packed with nutrition, and it contains substances that inhibit cancer and lower cholesterol. You can use soy milk instead of cow's milk, you can eat tofu with just about anything, you can eat miso soup, or you can use tempeh as a meat substitute.

Exercise Your Body to Rev Up Your Sex Life

Having sex takes a lot of energy, and the better shape your body is in, the better shape your sex life will be in. Exercise improves circulation, strengthens the heart and muscles, lowers blood pressure and cholesterol, helps the body rid itself of toxins, increases lung capacity, improves endurance, and gives you an overall feeling of well-being and energy. People who exercise tend to be bright-eyed and bushy-tailed, with a twinkle in the eye and a bounce in the step. Because I travel so much, my favorite form of exercise is brisk walking. I can do it anywhere, and 30 minutes a day four or five times a week keeps me fit and trim. You can ride a bike, weed the garden, rake the lawn, swim, take an aerobics or dance class, or do just about anything else that's enjoyable. Any type of moderate exercise that gets your heart going and makes you sweat a little will work fine.

Research supports the exercise-and-better-sex connection. In one study, a group of seventy-eight previously sedentary but healthy men (average age forty-eight) jogged or bicycled for an hour a day, 3.5 days per week. A control group of seventeen men did not get any regular strenuous or aerobic exercise. After just nine months, the exercise group had a 30 percent increase in the amount of time they had intercourse, with a 26 percent increase in their frequency of orgasms. The control group's rate of intercourse dropped in the same time span. Chances are, the exercise had myriad effects on these men, including an increase in self-esteem. They looked better and felt better; their blood pressure and cholesterol dropped; and they cut their body fat by 19 percent. Speeding up their metabolism with exercise may have also increased their testosterone levels.

Exercise is an excellent stress buster, and stress can put a real damper on your sex life. When you're under chronic stress, your body releases adrenal hormones that over time will throw your body chemistry out of balance. Adrenal hormones are meant for occasional use only—say, when a saber-toothed tiger is chasing you. When you call on them constantly, with no physical outlet, you're heading for trouble. Exercise is one of the best ways you can neutralize the physical damage stress can do, and it is also a powerful relaxant. However, if you overdo the exercise, it will affect your libido. Moderation is the watchword here.

If exercise isn't enough to de-stress your life, take classes in one of the Asian movement disciplines such as yoga, chi gong, or tai chi, which are easy to find these days nearly everywhere in North America.

Learning a form of meditation can also help in coping with stress.

HERBS AND SUPPLEMENTS FOR SEXUAL HEALTH

There is plenty you can do with herbs and supplements to spark your sex life. Sometimes a lack of libido can be caused by a simple nutritional deficiency or chronic dehydration. Something as simple as a vitamin E or zinc deficiency can contribute to low sex drive. In fact, having too much sex can deplete a man of zinc, which will in turn reduce sex drive. This seems to be nature's built-in mechanism for moderation.

Of course, my first recommendation for a healthy sex life is to follow the dietary and lifestyle changes discussed previously. But if you need a little extra jump start, something in the vitamin, mineral, amino acid, or herb department might be just the ticket.

Supplements for Sexual Health

As mentioned previously, stress will lower sex drive in even a physically healthy man. Constantly releasing stress hormones from the adrenal glands will deplete sex hormones. Both stress hormones and sex hormones, called steroid hormones, are made from cholesterol and use the same biochemical pathways. If adrenal hormones become exhausted, the sex hormones aren't far behind. Stress also interferes with digestion, making your body less able to absorb and utilize the nutrients you are getting from food and vitamins. And meanwhile, the stress hormones raise LDL cholesterol levels, adding insult to injury. You can support your adrenal glands by reducing stress, exercising, getting plenty of sleep, eating properly, and taking some vitamins.

There are many steps along the pathway to manufacturing your steroid hormones, and each one requires very specific vitamin and mineral cofactors. Some of the most important cofactor vitamins and minerals are the B vitamins, vitamins C and E, magnesium, and zinc. Also necessary, although in small amounts, are iron, molybdenum, and manganese.

Vitamins C and E

One researcher gave thirty-five infertile men 1,000 mg of vitamin C daily. Just the addition of this vitamin significantly increased their sperm counts. Vitamin E is the antioxidant of choice in the reproductive organs, protecting them from oxidation reactions.

Zinc and Selenium

A man's semen contains very high concentrations of zinc. It is estimated that when a young man ejaculates, he loses 1.4 mg of zinc. Low levels of zinc are correlated with infertility and low sex drive. The mineral selenium works with zinc in the male reproductive system, and low selenium is correlated with a low sperm count. Americans are chronically deficient in selenium because of our mineral-depleted soil, so this is an important mineral to be taking every day as a vitamin. Selenium is found naturally in deep green vegetables, onions, tomatoes, and whole grains.

Lecithin

Another nutrient found in high concentrations in semen is lecithin, an essential fatty substance found in the membranes of every cell in the body. Lecithin protects cells from oxidation, keeps them flexible, and helps dissolve cholesterol in the blood. It is a primary component of brain cells, nerve cells, and muscle cells. High concentrations of lecithin are found in the testicles. Lecithin is made of the B vitamins choline and inositol and also linoleic acid, an essential fatty acid found in olive, canola, and soy oils. Lecithin is found in meat, egg yolks, whole grains, seeds, and soy. You can buy lecithin as granules or in capsules at your health food store. The granules can be eaten plain or sprinkled on cereals, on salads, and in casseroles (after cooking). Avoid buying rancid lecithin, which will do you more harm than good. Lecithin should have a pleasant, nutty smell. I recommend 1 or 2 tablespoons of lecithin daily.

Magnesium

This mineral plays many diverse and important roles in the body, from acting as a cofactor for hundreds of biochemical reactions to regulating fluid balance within the cells. Magnesium is important in the production of steroid hormones, including testosterone. Americans tend to be chronically deficient in magnesium (and many other minerals) thanks to processed foods and depleted soils. I recommend that unless you're eating plenty of fresh, organic vegetables every day, you take 300 mg of magnesium daily. It's best taken in a buffered form, with food, or it can cause diarrhea.

Vitamin A

Vitamin A is so important to a healthy male reproductive system that a deficiency is actually known to cause shrinkage of the male sex organs. Vitamin A is essential in maintaining healthy tissues and acts as an antioxidant. Furthermore, you have learned how important the B vitamins are to male health, and most of our B vitamins are derived from protein. Without vitamin A, the body is unable to properly utilize protein. Because vitamin A as a supplement can accumulate in the body and become toxic, most people get their supply by taking beta-carotene, a precursor to the vitamin. You should be getting 15,000 IU of beta-carotene daily, which is about equal to one carrot. Most yellow and orange vegetables contain plenty of beta-carotene. Vitamin A is found in most fruits and vegetables, fish liver oil, and animal liver.

Coenzyme Q10

Coenzyme Q10 (CoQ10), an enzyme found in the body, can significantly raise your energy levels as well as protect and strengthen your heart, lower your blood pressure, and strengthen your immune system. CoQ10 is vital to the production of energy in our cells. Its chemical name is ubiquinone—it is ubiquitous, or everywhere, where there is life. Its levels in the human body are highest in the heart and liver. When we are ill or stressed, and also as we age, our bodies are less able to produce CoQ10. Many older people whose heart function has degenerated and who try CoQ10 report an almost immediate boost in their energy levels.

CoQ10 should come as a powder in a capsule and be a deep yellow color. The purity and quality of

CoQ10 does vary, and since it's not a cheap supplement, it pays to get a high-quality brand. I recommend 30–80 mg a day to boost energy and strengthen the heart.

Herbs for Sexual Health

There are three major categories of herbs for male sexual health. The first category consists of herbs that tone, strengthen, and rejuvenate the male reproductive system and bring an overall sense of energy. In Chinese medicine, these are called *yang* herbs. Yang is a way of describing male energy. These herbs can be thought of as tonic herbs. The second category of herbs consists of those that directly stimulate sexual energy and erections, which I'll call stimulatory herbs. The third category consists of those herbs that improve blood flow and circulation in general.

Tonic Herbs

Ashwagandha

Ashwagandha, an herb used in Ayurvedic medicine, is often called Indian ginseng. As well as being an immune system booster and improving memory and learning ability, it is used specifically to treat male impotence and infertility. In Ayurvedic medicine, it is taken as a root powder in warm milk.

Astragalus

Astragalus is widely used in China as a tonic herb that brings up the energy and increases metabolism. It strengthens the body, increases appetite, builds immune function, improves endurance, improves digestion, and supports such important organs as the adrenals, kidneys, and liver. In studies, astragalus was shown to improve sperm motility in a test tube. It can be taken as a tincture, as a tea, or in capsules, 500–1,500 mg daily.

Ginseng

Ginseng root is another plant medicine widely used all over Asia, especially in China and Korea. It has been extensively studied, and its properties are so unique that a new term was coined to describe it: "adaptogen," meaning an herb that balances whatever is out of balance in the body. If blood pressure is low, ginseng is a very stimulating herb, but without the "buzz" associated with caffeine and ephedrine, which also have the effect of constricting blood vessels. Ginseng helps stabilize blood sugar, lowers cholesterol, improves liver function, and is used extensively in China to support people who have been weakened by illness. Some studies show that ginseng increases sperm production and the production of testosterone and promotes the growth of the testes.

There are many types of ginseng, but the one most studied and widely available is *Panax ginseng*, originally from China. Siberian ginseng has similar properties. The major active ingredient in ginseng is a group of steroidlike substances called ginsenosides. The amount of ginsenosides in different ginseng preparations varies considerably. Look for a standardized product or one that guarantees its ginsenoside content.

Stimulatory Herbs

Yohimbe

Yohimbe is the only herb known to have a direct aphrodisiac effect, but it should be used with caution. The yohimbe tree is the source of an extract called yohimbine, the only herbal substance available by a doctor's prescription for treating impotence. However, this does not mean that it is safe or effective for everyone. Yohimbe can raise blood pressure and can interact with many types of drugs, including antihistamines, alcohol, tranquilizers, and sedatives. Some herbalists believe that it can aggravate an inflamed prostate gland. If you decide to try yohimbe, I suggest you do it under the supervision of a health care professional and be very cautious. It could be good for what ails you, or it could do more harm than good. If you purchase it at a health food store, buy a reputable brand, because its quality can vary widely. Follow the directions on the bottle.

Damiana

The leaves of the damiana plant have a long history of use as an aphrodisiac in Central America. It is thought to strengthen the nervous system, support the manufacture of hormones, and act as an antidepressant. Some researchers believe that damiana irritates the urethra slightly, thus sensitizing the penis and making it more responsive to stimulation. Its aphrodisiac action may also have to do with stimulating the production of testosterone or mimicking the action of testosterone. In Mexico, damiana is sold as a liqueur called Creme de Damiana. A tea made from damiana is a common drink in Central America.

Herbs That Improve Circulation and Blood Flow

Ginkgo Biloba

Ginkgo biloba is an ancient Chinese herb that comes from one of the most ancient species of trees on the planet. The Chinese have been using ginkgo leaf medicinally for at least five thousand years. They prize ginkgo leaves for their ability to improve blood flow to the brain, open up congested lungs, and improve blood flow to the extremities.

In the past decade or so, ginkgo has been the subject of over three hundred scientific studies. It is one of the most popular medicines in Europe, sold to an estimated ten million people there every year. GBE, a standardized ginkgo biloba extract, is a government-approved medicine in Germany and is covered by health insurance there. In general, ginkgo's healing abilities have to do with improving circulation and increasing the flow of oxygen to the brain and extremities.

In addition to promoting circulation to the extremities, ginkgo improves microcirculation, which is the blood flow into the tiny capillaries. Ginkgo relieves the symptoms of peripheral vascular disease, such as pains in the legs at night, cramps, numbness, and impotence.

The effects of ginkgo do not generally show up after a single dose. It is not used in massive quantities but in repeated doses that can produce beneficial effects over a relatively long period of time. The best way to take ginkgo is in a standardized liquid extract. GBE is a concentrated and semipurified extract designed to enhance ginkgo's health benefits and provide a consistent level of ginkgolides, the most active principles.

I recommend that you find a GBE extract with at least 24 percent ginkgo flavoglycosides. You can take two to three tablets daily with food or use the liquid preparations and take one to three dropperfuls up to three or four times a day, but check the label for recommendations.

Cayenne

Cayenne is one of those versatile herbs that serves as a wonderful spice, a good source of nutrition, and a powerful healing agent. Capsicum peppers and chili peppers have similar properties. The ingredient in peppers that makes them hot, called capsaicin, is widely used in alternative medicine and in Asian medicine.

Chili peppers are also high in vitamin A, the carotenoids such as beta-carotene, calcium, phosphorus, iron, potassium, thiamine, riboflavin, and niacin. It is helpful for male sexual health because it effectively stimulates circulation.

As a bonus, regular use of cayenne can reduce levels of "bad" LDL cholesterol and relieve the pain of arthritis. Studies have shown that capsaicin also reduces triglyceride levels, lowers blood pressure, and raises metabolism, making it easier to burn fat and lose weight.

You can add cayenne to your food or take it in capsule form.

IS YOUR PROSTATE HEALTHY?

After leading a prostate-healthy lifestyle, the next most important part of good prostate health is knowing when you're having prostate troubles. There are three basic types of prostate disease: benign prostatic hypertrophy or enlargement (BPH), prostatitis, and cancer of the prostate. You can self-diagnose up to a point, but only a thorough medical examination can precisely determine the condition of the prostate. However, when you go to a mainstream doctor for a medical exam of your prostate, you should be thoroughly versed on the subject, or you may wind up getting more treatment than you need. Your best bet is to find a naturopath, an MD with a focus on natural health, an osteopath, or a chiropractor.

Mainstream doctors in the United States are only just beginning to accept findings that show the role of nutrition, lifestyle, and environment in prostate gland health. Therefore, it is in your best interest to find a doctor you trust who does keep up with the latest data. A good doctor will agree that prostate trouble is not an inevitable part of growing old and that a conservative approach is the best approach nearly all the time.

A Brief Review of Prostate Anatomy

The prostate is a gland in men located at the neck of the bladder and urethra (the tube through which urine and semen pass on the way out of the body). When a male is born, the prostate is about the size of a grain of rice, and by the time he's in his twenties, it's about the size and shape of a chestnut. Starting at puberty, the gland produces a milky fluid that mixes with semen during ejaculation. The fluid is designed to prevent infection in the urethra, increase sperm motility (movement), and increase the alkalinity of the vagina.

The prostate stays about the same size until the age when some male hormones begin to decline (in most men, their fifties), and then the prostate begins to grow again. This is called benign prostatic hypertrophy (BPH). If the gland grows too much, it can begin to create problems.

How the Prostate Gland Causes Urination Problems

You used to be in line at the urinal wondering how that guy at the trough could take so long. Now you're the one holding up the line while your prostate is holding up the flow. The prostate is well positioned to pile on this kind of pressure. Nestling at the base of the bladder, the prostate encircles the urethra, the tube leading from the bladder. Prostate gland enlargement squeezes the urethra, blocking

---

Do You Have Any of These Symptoms? You May Have Prostate Trouble

- Coaxing, waiting—it takes a while to get the stream started.
- Weak flow, some stopping and starting—the stream is not very strong, drying and starting up again on its own, a condition known as *intermittency*.
- Dribbling—at the end of urination, a little involuntary flow continues.
- Frequency—the need to urinate often, even shortly after urinating, especially at night, when it is known as *nocturia*.
- Lack of relief—often the bladder feels unemptied, as urination fails to bring complete relief.
- Urgency—the need to urinate is strong, particularly at night.
- Swollen bladder—often noticeable when it causes abdominal swelling.
- Burning sensation on urination—a possible sign of infection, often stemming from prostate-caused bladder restriction.

---

the flow of urine and creating a list of possible symptoms. Half of all men in the United States over the age of forty will experience prostate enlargement. In some men it goes virtually unnoticed; in others it causes some or all of the symptoms of prostrate trouble.

Problems with urination can occur even without any prostate involvement. Inhibition about urinating in public, kidney trouble, and simple bladder infections can all cause difficulty. There is a very good chance that the prostate gland is a factor in persistent problems, however, once middle age is reached.

The overgrowth of prostate tissues means that the gland begins to push against the structures nearest to it. The inner prostate tissues begin to choke the neck of the urethra, restricting the flow of urine from the bladder. This eventually results in difficulty starting the flow of urine. It can also bring about a stop/start, weak flow of urine.

Growth of the outer or inner tissue of the prostate often leads to overall enlargement, causing the gland to begin to push against the bladder itself. This pressure can trigger the urge to urinate. Pressure leads to blockage of the bladder. The bladder fails to empty completely, urination feels unsatisfactory, and the need to urinate becomes frequent. The conditions are compounded, since the inner prostate is restricting urine flow, also making it difficult to empty the bladder.

When urine is trapped in the bladder, it becomes a breeding ground for bacteria, and infection can result. Infection produces a burning sensation on urination and bladder pain. Aside from infection, the bladder can swell, often seen as abdominal swelling. Blockage of the bladder can also lead to stiffening of its muscular wall as it compensates for the pressure exerted by the prostate gland. If the bladder wall becomes less flexible, then the volume of urine exerts a greater pressure than usual, creating another reason why the urge to urinate is felt more often, particularly at night.

Some men resort to diuretic drugs in an attempt to resolve urinary problems caused by prostate enlargement. This is a bad idea, since the trouble is essentially a blockage that cannot be flushed away. In fact, diuretics usually aggravate the condition, as the poor bladder is put under even greater pressure with no relief possible. That said, there are specific diuretic herbal remedies that also have other healing properties that can be of help in the case of an inflamed prostate. For straightforward urinary trouble, stick to healthy food and selected supplements.

The average man can go 4 to 5 hours between trips to the bathroom, for a total of five or six trips in 24 hours. Men who drink diuretics such as coffee or who take in a lot of fluids urinate more frequently. Cold weather causes increased frequency as blood vessels constrict and less blood circulates, creating less demand for water, which is therefore excreted. Cold also makes bladder muscles constrict, which increases the pressure of its contents, producing the urge to urinate at smaller volumes than usual.

Age can also bring increased frequency as the kidneys require more water to flush out excess salt.

Old age can also bring a slower flow if musculature becomes "baggy" or weakened.

Other Symptoms of Prostate Problems

Aside from urinary problems, enlargement of the prostate gland is usually pain free. However, there are a few other symptoms that can indicate prostate problems, and every man should be aware of them.

If the prostate itself becomes inflamed, it can cause a dull, constant ache between the anus and the back of the scrotum. Pain can also radiate to the groin, the back, and the legs.

Prostate blockage can cause infection in the urinary tract. The infection can be carried to a kidney, which will cause pain in one side of the back below the kidneys. Pain from a kidney infection can also be felt in the testicle on the same side. Painful testicle infection itself can occur when infection travels from the prostate gland.

Prostate or bladder infection can cause pain in the lower abdomen. Most lower abdominal pain associated with the prostate gland occurs with retention of urine. The bladder becomes overfull and painfully distended over the course of a few days.

Blood at the beginning or end of the urinary stream is often due to problems with the prostate or urethra. Conditions arising with the kidneys or bladder tend to cause blood in the entire urinary stream. Blood is also sometimes seen in semen and usually stems from infection of the seminal vesicles or prostate.

Always seek medical advice for these sorts of symptoms as soon as possible. A good doctor will investigate possible prostatic origins as an underlying cause.

BENIGN PROSTATE ENLARGEMENT

Thomas Jefferson and Benjamin Franklin were both reportedly afflicted with prostate enlargement, also known as benign prostatic hypertrophy (BPH). No matter who you are, if you're a man and you live long enough, your aging prostate gland will grow. Commonly called prostate enlargement, this condition is the most common one afflicting the prostate gland. The technical term is benign prostatic hyperplasia (or hypertrophy), meaning abnormal, nonmalignant overgrowth of the prostate gland.

BPH means what it says. The condition is benign, or not harmful. It is not cancer. If the condition does not cause other problems, it might even pass unnoticed. BPH can cause urinary problems and it can be a precursor of prostate inflammation and prostate cancer, so it's worth paying attention to and treating if you begin to have symptoms.

In BPH, glandular cells in the inner portion of the prostate, called the transition zone, begin to live longer than usual and develop lumpy nodules. At the same time, the muscular tissue surrounding the gland begins to tighten. Because the prostate gland surrounds the urethra, the tube from the bladder, the nodules can obstruct the flow of urine. The urethra is further squeezed by the tightened prostate muscle.

About 20 percent of men with BPH do not experience urinary trouble because the inner nodules are lateral; that is, they grow sideways into the gland. This "silent" development of BPH may continue until the exterior of the prostate has enlarged to the point where it obstructs the bladder itself. Another 50 percent of men with BPH suffer with middle-lobe enlargement, the term for the growth of tissue outward, exerting pressure all around the urethra. Middle- and lateral-lobe growth is seen in 30 percent of men with BPH. These differences in the way the prostate gland enlarges are the reason why the actual size of the gland is often unrelated to the seriousness of symptoms.

Causes of BPH

The biochemical processes that result in BPH are quite involved and the subject of considerable research. Most researchers speculate that as men age, testosterone levels fall, while levels of other hormones, including estrogen, increase slightly, and the aging prostate gland becomes more hormone sensitive. Increased hormone sensitivity results in chemical messages to cells to live longer. Other chemicals, called growth factors, produced by prostate cells begin to send messages that encourage glandular cells to grow, form lumpy tissue, and secrete less, while the signal to muscle tissue is to tighten.

In addition, prolactin, a hormone secreted by the pituitary gland in the brain, increases the uptake of testosterone. Prolactin also stimulates the action of the enzyme that converts testosterone to a more powerful form. The converted testosterone then triggers unwanted messages to prostate cells. Prolactin levels increase with beer consumption and stress, which is why it is advisable to reduce both to prevent or reduce BPH.

BPH is seldom seen in men before the age of forty or in men who lose their testes (which produce testosterone) before puberty. And studies at Johns Hopkins University indicate a genetic factor at play in about 7 percent of BPH cases. The researchers looked at men aged sixty-four and younger with notable prostate enlargement. It was found that relatives of men with early-onset BPH were four times more likely to need prostate surgery. For brothers, the rate was six times.

A major five-year Harvard Medical School study of 25,000 men revealed that a large waistline goes along with a 75 percent increase in urinary symptoms after the age of fifty. Adding 7 inches around the waist was enough to cause problems. The researchers believe that excess abdominal fat can press against the prostate gland, which in turn chokes off urine flow. The scientists also suggest that since getting fat raises estrogen levels and lowers testosterone levels, the extra fat could also influence BPH directly.

A growing body of evidence shows that BPH is affected by nutrition. Studies show that a healthy, high-fiber diet and specific supplements can hold off or relieve BPH. If you apply proven natural approaches to BPH, you may well avoid the possibility of considerable trauma from surgery and the side effects of drugs used to treat prostate enlargement.

The Surgical "Solution"

Since the beginning of the twentieth century, men in their mid- to late forties have been running a 20 percent risk of BPH. One in two men aged sixty or over suffers prostate enlargement, and an estimated 80 percent aged eighty and over have developed the condition. Over $3 billion a year is spent on hospital care and surgery for prostate problems in the United States.

For many men, though, BPH is highly preventable and treatable without surgery or hospitalization. Research and clinical trials continue to prove the effectiveness of nutritional treatment and simple therapies. Surgery is not the inevitable fate of someone with BPH. What's more, your risk of developing problematic BPH doesn't have to be the luck of the draw. Good diet, exercise, and sensible use of supplements can help you buck recent statistical trends.

It's important to keep in mind that simple enlargement of the prostate gland does not need treatment. Treatment for BPH is recommended by doctors only when it causes serious problems. Surgery to remove excess tissue has so far been the most common course taken when symptoms are serious or related conditions develop. The technical term for any procedure that cuts away prostate gland tissue is *prostatectomy*, and it can take the form of several types of surgical operation. The average age of men who have a prostatectomy is seventy, showing again that prostate trouble is a disease associated with longevity.

Because most prostate patients are elderly, they frequently suffer from other conditions that limit the types of treatment that may be applicable. Sometimes physicians will advise the use of catheters or stents to relieve a bladder problem caused by BPH rather than operate on the prostate itself.

For the vast majority of men, symptoms are mild enough that even if BPH is diagnosed, the course advised is just watchful waiting. Your physician may advise limited fluid intake before bed and steer you away from certain drugs such as decongestants, which can worsen BPH. But there is more that you can do, which I'll tell you about shortly.

Drugs for BPH

Drugs developed for prostate enlargement are not very effective and tend to have unpleasant side effects. BPH drugs work in two ways: They either interfere with the hormones that trigger prostate cell growth or they relax prostate muscle tissue to relieve its pressure on the urethra. Neither of these

---

Possible Side Effects of Prostate Surgery

- "Dry" ejaculation (which does not affect the pleasure of an orgasm) occurs in about 75 to 90 percent of patients.
- Failure of symptoms to improve is seen in about 10 percent of cases.
- Infections occur in about 10 percent of men.
- About 5 to 10 percent of men have a loss of erection or impotence.
- Transfusions are needed in about 5 percent of cases.
- Urethral scarring happens in about 5 percent of patients.
- Serious or permanent incontinence occurs in 1 percent of patients.

---

approaches tackles the underlying causes of the hormonal action seen in BPH, which is why they do not cure the condition.

Herbal Remedies for BPH

Thanks to the wisdom and practices of native peoples of Africa and America, several effective herbal treatments exist for BPH. These plant-based remedies have been shown in studies to be more effective, safer, and cheaper than modern BPH drugs. Your pocketbook and your prostate will benefit when you use these simple, yet powerful extracts. Backed up by sensible diet and supplements, herbs are a valuable part of a comprehensive BPH treatment plan.

Herbs make powerful medicine. If you are taking any medication or have been diagnosed with cancer, heart problems of any kind, hypertension, impotence due to nerve damage, or any other major condition, always check any form of self-treatment you are considering with your physician.

Saw Palmetto (Serenoa repens)

According to folk history, the small, wrinkly, reddish brown to black berries of the saw palmetto tree make a good aphrodisiac. In fact, it is an overall tonic for the male reproductive system and formed part of the diet of some Native Americans. Early herbalists used saw palmetto berries to increase testicle function and to treat prostate conditions. The tree itself is a palm tree but grows only 6 to 10 feet tall. It is native to the dunes and coasts of Florida, Texas, and Georgia.

Several clinical studies published in the 1980s demonstrated the value of saw palmetto extract in treating almost 90 percent of the BPH patients studied. One trial compared men with BPH taking saw palmetto extract with other BPH patients taking a placebo. After just twenty-eight days, of the 110 men studied, those using the extract saw a 40 to 50 percent improvement in symptoms. Those on a placebo showed no significant improvement. The results were supported in ratings by both patients and doctors.

A three-month study of 350 men taking 160 mg of saw palmetto extract twice daily showed an 88 percent improvement in symptoms within ninety days. This favorable result was echoed in the objective findings. Remarkable improvements were obtained in all measurements, including urinary flow, flow rate, and prostate size. Another important finding was the self-rating for quality of life. The number of men who considered themselves unhappy dropped from 18.5 percent to 2.4 percent; and those who felt satisfied with life numbered only 9.7 percent at the beginning of the trial but jumped to 36.8 percent by the end. As well as demonstrating the value of saw palmetto extract, these findings show just how much BPH symptoms can badly affect mental outlook. Relieving the condition can make a big change for the better in a man's life.

The good results with saw palmetto for almost all patients in clinical trials are also encouraging because they were achieved without any side effects or toxicity. Safe use goes for both the extract and for eating the berries themselves. This is in contrast to Proscar (finasteride), a prescription drug approved by the FDA for use in 1992 to treat BPH. A year's course of Proscar has been shown to work in less than 50 percent of patients. When trial results are compared, patients using saw palmetto extract show greater improvement in symptoms at three months than men using Proscar. Furthermore, the results of

these studies showed that Proscar caused impotence in 3.7 percent of men and decreased libido in 3.3 percent. Pregnant women are advised not to handle the drug or expose themselves to the semen of men who are taking it. Proscar is also four times more expensive than saw palmetto. It's clear that natural saw palmetto is a much safer and effective remedy for BPH than this expensive drug.

The compounds in saw palmetto extract are known as antagonists to the effects of the form of testosterone that initiates BPH. They work in two ways: by inhibiting the formation of the converted testosterone (dihydrotestosterone, or DHT) and by helping to block it from binding to receptor sites on cells. By inhibiting the binding of DHT, saw palmetto also encourages its breakdown and excretion—good news for the aging prostate. Herbalists have also found that saw palmetto has a mild sedative effect, which is helpful to patients getting over nighttime urination problems.

If you take saw palmetto in a tincture form, be prepared for the strong taste, which is disagreeable to many. At least 10–20 g of the raw fruit would have to be eaten twice a day to take in enough of the active chemical. You can also take it in capsule form.

Take 160 mg of liposterolic (85 to 95 percent) extract twice daily (equivalent to about 10 g of raw berries twice daily). If no result occurs from using saw palmetto alone for three months, pygeum can be used instead, or you can try taking them together.

Pygeum africanum

An evergreen, pygeum grows to more than 100 feet tall in Madagascar and on the high plateaus of central and southern Africa, where it is native. The tribes of Natal create infusions of the dark brown or gray pygeum bark to treat bladder pains and urinary difficulty, familiar symptoms to men with BPH. Other countries have been slow to catch on. The herb was only introduced to Europe in the 1960s after researchers observed its effectiveness among native peoples. It wasn't long, however, before European journals began to publish exciting studies verifying pygeum as a valuable BPH treatment. European men have benefited, as now 81 percent of all doctors' prescriptions for BPH in France are for extract of *Pygeum africanum*, where it relieves symptoms for more than half of all BPH patients. Yet in the United States, where it has been viewed only as a "health food," doctors are only just beginning to learn about pygeum.

Like saw palmetto berries, the bark of pygeum contains fatty acids and sterols, which act to inhibit the formation of the prostate growth stimulant DHT. They also help to balance prostate testosterone levels, and the sterols help to reduce prostate inflammation. The compounds in pygeum act in a slightly different way from those in saw palmetto. They are not quite as good at reducing symptoms, and some men do not tolerate them as well, experiencing nausea or stomach pains. Moreover, there is not as much information about objective measurements of symptoms as there is for saw palmetto. However, the biochemical actions of pygeum appear to be complementary to as well as overlapping those of saw palmetto, and the two herbs are often taken together. This is advisable, since pygeum also improves the quality and quantity of prostate secretions, which is something saw palmetto does not accomplish.

Analysis of the studies of outpatients since the mid-1970s shows that pygeum lessens symptoms and clinical signs of BPH, particularly in cases detected early on in their development. Look for extracts standardized to 14 percent sterols.

Take 50–100 mg of extract twice daily (almost always available as a pill). The most potent form is a 70:1 extract, but many men see good results with just an 8:1 extract. Studies show that saw palmetto has a slightly stronger effect on symptoms, but pygeum also improves prostate secretions. For this reason, the two can be used in combination.

Flower Pollen Extract

In Europe, flower pollen extract has been used to treat BPH and prostate inflammation for over twenty-five years. The main product used is called Cernilton, produced in Sweden and available in health food stores in the United States. Published clinical studies show that Cernilton is probably most effective in the treatment of prostate inflammation but can also be helpful in treating BPH. A report in the *Swedish Medical Journal* described a small one-year trial using Cernilton that resulted in the prostate returning to normal size in five out of ten patients. The most improvement was seen in patients with inflamed prostates. None of the studies reported any side effects.

Pollen is a rich supply of vitamins and minerals, trace elements, and carbohydrates. It also contains fatty acids, flavonoids, and protein. The mechanisms are unclear, but the effects of these agents are to reduce inflammation, contract the bladder, and relax the urethra. The result is less pain and eased urinary symptoms. Use pollen with care, as some people are allergic to different types. Take two tablets of Cernilton or a similar product three times daily.

Panax ginseng

Ginseng is an ancient Asian herb, used for centuries as a male tonic. A study of male rats showed that ginseng increased testosterone while decreasing prostate gland weight. One of the effects of lowered testosterone levels seen in the aging male body is a decreased uptake of zinc. Increasing testosterone would in theory lead to higher levels of zinc, which has been proven effective in reducing the size of an enlarged prostate.

If you decide to use ginseng, be careful to select a genuine *Panax ginseng* product standardized for ginsenoside content, as ginseng quality is highly variable. Take the dried root, 2–4 g three times daily, or extracts equivalent to 25–50 mg ginsenosides daily.

PROSTATE INFLAMMATION

There are other prostate problems that don't fit under the BPH category but which can usually be treated successfully with noninvasive, natural methods. First, do not be confused by the term *prostatosis*. This is medico-speak for "a condition of the prostate," often used when a doctor does not know what is wrong.

Prostatitis means inflammation of the prostate gland. It is a common ailment of young men prone to urinary tract infections, while older men are prone to prostate enlargement. The usual symptoms of an inflamed prostate include discomfort in and around the gland, usually accompanied by acute urinary symptoms, such as burning and increased and urgent need to urinate. Pain from an inflamed prostate gland can be transmitted around the anus and scrotum, the groin, the lower back, the lower abdomen, and the legs. Prostatitis can also cause pain on ejaculation.

Nonbacterial prostatitis, the term for prostate inflammation not caused by bacteria, is the most common type of prostatitis, but it has doctors puzzled. Patients suffer the same symptoms as chronic bacterial prostatitis, but their urine shows no sign of infection and antibiotics have no effect. In addition, most sufferers have never had a urinary tract infection. The pain involved and white blood cells in the prostatic fluid are the main signs of prostatitis.

Supplements to Treat Prostate Infection and Inflammation

Zinc dissolved in prostate fluids exhibits antibacterial action, and levels have been found to be as low as one-tenth of normal in men with prostatitis. It's not surprising, then, that studies show that prostatitis symptoms can be resolved with zinc supplementation. Zinc should be taken in a readily absorbable form such as zinc picolinate, and not for too long at high doses. To prevent and relieve prostatitis, consumption of foods rich in zinc, such as herring and pumpkin seeds, is a good idea.

A mainstream treatment of prostatitis can be problematic, because even a normal prostate gland is poorly supplied with blood, making it a tough site for the immune system to defend and for antibiotics to reach. For this reason, recurrences of this type of infection are common. Some mainstream urologists have resorted to prescribing a long, six-week term of antibiotic treatment. Such a long course of antibiotics is hard on the body and ignores probable contributory nutritional deficiencies that leave the immune system underpowered. A better path may be a more standard two-week course of antibiotics backed up by supplements, including vitamins C and E and zinc. Also, ensure that your diet is high in fiber and nutrients. Cut out coffee and other prostate irritants, and drink plenty of clean water. Vitamin B complex and probiotic supplements like acidophilus are also a must with antibiotics.

Herbs to Treat Prostate Infection and Inflammation

Here are some herbs that are useful for relief of uncomfortable prostate and urinary tract conditions.

Bearberry (Uva-Ursi)

This herb has traditionally been used as a diuretic, but because it contains flavonoids and a substance called arbutin, which converts in the human body to hydroquinone, it is also a urinary disinfectant. Hydroquinone is poisonous at high doses, but bearberry is safe for short-term treatment of prostate gland infection.

Couch Grass

Also known as witch grass, among other names, this herb is used specifically to treat prostatitis as well as urinary tract infections and urinary stones. Couch grass is rich in oils and contains vitamins A and B and other valuable compounds, such as iron. It is a soothing diuretic with antibiotic properties.

Echinacea

Known for its immune-boosting properties, which are due to its mix of essential oils and other potent plant chemicals, echinacea is used in the treatment of infections generally.

Goldenseal

This herb is effective in treating urinary and kidney infections and stones. Goldenseal has cleansing actions that stem from its mixture of essential oils, flavonoids, tannins, and saponins.

Horsetail

This herb offers a storehouse of minerals useful in treating prostatitis, BPH, cystitis, and urinary stones. Saponins are also found in this herb, probably contributing their antimicrobe and hormone-mimicking properties when horsetail is used as a remedy.

PROSTATE CANCER

Fear and confusion surround the topic of prostate cancer for many men. However, the statistics and research provide a great deal of reassurance. Even though more than half of all men experience prostate enlargement, only 13 percent of men develop threatening cancer of the prostate gland and only 2 to 3 percent will die of the condition. Prostate cancer is age related, developing almost exclusively in men over fifty years of age. More than 80 percent of men diagnosed with prostate cancer are over the age of sixty-five.

An analysis of population studies and experimental evidence shows that several dietary factors increase the risk of developing prostate cancer. A high intake of refined sugar, animal protein, and animal fat and a lack of carotenes, also known as carotenoids (found in carrots and other orange and yellow vegetables), are the most significant. Clearly, then, a diet rich in fruits and vegetables and low in meat and animal fat should offer some protection against prostate cancer.

Heredity can confer up to a 50 percent risk of developing prostate cancer. This risk is seen when prostate cancer has occurred in three generations, or when three or more close relatives (such as father or brother) suffer from the disease. But this accounts for only about 5 percent of prostate cancer.

Prostate cancer is the most common form of cancer in men, but it lies behind lung cancer as their main cause of cancer deaths. Only 2 to 3 percent of men in the United States die of prostate cancer. Compare that to the 47 percent of U.S. men who die of heart disease. Any man can lessen his risk of prostate cancer by adopting a healthy lifestyle. Diet is almost certainly a major reason why there is less incidence of prostate cancer in countries like Japan, particularly since rates of this condition increase in Japanese men whose diet becomes more westernized.

The Two Forms of Prostate Cancer

Like all cancers, prostate cancer consists of undifferentiated cells that grow out of control. Normal growth checks have little or no effect on cancer cells, which can invade and destroy normal cells. A study of 100 tissue samples removed in surgery shows that the size of a prostate tumor is related to how dangerous it is. Scientists found that tumors less than 1 cm^3 (just under half an inch) rarely spread; in fact, most tumors under 3.5 cm^3 remain inside the prostate. The bigger a tumor, however, the more aggressive it becomes. Tumors over 5 cm^3 are more difficult to treat.

Early prostate cancer is slow growing, often taking two to four years or longer to double in size. To reach 1 cm^3, a tumor has to double at least thirty times, and it would be at about this point that a tumor could be felt by a doctor. Due to this growth pattern, prostate cancer is considered to exist in two forms: incidental and clinical.

Incidental, *histological*, and *latent* are terms for microscopic cancers seen on slides, usually at autopsy. This form is thought to affect about 60 to 70 percent of all men over eighty years old, going undetected in most. This gives physicians the problem of whether or not to treat incidental cancer when discovered, since it could easily continue to exist without causing any problems. In the younger man, early development of a tumor is believed to be a sign that the cancer is likely to evolve into a threatening form. Older men may well die of other causes long before their prostate cancer becomes a problem.

The second type of prostate cancer is called *clinical*, *clinically significant*, *advanced*, or *malignant*. These terms refer to cancer that may spread to other parts of the body. The nearby seminal vesicles, bladder, urethra, and pelvic side walls are common sites for prostate cancer that has begun to spread. From these sites it can be carried via the lymphatic system and the bloodstream to sites such as bones and lungs. It can grow "silently" or cause symptoms. Clinical prostate cancer is 2½ times less common than the incidental kind. There is a genetic connection for clinical prostate cancer. Having a father or brother with the disease means that a man's risk of developing it is two times greater than normal and often leads to earlier affliction. Prostate cancer in three generations of either parent's family brings a one-in-two risk of its development.

Another term used in relation to prostate cancer is *localized*. This refers to cancer that has not developed beyond the prostate gland. Prostate cancer can remain in the gland indefinitely, which is why many elderly men can have prostate cancer but die of other causes. Removal of the prostate gland is the most extreme treatment for localized prostate cancer and is termed a *radical prostatectomy*. Localized cancer usually takes two or three years to double in size.

The environmental factor is important when considering the two forms of prostate cancer. This is shown in studies of Japanese and American men. Incidental prostate cancer is as common in both groups of men, and both groups have the same life span of seventy-four years. Yet far fewer men in Japan die of prostate cancer. However, rates of prostate cancer death in Japanese men who move to Hawaii or California shoot up to American levels. The major variable here seems to be diet. Nutrients and other agents in the Japanese diet are thought to inhibit the growth of cancer beyond its first stage, called initiation. It is the further stages of cancer—promotion, progression, and metastasis—that are seen less commonly in Japanese men.

Symptoms of Prostate Cancer

Most prostate cancers, about 72 percent, begin in the outer, peripheral zone of the gland, and 8 percent start in the central zone. The remaining 20 percent begin in the transition zone, which is where prostate enlargement originates. For this reason and because it is slow growing in its early stage, prostate cancer, unlike BPH, does not at first cause pressure on the urethra and related urinary problems. Silent development is typical, and the cancer is often quite advanced once it causes symptoms. Such symptoms include signs of BPH, blood in the urine or semen, less ejaculated fluid, less rigid erections or impotence, and severe pain in the back, pelvis, hips, or thighs. It's important to remember that all of these problems can have other causes. If you are experiencing prostate problems, get a thorough prostate checkup.

Diagnosis of Prostate Trouble

Debate is heated on the subject of diagnosis of prostate gland problems, cancer in particular. Doctors dis-

agree about methods of diagnosis, test results, and the significance of physical signs. Some physicians look for BPH earlier than others, some pathologists have seen cancerous cells where others have not. Studies are ongoing to determine the value of different tests and the way they are used. One of the most important prostate diagnostic tests is the DRE, or digital rectal exam.

Yes, it's time for all those rubber-glove jokes. Women in our culture have long been used to pelvic examinations. Men, on the other hand, tend to have relatively little experience of a physician inserting things into their lower regions. In fact, a digital rectal exam uses a surgical-gloved finger to conduct a basic but effective test of prostate health.

The digital rectal examination is a subjective test and is best performed by a doctor experienced in the procedure. The message on diagnosing prostate trouble is to seek out a good, likable physician. It is also important to note that as many as 40 percent of prostate cancers begin in a spot that is inaccessible through this procedure. In some cases, disease can be advanced by the time it is detected through a digital exam. Make sure your physician uses this diagnostic tool with a PSA test. The PSA test and digital rectal exam were almost equal in their ability to detect cancers in a study of 2,634 men. However, the different tests did not always find the same tumors. If only one had been used, some cancers would have been missed.

Healthy prostate tissue feels much like the flesh between the first finger and thumb when a fist is made. It is firm and smooth without being solid. The length of tissue felt by the doctor should be no more than about 1.5 inches long. The physician will check if the prostate tissue feels hard and lumpy or soft and mushy. The physician will also be alert for any enlargement of the gland, which can grow to the size of an orange in some cases. Often, however, the inner prostate tissue has enlarged without causing any external expansion of the gland. For this reason, the digital rectal exam is not a surefire way to diagnose BPH.

A physician may also "milk" the prostate gland during a DRE. Pressure on the gland can push a drop or two of prostate fluid into the urethra. Such drops can be collected when passed through the urethra and checked microscopically for signs of bacterial infection.

It is well worth overcoming any embarrassment or distaste for this simple procedure. It is a useful aid in assessing prostate health.

The Prostate-Specific Antigen (PSA) Test

This test has become highly controversial in recent years. It has a high rate of false positives—up to 75 percent—meaning that up to 75 percent of the time it will show that a man has prostate cancer when he doesn't. It also has a high false negative rate, meaning that it fails to indicate the presence of a cancer. It can also indicate the genuine existence of prostate cancer in elderly men, who are unlikely to survive to see the cancer become problematic. Doctors and patients then cannot be sure that treatment would ultimately improve health or life expectancy.

An antigen is a substance that stimulates the production of antibodies by the immune system. Often an antigen is something foreign to the body. Prostate-specific antigen (PSA), however, is a protein secreted almost exclusively by cells of the prostate gland. Its role is to break down coagulated semen. Normally, very little PSA leaks into the blood. Elevated PSA levels can be a sign of BPH, infection, and prostatitis. High PSA levels are mainly associated with cancer because cancer often makes prostate cell walls leaky. However, PSA is prostate specific, not cancer specific, so the PSA could be high for any number of reasons besides the presence of cancer. To complicate matters even further, about one-quarter of men who turn out to have prostate cancer have *low* PSA levels. In men with PSA levels between 4 and 10, about a quarter have cancer. About 65 percent of men with PSA levels over 10 turn out to have cancer. PSA readings alone should not form the basis of prostate cancer diagnosis. In fact, older men who get PSA tests and then allow themselves to undergo surgery have a higher death rate than men who do nothing. Because prostate cancer is such a slow-growing cancer, watchful waiting has been recommended by many highly respected physicians. And while you wait watchfully, there's plenty you can do with nutrition and lifestyle to reduce your chances of a serious prostate cancer.

A University of Chicago study published in the *New England Journal of Medicine* gives evidence regarding treatment of prostate cancer in men with overall short life expectancy. The study found that those expected generally to live only ten years or less at the time their cancer is detected (that is, men in their seventies and eighties) are much more likely to die of a cause other than untreated prostate cancer. Since prostate surgery can cause incontinence, impotence, and general weakness, it's highly debatable whether it will do more harm than good in most cases.

Unless it becomes possible to refine PSA testing, different tests are advisable to see if results are consistent. The combination of a PSA test with a digital rectal exam is recommended. Ultrasound and needle biopsy can also be used. Each of these tests can pick up cancers that the other tests missed. Surgery should only be undertaken if serious cancer is almost certain.

Ask if your doctor is aware of the latest information about PSA testing. Does your doctor monitor PSA velocity and calculate PSA density? Has your doctor heard of PSA level age ranges? See if the response you get is positive, open, and well informed. If it's not and if he or she seems overeager to perform surgery, run the other way and find another doctor!

Remember, only 13 percent of men are diagnosed with prostate cancer, and only 2 to 3 percent die of it. What's more, 80 percent of men with prostate cancer are over sixty-five, and most of them die from other causes. Less than 1 percent of prostate cancers have been found in men younger than fifty and only 16 percent in men between fifty and sixty-four. The average age of prostate cancer diagnosis is seventy-two. Confusion arises because although incidental prostate cancer is believed to exist in about two-thirds of all men over eighty years old, wherever they live, diagnosis of advanced, clinical cancer occurs for only 13 percent.

Prostate enlargement, or BPH, is much more common, affecting half of all men aged sixty. If men took better care of their prostate glands, would these statistics improve? The studies of Japanese men as well as those on particular nutrients and herbs indicate that they would. Sound nutrition and a healthy lifestyle can only help guard against prostate trouble.

NUTRITION AND THE PROSTATE

Are you a hunter-gatherer, driving herds of game, fishing, and harvesting your way through life? Or do you drive a car, graze the Internet, and hunt down bargains? Along with twentieth-century changes in the lifestyle and diet of modern man has come a staggering increase in the incidence of prostate trouble. The medical establishment has held that prostate gland trouble is an inevitable consequence of aging, and more than $3 billion is spent annually on prostate-related surgery. Look to Asia, however, and you'll find a much lower incidence of prostate problems. Even in the Far East, though, rates of prostate disease have risen at the same time as the Asian diet has become increasingly westernized.

Nutrients for Prostate Health

While doctors debate the causes of BPH, more and more research points to nutritional connections. Numerous studies show that good nutrition plays an important role in the prevention of and relief from prostate disease. It's a wise prostate health maintenance move to make the dietary changes needed and take supplements selected for their proven effects.

Amino Acids

Amino acids have been shown in several studies to relieve many of the symptoms of BPH. For instance, an American study of 45 men with BPH showed that 95 percent of those using three amino acids found relief from or reduction in nighttime urination, with a high percentage of alleviation of other symptoms also being achieved. The three amino acids found to be effective are alanine, glycine, and glutamic acid. However, the mechanisms at work are unclear, and many researchers believe that amino acid treatment only reduces symptoms without curing prostate problems.

Carotenes

Some studies show that a low intake of carotenoids, particularly beta-carotene, significantly increases the risk for prostate cancer. Carotenoids are red-to-yellow plant pigments best known for their antioxidant activity and anticancer properties and their conversion to vitamin A in the body.

Vitamin A helps the prostate overcome and resist infections by keeping its mucous membranes functioning well. It aids the production of cells that grow tiny hairs called cilia, which trap and sweep out germs and other foreign matter. To increase your intake of these helpful substances, eat lots of yellow-orange fruits and vegetables like carrots, apricots, sweet potatoes, yams, and squash. Dark green leafy vegetables, such as kale and spinach, are also excellent carotene sources. Taking a beta-carotene supplement is not a substitute for eating plenty of carotenoid-rich fruits and vegetables!

Vitamin B_6

Bladder stones are seen more commonly in parts of the world where a vitamin B_6 deficiency is found. A lack of this vitamin increases the excretion of oxalate in urine. Oxalate tends to crystallize easily, forming stones. Because BPH often leads to the retention of urine, there is an increased likelihood that stones will form. Taking a good B-complex supplement is wise insurance against this condition. It also indirectly aids the prostate through the involvement of vitamin B_6 in the synthesis and management of hormones and as an aid to the absorption of the critical prostate mineral, zinc.

Vitamin C

This is one case where flushing a vitamin down the toilet actually does you good—as long as it's passed through you first! Up to 60 percent of the vitamin C consumed ends up in urine. Owing to its beneficial effects on the urinary tract, however, this apparent loss is not a waste at all. Authorities in the United States report that vitamin C is effective against inflammation of the urethra. The body requires higher levels of vitamin C at times of any infection, but it is thought that its beneficial effects in the urethra are also due in part to the way high doses of vitamin C increase the acidity of urine. Retention of urine is a common result of BPH that can lead to infection of the bladder and urethra. Retained urine begins to decompose, becoming less acidic. This can also lead to the formation of tiny crystalline stones in the urine that cause pain and irritation. Of course, tackling infection in the urinary tract keeps down the risk of the condition spreading to the prostate and causing prostatitis. Vitamin C as a powerful anti-infectant is also definitely recommended for prostatitis itself.

Include zinc on your supplements list, too, since vitamin C works more effectively with zinc. The two substances create a very good anti-infection double act for the prostate gland and urinary tract.

Vitamin D

A study published in the journal *Cancer* found that deaths from prostate cancer in white men were more common in northern areas of the United States. Those areas with greatest sunlight saw the least prostate cancer. These findings also correlate with the fact that prostate cancer rates are lowest in Japan and Hong Kong and highest in the United States, Canada, and Scandinavia. The study suggests that ultraviolet radiation may protect against clinical prostate cancer.

There may also be a link to vitamin D, which is mainly synthesized by the body as a result of exposure to sunlight. Vitamin D is known to inhibit the growth of tumors, preventing them from progressing past the incidental stage.

Not only is Japan exposed to more ultraviolet light, but the Japanese diet is rich in fish with a high vitamin D content. Research into the ultraviolet connection and prostate cancer has only just begun, and much more work needs to be completed before anyone can definitely say that a lack of vitamin D increases the risk of prostate cancer. Of course, overexposure to ultraviolet radiation brings a high risk itself of skin cancer. There would be no harm, though, and possibly some insurance against prostate cancer, in taking a daily 10-minute walk without sunscreen and returning to a grilled fish dinner!

Essential Fatty Acids

Pumpkin seeds for virility? There is some truth to folklore from Eastern Europe, where pumpkin seeds have long been used as a prostate tonic and remedy. It took until the late 1920s, however, for scientists at the University of Vienna to discover that men in countries like Bulgaria, the Ukraine, and Turkey really did have much lower rates of prostate enlargement.

As well as being an excellent source of zinc, pumpkin seeds are rich in essential fatty acids (EFAs). A study from a nutritional research foundation in Milwaukee has shown that supplementation with EFAs alone for several weeks reduced or completely relieved prostate enlargement symptoms.

Flavonoids

When you eat plenty of fresh fruit, you increase the concentration of flavonoids in your blood. The berries and citrus fruits have the highest concentration of flavonoids. Flavonoids—including bioflavonoids and isoflavonoids—are found in the pigmentation of plants and act as powerful antioxidants.

A small study published in *The Lancet* compared the levels of isoflavonoids in the blood of Finnish and Japanese men. Levels in the Japanese men were 110 times higher than those in the Finnish men! The researchers observed that lifelong high blood concentrations of isoflavonoids may explain the low incidence of clinical cancer in Japanese men. One notable ingredient of Japanese traditional diet is soy. Eating soy is one of the best ways to ensure a high intake of flavonoids.

Saponins

Saponins are yet another plant ingredient that may contribute to the differences in cancer rates between countries with very different diets. Saponins mimic precursors to steroid hormones. Research at the University of Toronto is showing that the rates of prostate and other cancers are lower where people eat foods richest in saponins. Saponins may well be a supplement of the future. In the meantime, it can only pay to eat plenty of saponin-rich vegetables like beans, spinach, tomatoes, potatoes, alfalfa, and even oats.

Zinc

Folklore about the aphrodisiac effects of oysters is more than just a myth. Oysters are high in zinc, which is essential to the workings of the male reproductive system.

Zinc is a mineral that inhibits the activity of the enzyme that converts testosterone to its more powerful form. The converted testosterone triggers prostate cells to grow abnormally, resulting in an enlarged prostate. Zinc has also been shown to inhibit the activity of prolactin, the hormone that also stimulates the testosterone-converting enzyme as well as increasing the uptake of testosterone itself.

Most American men are deficient in zinc. You may read in some publications that zinc supplementation does not result in higher levels being found in the prostate. In some cases, this may be true. BPH is an older man's disease, and increasing age often brings a lessening of pancreatic function, which is necessary for the absorption of zinc. What's more, the lowered testosterone levels seen in the older man lead to less absorption of zinc in the intestine. Adequate levels of vitamin B_6 are needed, too, for the uptake of zinc. What is certain is that there have been many studies showing that zinc does indeed reduce the symptoms of BPH. Measurements by digital rectal exam, endoscopy, and X ray have all shown that treatment with zinc reduces the size of prostate enlargement. It's essential, however, that zinc be taken in a readily absorbable form, usually zinc picolinate, and to ensure sound nutrition in general.

Zinc also fights infection and boosts the efficiency of vitamin C. Cut down on alcohol to keep levels up. Eat lots of nuts and seeds, especially pumpkin seeds, and be sure that this is one substance on your prostate health supplement list!

How Much of Any Supplement Should You Take?

It does not follow that, because a substance is beneficial, more is better. Taken at high levels for too long, zinc, for example, will depress the immune system. Illness usually produces an increased need for various nutrients. Individual requirements vary, too, so be prepared to monitor your progress and seek advice from a knowledgeable health care professional.

Supplements are just that! They are not a substitute for a good, healthy diet, but *are* useful support for one that is not ideal, as well as for modern, fast-paced, highly stressed lifestyles and environments. Note, too, that nutritional substances work in balance with each other, becoming most efficient when general nutrition is sound. Partly in keeping with this principle, and partly for convenience, formulas have been developed that combine supplements that specifically address prostate trouble. The following quantity guidelines are frequently recommended:

- *Zinc picolinate*. Take 15–30 mg daily (increase to 60 mg for prostatitis until symptoms subside).
- *Vitamin B_6* (pyridoxine). Take 50–100 mg daily. Always take vitamin B complex, too, when you take a B vitamin supplement. Some B-complex "stress" formulas include higher amounts of B_6 and B_5.
- *Alanine, glycine, and glutamic acid*. Take 200 mg daily of these amino acids. I prefer you take your glutamic acid in the form of glutamine, which the body will convert to glutamic acid as needed.
- *Vitamin C*. Take 1,000 mg three times daily. Increase this triple dose to 2,000 mg at the onset of prostatitis. Vitamin C intake can be increased until it causes diarrhea (then lower the dose), as the body's requirement for this vitamin varies considerably with illness and stress.

Foods for a Healthy Prostate

One thing for certain is that a lot of red meat, animal fats, butter, mayonnaise, and creamy salad dressings are not food for a healthy prostate gland. A Harvard Medical School study showed that these foods were most closely linked to a risk of advanced, fatal cancer. Analysis of dietary and blood sample data from 300 cases, including 126 advanced cases of prostate cancer, was compared with that from a comparable group of healthy doctors. Analysis showed that eating meat just once a week, instead of five times, could lower your risk of advanced cancer by two to three times. However, consuming high amounts of any of the offending foods raises blood levels of a type of fatty acid called alpha-linolenic acid, or ALA. It was this fatty acid that seemed to cause the increased risk, probably through its enzyme-related activity in the prostate.

Evidence that high-cholesterol levels are bad for the prostate comes from the fact that anticholesterol drugs have been shown to relieve BPH. In addition, a study from the Metropolitan Hospital in New York found that men with BPH had 80 percent more cholesterol in their blood than men without BPH. Harmful substances are produced when cholesterol breaks down. If the body is deficient in nutrients like vitamins C and E and essential fatty acids, then the harmful cholesterol by-products are not cleared out of the body. Some accumulate in the prostate gland, where they promote BPH. This rules out processed and refined foods, including sugar, and saturated fats in large amounts if BPH is to be avoided.

If fatty, mainly animal-based and refined foods are out, what's in? It makes sense to look for examples in countries like Bulgaria and Japan where rates of BPH prostate cancer are low. The following foods will help you keep your prostate in good shape—literally!

Soy

Soy is a plant source of complete protein and numerous other valuable nutrients, such as flavonoids (plant hormones) and essential fatty acids. Try the different varieties, from tofu to tempeh and soy flour to soy drinks. There are lots of different recipes.

Cold-Water Fish

Salmon, sardines, and tuna are excellent sources of vitamin C and essential fatty acids, both of benefit to the prostate. Herring is also high in zinc.

Fresh Vegetables

From dark green and leafy to yellow and red to white and creamy, all will keep you well supplied with carotenes, flavonoids, and saponins, as well as lots of vitamins and fiber. Fiber is particularly helpful in keeping cholesterol levels down, which is important for the prostate gland.

Fresh Fruit

The best fruits for the prostate are the red and yellow kinds, from tomatoes (yes, they're a fruit, not a vegetable!) and apricots to strawberries and oranges. A good source of vitamin C, many fruits are high in the plant pigments called flavonoids and carotenoids, which are nutritional powerhouses.

Nuts and Seeds

A daily handful of nuts and seeds is a good source of protective minerals and essential fatty acids. Pumpkin and sunflower seeds especially will help keep you topped up with zinc, which, like essential fatty acids, is involved with hormone regulation, so important to prostate health. Zinc also fights and resists prostate-related infections.

Whole Grains

Wheat, oatmeal, brown rice, and other complex carbohydrates help keep your cholesterol levels low and fiber up, both significant aids to the prostate. Oatmeal and wheat bran are also both fairly good sources of zinc, and oatmeal is also rich in saponins and the hard-to-get GLA, an essential fatty acid.

Organic Live Yogurt

Organic live yogurt a few times a week is a good source of beneficial bacteria for the digestive tract. Keeping the bacterial balance right will help keep the urinary tract free of infection. Eat only "live" yogurts made from the milk of organically reared animals to avoid encountering hormones, antibiotics, and other chemicals added to animal feed.

Cranberry Juice

Cranberry juice keeps bacteria from sticking to the urinary tract, so a daily glassful is a precautionary measure against infection if you have a tendency to get urinary tract infections. However, please don't drink the sugar-laden varieties.

Water, Water, Water!

This is an essential but often forgotten nutrient required for the processing of all the others. Dehydration stresses the prostate, while about eight glasses of clean water a day will keep your system well supplied. Mild herb teas make a pleasant variation and a worthwhile switch from coffee, a prostate irritant.

Substances to Avoid

On top of poor foods, it's easy to give your prostate a hard time by exposing it to certain other substances. The following substances are all likely to keep the prostate gland working hard and under pressure.

Beer

This and other alcohol sources stimulate the growth-triggering mechanisms in BPH.

Caffeine

Even decaffeinated coffee has enough irritants to prove harmful to an aging, sensitive prostate. Sodas are another common source of caffeine, and chocolate contains a little. Go very easy on all sources. Herb teas are a much healthier beverage than coffee, and since many, such as chamomile, are calming, they can help alleviate stress, which also contributes to

harmful prostate chemistry. Try some ginseng tea to perk you up and support your reproductive system at the same time.

Tobacco

Never good for you! Smoking and other tobacco habits bring all kinds of toxins into the body, from nicotine to cadmium. Studies show that there may be a greater risk of developing prostate cancer if you smoke, and at least one study has shown a definite risk if smokers are exposed to other sources of cadmium. (Occupations such as welding and electroplating can lead, over time, to high levels of cadmium exposure.)

Environmental Toxins

These include contaminants such as pesticides, dioxins, and heavy metals. Synthetic hormones, too, should be avoided by consuming only whole, organic foods. Most livestock are fed hormones for fattening and antibiotics for disease prevention. Residues of these substances are found in foods. Even plastic can linings and butter wrapping can contain traces of synthetic estrogens. Contaminants like these become concentrated in the prostate gland, where they can lead to BPH by increasing the conversion of testosterone. The large increase in the incidence of BPH in the last few decades may in part reflect the increasing effect of toxic chemicals on human health.

9 NUTRITION FOR ACTIVE LIFESTYLES ~

STAYING HEALTHY WITH AN ACTIVE LIFESTYLE

If you want to live life to its fullest, you need to maximize your energy and minimize the impact that stress has on your life. I often refer to stress as "crunch times." We all have crunch times, and not always for negative reasons. My annual book tours, for example, are a positive but hectic experience. The goal of getting through a book tour with my health intact inspires me to pull out all of my antistress tricks. I'm happy to tell you that they work. I accomplish a tremendous amount in a very short time, working from the wee small hours until late at night, and stay healthy and energetic throughout.

Stress can also come in bad packages. Disease, holidays, anxiety, and even moving can burn you out before you realize it. The problem for many people during crunch times begins when they start to feel overwhelmed by life's demands and don't do anything to remedy it. It's at this point that they start to feel serious stress and suffer the physical and emotional consequences, like inability to sleep, gaining or losing weight, exhaustion, irritability, depression, and loss of emotional control. Physical symptoms can range from minor aches and pains to considerable chronic and acute conditions.

Physicians in general practice have reported that at least 75 percent of their patients have problems with an emotional beginning. High blood pressure, colitis, heart disease, even cancer have been attributed in large part to poorly managed chronic stress.

I'm not saying to avoid stress—you can't. It shows up in all our lives. And since there's often not much we can do to prevent stressful events from occurring,

the best possible strategy is to expect and be prepared for stress and know how our own personal system reacts to it. This chapter is about maintaining an active lifestyle while you maintain your health and manage stress effectively.

Five keys to maintaining your health are to get plenty of sleep; get plenty of exercise; drink plenty of clean, fresh water; fill your body with delicious, nutritious food; and follow a sensible program of herbs and supplements to support your body and especially your immune system.

There are a few don'ts, too. It's best not to eat a lot of sugar or fats, not to eat just before bedtime, not to drink too much coffee or alcohol, and, of course, not to smoke or spend much time breathing polluted air. Finally, don't expect yourself to be perfect.

If a crunch time hits you, one of the worst things you can do is resort to a prescription drug. There is plenty of well-documented research showing that popular prescribed drugs like Valium are extremely addictive and can actually increase depression. Prozac and other antidepressant drugs in the same family (Paxil and Zoloft, for example) can cause very erratic responses in some people, including increased irritability, withdrawal from loved ones, and even violent or suicidal behavior. The side effects of these drugs are potentially so damaging that using herbal and nutritional methods to reduce the anxiety and depression that often accompanies chronic stress is most often the preferred method of treatment.

There are an almost infinite variety of ways that we can respond to stress and cope with it. Rather than using this chapter as a formula approach to maximizing your energy and minimizing stress, think of it as a resource with which you can discover your own personal path to an optimal high-energy lifestyle.

RECLAIMING YOUR ENERGY BY BALANCING YOUR HORMONES

While your body's source of energy is food, and nutrients are transformed into energy within your cells, certain of your hormones play a vital role in regulating and synchronizing when, where, and how your energy is used. When your hormones are out of balance or depleted, your energy levels can suffer. In fact, I suspect that much of what is identified as chronic fatigue syndrome is really a depletion of adrenal hormones by years of chronic stress.

Along with brain hormones and neurotransmitters, the steroid hormones are your most important energy regulators. They regulate and play a part in a seemingly endless list of functions in the body, including sex characteristics, sex drive, thyroid metabolism, insulin regulation, blood pressure, behavior and moods, inflammation, and allergic reactions.

The steroid hormones include those made in the adrenal glands, such as cortisol and DHEA (dehydroepiandrosterone), and the sex hormones made in the ovaries and testicles, such as progesterone, testosterone, and estrogen. These hormones all work in synchronization with each other, and when one is depleted or excessive, it throws the rest out of balance.

All of these hormones are made in the body from cholesterol, and they all need vitamins and mineral cofactors to be produced. In other words, it takes cholesterol plus enzymes plus specific vitamins and minerals to produce each of the steroid hormones. Both men and women can suffer from hormone imbalance, but since women's hormones are complicated by the fact of menstrual periods, pregnancies, and menopause, they tend to suffer more from imbalances.

I think that hormone replacement therapy can be very useful for many women as long as the hormones are in their natural form and the primary hormone used is a natural progesterone cream. I've been saying for years that synthetic hormone replacement therapy has way too many risks and side effects to be worth using, and some of the top researchers in the world continue to present evidence backing me up on this view. I'm not against hormone replacement therapy by any means. I just want you to use natural hormones and to start with the safest ones.

Don't Let Your Doctor Put You on Synthetic Hormones

Mainstream medicine is promoting synthetic estrogens as if they will stop a woman from aging and return her to her youth. In fact, nothing could be further from the truth. I call estrogen the grim reaper. Estrogen in excess, or in excess relative to a shortage of progesterone, causes weight gain, bloating, headaches, irritability, depression, tender breasts, fatigue, thinning of scalp hair, foggy thinking, decreased libido, and, most life threatening, an increased risk of strokes and cancers of the breast and reproductive organs. I believe that much fatigue in women over the age of thirty-five is caused by a combination of excess estrogen (relative to a deficiency of progesterone), and exhausted adrenal glands.

Every risk associated with breast cancer is directly or indirectly related to estrogen, and cancers of the cervix and uterus are directly related to estrogen excess. So are fibroids, fibrocystic breasts, and many of the other complaints that women have as they approach menopause.

Mainstream medicine, backed by the big drug companies, strongly pushes synthetic estrogen (Premarin, Prempro) and the synthetic progesterones called progestins (Provera, Prempro) on women of menopausal age, supposedly to reduce the risk of heart disease and osteoporosis. But the evidence for both of these claims is scanty and, as far as I'm concerned, based more on fancy juggling of statistics than reality. The fact is that estrogen will only slow bone loss for a few years around the time of menopause, and then there is no benefit. And as for the claims that it reduces heart disease—well, the truth is that estrogen greatly raises your risk of stroke, one of the major causes of death among women.

Adding progestins to the hormone replacement mix gives some benefits, but because they are a synthetic version of progesterone, side effects include bloating, headaches, weight gain, breast tenderness, and depression. Women on progestins may also suffer from migraines, asthma, breakthrough bleeding, liver damage, decreased glucose tolerance, excess hair growth, and an increased risk of stroke. Some elixir of youth!

Natural Progesterone May Be Your Answer to Menopause Symptoms

Next time your doctor suggests that you take Premarin or Provera for menopause, ask him or her about natural progesterone. Somehow this important hormone has been all but forgotten. And yet progesterone levels can drop to near zero at menopause, while estrogen levels only fall by 40 to 60 percent, just enough to stop menstrual periods and, for many women, PMS. This dramatic drop in progesterone, combined with a relatively higher level of estrogen, is responsible for most menopause symptoms.

Mainstream medicine rarely distinguishes between the synthetic progestins and natural progesterone as made by the ovaries. And yet the progestins have a long list of negative side effects, including possible miscarriage and fetal malformation, while progesterone is essential for a successful pregnancy. This alone should be a major clue to physicians and their patients that these two substances are very, very different. Sadly, very few studies have been done with progesterone, as it is a natural substance and therefore not patentable and profitable. Those studies that have been done show no side effects aside from some sleepiness at very high doses, and they show many benefits, especially for menopausal women.

Meanwhile, the latest marketing salvo from the makers of Premarin, a conjugated estrogen, is that it's a "natural" hormone. I'm afraid that Premarin is only natural if you're a horse. It is made from pregnant mares' urine. And those poor horses spend their lives standing in narrow stalls with catheters attached to them to collect their urine. When their foals are born, they are soon taken away (and usually killed for pet food) so the mare can be impregnated again right away. These animals suffer needlessly so that the manufacturer can produce a synthetic and therefore patentable and therefore more profitable hormone, when all along the natural hormones, identical to the ones made in your body, are cheaply and easily made from plant sources.

The Hormone Balance and Antiaging Solutions for Women

All the maladies for which doctors are prescribing estrogen can be prevented and reversed with diet and lifestyle changes and, when necessary, with some natural progesterone cream (not the synthetic progestins), which has no side effects and all of the benefits attributed to estrogen. Some women who have persistent hot flashes and vaginal dryness may benefit from a natural estrogen cream, but most women can do just fine without it.

It is well known now that heart disease is one of the most preventable of all chronic diseases with diet and lifestyle changes. Why should a woman suffer from all the estrogen and progestin side effects when she can achieve the desired goals naturally and increase her quality of life in every way?

Women who keep their weight within reasonable limits, who keep their fat intake low and their vegetable intake high, and who get some regular exercise rarely suffer from distressing menopause symptoms. Those who add soy products, such as soy milk and tofu, to their daily diet are even less likely to complain about menopause symptoms.

Women at risk for osteoporosis can prevent it with a combination of diet (not too much protein, a minimum of carbonated beverages, and plenty of fresh vegetables), weight-bearing exercise, and some progesterone cream, which has been convincingly shown by Dr. John Lee to stimulate bone growth and reverse osteoporosis. I've covered the topics of progesterone, estrogen, osteoporosis, and other women's health concerns in depth in chapter 7. Refer back to find out more about women's hormone balance and how to find a good source of supplemental progesterone.

Getting Your Adrenal Glands Back in Balance

As I mentioned earlier, much of what is identified as chronic fatigue may really be depletion and exhaustion of the adrenal glands caused by chronic stress.

People who have tired adrenal glands don't have any get-up-and-go. They go to bed exhausted, wake up tired, and drag through the day trying to pump up their energy with sugar and caffeine. They gain weight because their metabolism slows down to a crawl, and they tend to complain of brain fog and muscle weakness. Their blood sugar is usually out of balance, and exercising can wipe them out for two or three days. Because the production of adrenal gland hormones is intimately tied to ovarian and testicular hormone balance, their estrogen, progesterone, and testosterone levels are often way out of balance. They tend to be dizzy when they stand up suddenly and sometimes have a rapid heartbeat when they lie down. If this sounds like you, have your doctor check your adrenal function.

Chronic stress stimulates the release of adrenal hormones such as cortisol and adrenaline, which in excess, by themselves, can throw the rest of the body's hormones out of balance. These stress hormones are designed to be released occasionally in response to extreme stress or danger; but in our fast-paced world, we tend to pump them out constantly. Eventually, the system breaks down, because it is not meant to be used that way.

Reducing stress, learning some types of meditation or yoga, getting plenty of sleep and rest, and eating nutritious foods will go a long way toward restoring adrenal function. Some people with severe adrenal insufficiency may need small doses of natural hydrocortisone, which is *not* harmful the way the synthetic cortisones such as prednisone are.

Many people can restore their adrenal glands and thus their energy with vitamins, minerals, and herbs that nourish the adrenal glands.

Licorice Root

Licorice root (*Glycyrrhiza glabra*) is top among herbs that support the adrenals. We think of this plant as a candy flavoring (even though most licorice candy is actually flavored with anise oil); however, the root and constituents of this herb provide a tremendous number of valuable medicinal properties.

It is a component of licorice called glycyrrhizin that stimulates the secretion of the adrenal cortex hormone aldosterone and has a powerful cortisone-like effect. In fact, one study found that glycyrrhizin was as effective a cough suppressant as codeine, and safer. In Europe, this unique compound is used extensively for its anti-inflammatory properties, especially for Addison's disease (adrenal insufficiency) and ulcers.

Glycyrrhizin can cause high blood pressure when it is used in very high doses for many months, so some licorice preparations are deglycyrrhizinized. This is *not* what you want if you have adrenal exhaustion. Most people with depleted adrenal glands actually have low blood pressure, so it could be just what you need! (In fact, for some, just adding more salt to the diet is enough to raise blood pressure and alleviate fatigue.)

You can take licorice root in lozenges, capsules, or tincture form. Follow the directions on the container. You can increase the dose by half if it isn't having an effect. If you double the dose and it still doesn't have an effect, this may not be the herb you need.

Vitamin C

This is one of the most important vitamins found in the adrenal glands, and low vitamin C levels will cause lowered adrenal function. If your adrenal glands are tired, increase your vitamin C intake to bowel tolerance; that is, raise the dose until it gives you diarrhea, and then back off from that dosage level until the diarrhea goes away.

Magnesium

Magnesium is one of the key minerals for healthy adrenal glands because it plays an important role in regulating fluid balance in the cells and also is an important vitamin cofactor in the manufacture of adrenal hormones. I recommend a supplement of 300–800 mg daily for supporting tired adrenals. Unbuffered magnesium can cause diarrhea, so try it in the glycinate or citrate form.

Vitamin B₆

This vitamin can help restore and support the adrenal glands, especially in women. Although all the B vitamins are important to healthy adrenal function, people with adrenal insufficiency are often deficient in vitamin B₆. You can take 50 mg daily in addition to your multivitamin (assuming that it doesn't have more than 50 mg in it) to help replenish your adrenal glands.

Pantothenic Acid

Pantothenic acid (vitamin B₅) directly helps strengthen the adrenal glands because it plays a role in making some of the adrenal hormones. If you're bringing your adrenal glands back up to speed, take 500–1,000 mg daily. If you're suffering from stress-induced allergies, try taking 1,000–2,000 mg of pantothenic acid daily.

DHEA Can Work Wonders

DHEA (dehydroepiandrosterone) is an important hormone, mainly made by the adrenal glands, that tends to be an androgen, or male hormone, although it is also a very important hormone for women. In both sexes, DHEA is the most abundant hormone made by the adrenal glands. There is some evidence that supplementing with DHEA can reverse the drop in immune function that happens as we age.

DHEA is one of our most significant markers of aging. It begins to decline in our early twenties, and by the time we're sixty, blood levels of DHEA may be almost imperceptible. In animal studies, DHEA increases life span, lowers cholesterol, increases muscle mass, and stops tumor growth. Although many claims have been made for DHEA, the single most significant factor reported in the human studies of DHEA is that even in relatively small doses, people reported a greatly enhanced sense of well-being.

It is clear that some men can benefit from DHEA supplementation, as high as 100 mg a day, as they age. There is some indication that older women may also benefit from 25 mg a day of DHEA or 25 mg every other day, but unfortunately, very little research has been done with women and DHEA. Too large a dose in women can cause male pattern baldness, insulin resistance, and an increased rate of heart disease. If you are a woman, don't take high doses of DHEA for more than a few weeks. And please do not take diosgenin or "wild yam extract" thinking you are getting DHEA. As far as we know, that doesn't happen reliably. It's best to take the real thing so that you know what you're getting.

GETTING A GOOD NIGHT'S SLEEP

Lack of sleep is one of the most common causes of fatigue, and conversely, sleep is one of the most important keys to maintaining a high-energy lifestyle. Fortunately for most people, it's relatively easy to remedy restless nights. The most obvious sleep robbers are the most common ones: stress, lack of exercise, caffeine, and prescription drugs. Having to get up at night repeatedly to urinate can disturb sleeping patterns enough to cause problems. Don't drink a lot of fluids before bed, and if you're having prostate problems, use the herb saw palmetto. For details on treating prostate problems naturally, see chapter 8.

De-stress for Deep Sleep

Often when people are under stress and feel helpless to do anything about it, they lie awake at night tossing and turning with repetitive "tapes" going through their head, or they wake up very early in the morning and can't get back to sleep. Big decisions, the illness or troubles of a loved one, major life changes, financial difficulties, and any number of the other lumps and bumps that life hands out can all cause sleeplessness. Depression will often cause sleeplessness, which creates a vicious circle of more depression and more sleeplessness.

There are many, many positive ways to cope with stress. One of them is to try a form of meditation that focuses on becoming aware of the mind and of your "self-talk" as well as on breathing and chanting techniques that can help focus the mind. If you are unconsciously saying negative things to yourself all day long, it can be more than enough to keep you up at night. Many forms of meditation will assist you in replacing that destructive self-talk with something more positive. I'll discuss this in more detail later in the chapter.

Another way to cope with stress is to talk to a trained therapist. Just talking out loud about a problem to another human being willing to listen attentively can be enough to begin the emotional healing process. Often, when we talk about our problems out loud, resolutions begin to appear.

One technique I have found helpful when stress levels are high is to ask myself, "What is one step I can take to reduce my stress levels?" Most often for me that step is taking a walk in a beautiful place. Sometimes it's just a matter of getting to bed earlier or spending relaxing time with my family. For some it may be a hot bath or a meal at a favorite restaurant.

More than one or two drinks of alcohol a day is not a good remedy for stress. You may escape temporarily from your problems, but excess alcohol is more likely to keep you up at night than put you to sleep, and it robs your body of many nutrients.

And don't be fooled into thinking that the new class of antidepressants, such as Prozac, Paxil, and Zoloft, are a good solution for anything. They create a false sense of detachment and can lead to violence and suicide. Just a few of their many side effects include liver damage, depression, and insomnia. The companies who make these drugs are now finally being forced to admit to the FDA that they cause a withdrawal syndrome in people who stop taking them. The most common symptoms reported by people going through withdrawal are fatigue, moodiness, foggy thinking, headaches, dizziness, nausea, and depression.

In ten years, we will all be looking back at the "Prozac years," shaking our heads and wondering how so many people could have been so gullible to think that such drugs could be harmless. Meanwhile, countless people's lives have already been destroyed by them. Even though these drugs are being handed out like candy by many doctors, I urge you to resist the urge to change your personality with a pill. First try a balanced, moderate lifestyle, cutting down on stress, getting some exercise, getting plenty of sleep, and taking some nutritional supplements.

Exercise Can Be a Simple, Effective Cure for Insomnia

Exercise is by far my favorite sleeping pill and cure for the blues. I have seen many people suffering from mild depression or insomnia cure it simply by getting some exercise. Somehow we resist the simple cures to our problems, but exercise is one of your best bets for a good night's sleep. A brisk 20- to 30-minute walk daily can be just the sleeping potion you need.

As for maintaining peak energy, anyone who exercises regularly knows that you use energy or lose it. Working the body keeps its fuel systems active, bringing in oxygen used to burn the calories taken in from food, which produces energy. Energy is needed for every activity, even sleeping. When you have optimum fitness, you'll have optimum energy. The greater the energy, the more active you can be in every area of your life and the better you'll function on every level, including physical, mental, and emotional.

Is Caffeine Your Sleep Robber?

Too much caffeine, or caffeine too late in the day, can keep your eyes wide open for hours into the night. While this might be nice if you're working a night shift, for most of us it only leads to bleary eyes and fatigue the next day. Some people are so sensitive to caffeine that a cup of coffee at any time after noon will keep them awake at night. And let's not forget that green tea and black tea contain caffeine. If you're suffering from insomnia, your best bet is to drink nonstimulating herbal teas such as chamomile or mint in the evening. If you need a boost in the afternoon, try a cup of ginseng tea.

Are Your Medications Keeping You Up?

Many over-the-counter painkillers, cold and allergy remedies, and appetite suppressants contain caffeine and other substances that can cause insomnia. Some examples are Anacin, Extra Strength Excedrin, Bayer Select Maximum, Midol, and Vanquish.

Allergy and cold medicines may contain synthetic variations of ephedrine, such as pseudo-ephedrine (Sudafed), which can keep you awake. The asthma drug theophylline (Bronkaid and Primatene tablets, Tedral, and others) are stimulants that can make sleeping difficult.

The cortisones, such as prednisone, can also cause sleeplessness. The heart drugs, such as propranolol, furosemide, and lovastatin, may cause insomnia, as can too high a dose of thyroid medication such as Synthroid. Ironically, many of the antidepressants cause insomnia, which can cause depression due to lack of sleep!

Unfortunately, if one of these medications is keeping you awake at night, your doctor is most likely to write you out a prescription for a sleeping pill. In nearly all cases, that is the worst thing you can do for insomnia. Sleeping pills cause either dependence or outright addiction very quickly. Moreover, they tend to lose their effectiveness over time and have a rebound effect if you stop, causing worse insomnia than ever. They also tend to suppress your dream, or REM, sleep, sometimes resulting in severe mental disturbances and psychoses if used over a long period of time. If someone hands you a prescription for a sleeping pill, my advice is to run the other way.

If you're having trouble sleeping and you're taking any type of medication, including over-the-counter drugs, read the label or package insert to find out if it can cause insomnia, restlessness, or irritability.

Supplements for Sleep

A variety of supplements can help you sleep at night. A deficiency of B vitamins, calcium, or magnesium can keep you awake. As we age, our production of melatonin, a hormone that regulates sleep-wake cycles, declines. A simple melatonin supplement may be your ticket to a good night's sleep if you're a senior citizen. An amino acid called tryptophan also helps you sleep and soothes anxiety and depression.

The B Vitamins

The B vitamins together and separately play important roles in nerve and brain function and in relaxing muscles. If you are sixty or older and not absorbing nutrients as well as you might be, your body may not be able to utilize the B vitamins in your food. It's im-

portant to include the B vitamins in a multivitamin. If you're having trouble with leg cramps at night, an extra 50 mg of vitamin B_6 an hour before bed may help. I have heard many anecdotal stories of people curing restless leg syndrome by taking an extra 400 mcg of folic acid before bed.

Calcium and Magnesium

Both of these important minerals play a role in muscle relaxation, the prevention of muscle spasms, and the balance of fluid in the cells. If you tend to tense up physically when you're under stress or if you suffer from leg cramps at night, calcium and magnesium might be the supplements for you. These two minerals should be taken together, since calcium can't do many of its jobs in the body without magnesium. You can take 600–800 mg of calcium and 300–600 mg of magnesium about an hour before bedtime. There are many formulas that combine these two minerals in a ratio of 2:1 calcium to magnesium, and these are fine.

Using Melatonin to Improve Sleep

Melatonin is a safe, effective, natural sleep remedy that is free of side effects when used as directed. It is normally secreted by the brain in response to darkness.

Because it regulates sleep-wake cycles, melatonin can also be very useful for banishing jet lag by adjusting circadian rhythms to match your geographical location. You do this simply by taking melatonin about an hour before you want to sleep in your new location. It will give your brain the message that it's time to sleep, regardless of what time zone you're in. One or two nights of melatonin should put you back on the right track.

As for the claims that melatonin is an antiaging drug, we need to be cautious in making the leap from extending life span in a particular strain of mice to extending life span in humans. In some studies, mice that were given melatonin lived 20 percent longer, but other strains of mice in other studies died sooner. Younger mice given melatonin developed cancer, and melatonin in high doses suppresses sex hormones.

I use melatonin regularly to erase jet lag when I travel, and I recommend it for older people who are having trouble sleeping, I want to caution you, though, that we simply don't know the long-term effects of using melatonin every night. Whenever we take a hormone in higher doses than the body would naturally produce, we're asking for an imbalance.

If you are over the age of sixty-five and your melatonin levels have dropped so far that you can't sleep at night, *and* you have eliminated other possible causes of your insomnia, then by all means take 0.5–3 mg at night to help you sleep. In that case, you are correcting a deficiency. It is also perfectly safe to take melatonin for an occasional bout of insomnia. Melatonin is a natural hormone, so when it is used occasionally your body should have no trouble excreting any excess.

If you need melatonin, it only takes a very small dose to help you sleep better. If low melatonin levels aren't your problem, even a big dose won't make any difference.

The melatonin sold in health food stores is manufactured but is the exact molecular structure as the melatonin made by the body. Sublingual forms of melatonin are more expensive but act more quickly. Look for a reputable brand at your health food store. Take regular melatonin tablets about one hour before you want to go to sleep, and the sublingual tablets half an hour before you want to go to sleep.

Some drugs, including NSAIDs (nonsteroidal anti-inflammatory drugs, such as aspirin, ibuprofen, and acetaminophen), interfere with the brain's production of melatonin. In fact, just one dose of normal aspirin can cut your melatonin production as much as 75 percent. If you're taking these drugs, take the last dose after dinner. Other drugs that can interfere with melatonin production in the brain include the benzodiazepines (such as Valium and Xanax), caffeine, alcohol, cold medicines, diuretics, beta-blockers, calcium channel blockers, stimulants (such as diet pills), and corticosteroids (such as prednisone).

Tryptophan May Help You Sleep

The amino acid tryptophan, a precursor to melatonin, is a very safe and effective sleep remedy and can also be a wonderful remedy for anxiety and depression. Unfortunately, it was pulled off the market in the United States by the FDA when a contaminated batch from Japan made some people ill. This type of contamination could have happened in thousands of drugs, and the illness it caused had nothing to do with the effects of uncontaminated tryptophan. In truth, tryptophan is very safe—in my opinion far safer than sleeping pills and antidepressants, which it was competing with in a big way when it was pulled off the market. My guess is that tryptophan was removed from the market to protect the profits of the big drug companies, not to protect your health.

Tryptophan's effect on the brain is similar to that of drugs such as Prozac, except that it doesn't have the side effects, dangers, and withdrawal problems that those drugs have, it's much less expensive, and it's probably more effective. Tryptophan is trickling back onto the market in the United States, and it can be purchased almost anywhere outside the United States.

One of tryptophan's primary effects on the brain is to reduce anxiety, which is often the culprit in insomnia. However, even if tryptophan is unavailable where you live, there are some herbs that can work wonders to alleviate feelings of anxiety.

Calming Herbs

The herbs I recommend most often for treating depression and anxiety are St. John's wort and kava.

St. John's Wort

St. John's wort, which has been used successfully for many centuries by the Chinese, the Greeks, the Europeans, and the American Indians, is well known for its positive effect on anxiety, insomnia, depression, and a physical illness that has long been associated with stress: heart disease.

St. John's wort, which you can get easily both as a tincture and in capsule form at your health food store, has no known side effects in humans. (If grazing cattle eat huge amounts of fresh St. John's wort, they have been found to develop photosensitivity; but so far I've heard no reports of humans having this problem—and humans would be highly unlikely to eat a proportionate amount of St. John's wort or to eat it fresh.) These positive effects seem even more positive when weighed against the less dramatic side effects of pharmaceutical drugs, such as drowsiness, constipation, and dry mouth.

Take St. John's wort in the dose recommended on the container.

Kava

Kava is one of our most useful antianxiety herbs. Anyone who's been to the South Pacific, where it grows like a bush, has probably tried it. Its Latin name is *Piper methysticum*, and it's a member of the pepper family. Kava is described medically as a sedative and muscle relaxant. It's also a pain reliever, often working just as well as NSAIDs (drugs in the aspirin, ibuprofen, and acetaminophen family).

As a folk medicine, kava is attributed with the power to bring on well-being and to encourage socializing. Many studies, mostly done in Europe, have demonstrated how effective kava is in the treatment of anxiety and depression. It has worked as effectively as benzodiazepines, of which Valium, Librium, and Serax are examples. In many ways, kava's effects are preferable. Rather than causing lethargy, drowsiness, and mental impairment (which are common responses to benzodiazepines), kava improves concentration, memory, and reaction time for people with anxiety symptoms. And the best part is that no side effects have been noted, except with very large amounts taken over a number of years. However, kava is not recommended for people with Parkinson's or Alzheimer's disease.

Kava is best taken powdered in a capsule or as a liquid extract. Follow the directions on the container.

SUPPLEMENTS FOR A STRONG IMMUNE SYSTEM

The immune system, which protects us from harmful bacteria, viruses, fungi, and other so-called foreign invaders, makes its presence known in every system of the body. Unlike the circulatory system or the reproductive system, you can't see the immune system on an anatomy chart or remove it in surgery, and yet it is equivalent in size and daily activity to a large organ that produces billions of new cells each day. It rallies its defenses from the cellular level everywhere in the body, from deep within the brain and bone marrow to the adrenal glands, the thymus gland, and the skin. It courses through the blood and the intestines; its wastes are dumped into the lymphatic system, the kidneys, and the liver for detoxifying; and it relies on an intricate identification system to discriminate between the good guys and the bad guys. When this identification system goes awry, we get autoimmune diseases and allergies. We fall prey to infections, viral diseases, and cancers when we are unable to rally the vast armies of specialized cells designed to protect us from deadly threats we can't see. These immune cells go by such names as white blood cells, T cells, helper cells, lymphocytes, and macrophages.

Without a healthy immune system, it is impossible to lead a fully active, healthy lifestyle. Keeping the immune system on full alert and in balance is achieved by keeping all levels in balance—physical, emotional, mental, and spiritual. Our immune system balance is intricately tied to our thoughts and emotions, but is influenced as well by nutrition, exercise, and environmental toxins.

All nutrients are important to the immune system and have a direct effect on it. A study in Newfoundland found that senior citizens who consumed a multivitamin supplement for one year had many increased immune responses and fewer days of illness due to infectious diseases. Let's zero in on those supplements that affect your immune system the most.

Vitamins and Minerals

If you're catching every bug that comes along, the first thing you should suspect is that you need more of certain vitamins and minerals.

Vitamin A

Vitamin A is important in maintaining the integrity of the skin and mucous membranes, your frontline defenses against airborne and intestinal invaders. Your largest mucous membrane is in the intestines, which contain a wide variety of immune cells. Vitamin A has been shown to stimulate many immune processes. It helps fight infection, is antiviral, and is anticarcinogenic. A large supplemental dose of vitamin A can reverse the suppression of the immune system that occurs after surgery and can improve wound healing. On a day-to-day basis, you can get most of your vitamin A from carotenoids such as beta-carotene, from which the body will make vitamin A as needed.

In a study with AIDS patients, beta-carotene in doses of 180 IU created an increase in helper cells. If you are fighting an infection or a virus, you can take up to 50,000 IU daily for a week or two. Since vitamin A accumulates in the body and can be toxic in high doses, it's best not to take it in high doses for more than a few weeks. Pregnant women shouldn't take more than 10,000 IU of vitamin A in supplement form daily.

The B Vitamins

The B vitamins are essential immune system boosters. Both vitamin B_{12} and folic acid play a particularly important role in the production of white blood cells and lymphocyte response. Population studies show an association between low levels of folic acid (folate) and cancer of the cervix, colon, lung, esophagus, and brain. According to Dr. John Lee, folic acid supplementation can reverse a precancerous growth of the cervix called cervical dysplasia.

You should be getting 200 mcg of folic acid daily in supplement form, up to 600 mcg daily if you are battling illness, and at least 400 mcg daily if there is any possibility that you could become pregnant. (Folic acid deficiencies can cause birth defects.)

Since vitamin B_{12} is not well absorbed when taken orally, you can take it in the form of a nasal gel or sublingually (under the tongue), 1,000 mcg one to three times daily when you need a boost.

Pantothenic acid (vitamin B_5) supports adrenal and pituitary hormones and reduces the body's histamine response. Take at least 25 mg daily and up to 100 mg if your immune system needs to shift into high gear. Low vitamin B_6 levels have been found to correlate with a low T cell count. In one eight-week study, 50 mg of vitamin B_6 per day stimulated lymphocytes. Take 50 mg daily and up to 100 mg when stress levels are high. This vitamin is particularly important for maintaining hormone balance in women who are under stress.

Vitamin C

This vitamin is a primary weapon in the immune system's arsenal against bacteria and viruses. When you need an extra boost to your immune system from vitamin C, try taking 1,500–4,000 mg in a buffered powder form that includes calcium, magnesium, and potassium. At the same time that you take the vitamin C, take a bioflavonoid supplement, which will maximize your body's use of the vitamin C.

Vitamin E

Vitamin E is one of the superstars of the vitamin world when it comes to boosting the immune system. Studies show that it increases helper T cells and antibody response, both potent weapons of the immune system. A study of vitamin E with healthy people taking 800 IU per day showed that it enhanced immune responses. When you're looking for an immune boost, take 800 IU daily of *d*-alpha-tocopherol. For maximum absorption, take it in the dry, or "succinate," form.

Minerals

Minerals are essential components of a healthy immune system, and you should be getting them every day in a multivitamin. A deficiency of minerals such as zinc and selenium can lead to reduced cellular immunity and an increased susceptibility to infection. Selenium deficiency is common in AIDS and colon cancer patients, people with chronic diarrhea, and those with poor absorption of nutrients. Deficiencies of selenium and zinc can indicate a depressed immune system. One way selenium supports the immune system is by acting as an antioxidant, mopping up free radicals that damage cells. Zinc deficiency causes the thymus, one of our primary immune system organs, to shrink.

Low zinc levels also cause poor wound healing and decreased numbers of T cells, lymphocytes, and natural killer cells. Zinc works with vitamin A to maintain mucous membranes and is especially important in fighting off viruses. Iron deficiency can also result in a decrease in T cell–mediated immunity.

Manganese increases natural killer cell activity. It is depleted from most soils, so this is an important trace mineral to include in a daily multivitamin.

Other Immune Boosters

If vitamins and minerals don't boost your immunity enough, try these immunity-boosting supplements.

Probiotics

Probiotics, particularly *Lactobacillus acidophilus*, are "good" intestinal bacteria that support the immune system by bringing the intestinal flora into balance. *Prebiotics* are nondigestible "food" for probiotics, but not for harmful bacteria. Fructooligosaccharides (FOS) are prebiotics that are now included in many probiotic products. I recommend that you choose a probiotic-prebiotic combination that is dated and refrigerated. Follow the directions on the container.

Dehydroepiandrosterone (DHEA)

DHEA, which we looked at in relationship to hormonal balance earlier in the chapter, is an adrenal hormone that declines with age and any type of illness involving adrenal insufficiency. Studies have found low DHEA levels in people who have AIDS and leukemia, and some researchers theorize that the hormone plays an important role in regulating T cells. DHEA can be a very useful supplement for those suffering from chronic illness who have low levels of DHEA or for people over the age of fifty. Women should keep their dosage low, up to 20–25 mg daily or every other day, as DHEA is an androgen, or masculinizing hormone. Men can take up to 100 mg daily, but 50 mg is the usual maintenance dose.

Essential Fatty Acids

EFAs, oils found primarily in vegetables, nuts, seeds, fish, flaxseed oil, evening primrose oil, and borage oil, affect the balance of prostaglandins, hormonelike substances that play an important role in regulating the immune system. Supplementing AIDS and cancer patients with omega-3 fatty acids (fish oils, flaxseed oil) has been shown to improve a depressed immune system. Other studies have shown that fish oil supplementation has an anti-inflammatory effect, inhibits tumor growth, and speeds healing after surgery.

Linoleic acid, an omega-6 fatty acid found in many vegetable oils, is necessary for T cells to work properly. On the other hand, too high an intake of linoleic acid, especially relative to not enough omega-3 fatty acids, will suppress immune function. This may be useful in treating autoimmune diseases, but some researchers believe that the increase in consumption of polyunsaturated oils, such as vegetable oils and margarines, has contributed to the increase in asthma and other lung-related problems over the last three decades by blocking "good" prostaglandin pathways.

Glutamine

Glutamine is the most abundant free amino acid in the human body. While glutamine is not considered an essential amino acid because your body can make plenty of it under normal circumstances, it becomes essential when you're under physical stress. It plays a powerful and essential role in maintaining a healthy digestive system, a strong immune system, muscle strength, and chemical balance in the brain. Some researchers believe that glutamine is *the* most essential nutrient in the digestive tract. When you're under stress, particularly stress caused by surgery, illness, or injury, the levels of glutamine in your body can drop up to 90 percent.

Studies have shown that surgery patients who are given supplemental glutamine after surgery recover faster and have a shorter hospital stay. Glutamine has also been shown in animal studies to enhance the tumor-killing effects of chemotherapy and radiation and to reduce their side effects.

Glutamine is not recommended if you have severe liver disease or other illnesses that could involve an accumulation of ammonia in the blood. I recommend that you take this supplement in the L-glutamine form, as a powder, capsule, or tablet.

Glutathione

Glutathione is an antioxidant made in the body by three amino acids: cysteine, glucine, and glutamic acid. Its primary job is neutralizing and disposing of free radicals, in coordination with vitamins E and C. It's also crucial in protecting the lymphatic system, one of the body's primary weapons in fighting infection. Glutathione directly improves immune function and protects the body against free radicals and external toxins. If glutathione levels drop anywhere in the body, the burden of toxic stress goes up. T cells cannot function when glutathione levels are low.

Glutathione concentrations are high in healthy people. People with chronic conditions such as heart disease, arthritis, and diabetes have low glutathione levels. The best way to raise glutathione levels is by taking a cysteine supplement, 500–1,000 mg daily (the body uses cysteine to make glutathione). You can take it in the form of cysteine or *N*-acetylcysteine.

Echinacea

This herb acts as a powerful immune system booster. It can be very useful in preventing colds and flu or in shortening their duration. Don't take echinacea for more than two weeks at a time, or it will start to lose its effectiveness.

ARE ALLERGIES BRINGING YOU DOWN?

Spring is a fresh, exuberant time of year, with balmy breezes, green grass sprouting, and flowers blooming everywhere. But if you have allergies to pollens and grasses, as one in ten Americans does, spring may only mean fatigue, mental fogginess, sniffling, snuffling, and sneezing to you. The normal response to allergy symptoms is to take drugs such as antihistamines, but as most of us have discovered, they all have undesirable side effects.

Allergies in general can also be caused by food, food additives and dyes, chemical sprays and fumes, dust, pet hair and fleas, molds, medication, perfumes,

---

Ten More Natural Ways to Charge Up Your Immune System

1. Stretching helps your lymphatic system do its job of removing toxins from your body. Chi gong is an especially effective form of exercise for boosting the immune system.
2. Take a good multivitamin (see chapter 1).
3. Exercise keeps everything in the body shipshape, but if you feel weak or tired, don't push too hard; it will only make things worse. If you have a cold or flu, you need your rest.
4. Drink plenty of clean water, which will help your body keep itself detoxified.
5. Eat plenty of fiber to keep things moving through the digestive system.
6. Eat yogurt once a day for the calcium and beneficial intestinal flora. The friendly bacteria in your intestines are your best weapon against unfriendly bacteria.
7. Eat your vegetables—fresh and preferably organic. And I'm not talking iceberg lettuce here, I'm talking the real stuff, like carrots, broccoli, spinach, and beets.
8. Eat more complex carbohydrates and less refined white flour, which causes blood sugar jumps and constipation.
9. Try shiitake or reishi mushrooms with your veggies. The Chinese use them to bolster the immune system.
10. If you have a late night or stressful day, balance things out by getting extra rest.

cosmetics, feathers, and dozens of other environmental offenders. While avoiding the offender works in part, it is also important to support your immune system.

Why Do We Sneeze and Sniffle?

We get allergies to pollen when our immune system is reacting, or sensitive, to something in the environment that is actually harmless. It's helpful (although unpleasant) when our body fights off a real invader such as a virus or bacteria with an immune reaction, which we call a cold or flu. But when we react to pollens, it's annoying and can interfere with our enjoyment of life.

Once our immune system decides that a particular type of pollen is a hostile invader, it becomes "sensitized" to it and can react with allergy symptoms for years and perhaps a lifetime. When spring arrives and the pollen begins to fly, our sensitized body releases histamines, designed to fight the enemy pollen. In the process of attacking the invaders, the histamines cause inflammation and even damage tissues, causing sinus irritation, itchy eyes, and often lung irritation as well. Some people may even develop rashes, eczema, or hives.

The frequent accompanying headaches and mental fogginess are caused by sinus congestion. Sneezing is caused by irritated sinuses. Sore throats are caused by the mucus that runs down the back of the throat. Asthma can be triggered by an overload of irritants and mucus. If the body tries to rid itself of the invaders via the skin, rashes, eczema, and hives may result.

Allergy drugs work to suppress symptoms rather than treat the cause of the allergy. The consequences of this type of treatment are generally unpleasant side effects and often a rebound effect, where the symptom is worse if the medication starts to wear off or treatment is stopped.

Natural Remedies for Allergies

The simplest way to avoid allergy symptoms is to avoid the offending allergens, but if you're allergic to pollens and grasses, yet love the outdoors and fresh air, this isn't a practical solution. The next simplest

way to deal with allergies is to drink plenty of clean water. I recommend at least eight to ten glasses a day during allergy season. Water not only helps flush toxins out of the body and supports proper cell function, but as our water levels go down, our histamine levels go up. Drinking a couple of glasses of clean water can quickly reduce allergy symptoms.

The reason some people suffer from allergies and others don't certainly has to do with genetic predisposition but also seems to have to do with how well your immune system is working. If you already have a weakened immune system from chronic nutritional deficiencies, disease, lack of exercise, or other factors, you're much more susceptible to allergies.

Echinacea

Echinacea is a powerful immune system booster. Take two dropperfuls of the tincture (preferably the fresh extract) in water, or two capsules, three times daily. Don't take echinacea for more than two weeks at a time, or it will start to lose its effectiveness. Through allergy season, take it two weeks on and two weeks off.

Astragalus

This Chinese plant has been used by healers in that country for centuries to restore normal function to the immune system. Follow the directions on the container.

Shiitake and Reishi Mushrooms

These mushrooms are another Eastern remedy for the immune system. I like them best in a vegetable stir-fry or in an omelet. They're expensive, but you don't need to use much—one or two small mushrooms per serving should do the trick. During allergy season, add these to your diet at least once a week, or take them in capsule form.

Garlic

The more we study and research garlic, the better it looks. If you like the taste, make it a part of your daily diet; and if you don't like the taste, you can take it in capsule form. In addition to lowering cholesterol levels and blood pressure, killing intestinal parasites, reducing the risk of blood clots, inhibiting some cancer tumors, and aiding digestion, garlic is a potent antioxidant, helping the body to keep our cells healthy, intact, and functioning smoothly.

Yogurt

If you eat yogurt with live cultures daily, you may greatly reduce the severity of your seasonal allergy symptoms. A one-year study at the University of California at Davis showed that those who ate just under a cup of yogurt daily had significantly reduced hay fever symptoms as well as fewer colds. The researchers who did the study found that 2 cups of yogurt a day worked even better than 1.

Ephedra

Also called Mormon tea and ma huang, this plant contains ephedrine. Pseudoephedrine is the synthetic version of ephedrine and is commonly found in over-the-counter allergy drugs. It is widely used in diet pills because it's an "upper." However, the downside is that it can also make you "hyper," restless, irritable, and nervous and can cause insomnia. While it is effective in reducing the symptoms of congestion, I urge you not to use it over a long period of time. Work instead on the underlying causes of your allergies, and take the steps I recommend, reserving these types of drugs for occasional symptomatic use. And do not use ephedra at all if you have high blood pressure or heart disease.

Milk Thistle

Milk thistle, or *Silybum marianum*, is one of the hot "new" herbs that's been used in folk medicine for centuries and is now gaining respectability, thanks to scientific studies. It has been clearly shown in studies to greatly support the liver, even to the extent of regenerating liver cells. Because your liver is one of the main places your immune system dumps toxins, it pays to support it during allergy season. Take one capsule three times daily. Make sure your milk thistle product is taken from the seeds, which contain most of the active ingredient, silymarin. These seeds are also rich in linoleic acid, which supports the production of prostaglandins, another important hormonelike substance. Linoleic acid also appears to help regulate the female hormones.

Vitamin C

If I could recommend only one vitamin to help with allergy symptoms, it would be vitamin C. This essential vitamin, which many Americans are deficient in, works directly to lower histamine levels in the body and supports the immune system in many ways. During allergy season, I recommend that you take at least 1,000 mg three times daily; and if your symptoms continue or get worse, increase that to 1,000 mg every 2 or 3 hours.

Quercetin

This is a powerful antioxidant flavonoid that has been shown to fight cancer tumors and seems to be very effective in helping fight allergy symptoms. I like it combined with bromelain for better absorption.

Grapeseed Extract

The star of the antioxidant world is a complex of substances called proanthocyanidins, known for short as PCOs. I like the PCOs extracted from grapeseeds. They rank among our most powerful flavonoids, being fifty times more powerful at scavenging free radicals than vitamin E and twenty times more powerful than vitamin C. Furthermore, they enhance the potency of both these vitamins.

You can take 150–300 mg of PCOs daily to combat allergies. I recommend the grapeseed PCO extract that comes in a "phytosome" package, meaning the molecules are combined with phosphatidylcholine, a natural component of lecithin. This new process allows the body to absorb and utilize much more of the PCOs than it would otherwise.

Homeopathic Remedies

There are dozens of homeopathic remedies for allergies, with very specific applications. If you want to try that route, I recommend that you read one of these books: *Everybody's Guide to Homeopathic Medicines* by

Stephen Cummings and Dana Ullman (Tarcher, 1997); *Homeopathic Medicine at Home* by M. B. Panos and J. Heimlich (Tarcher, 1981); or *The Family Guide to Homeopathy* by Dr. Andrew Locke (Simon & Schuster-Fireside, 1983). For more in-depth treatment, find an experienced homeopathic physician. I've also devoted chapter 12 of this book to homeopathic remedies.

BOOSTING ENERGY AND BRAINPOWER NATURALLY

The most important thing you can do for your brain is to feed it well, which is the same as feeding the rest of your body. Everything you eat affects your brain to some extent. I can't emphasize enough how important a healthy lifestyle is to a healthy brain. Brain function is dependent on balanced nutrition and particularly on keeping your body's detoxification systems working effectively. The additives, preservatives, and dyes found in processed food only add to your body's detoxification load. Your load will have less to detoxify if you're careful about what you put in it.

Clean water is your most important detoxifier, and exercise is your second most important detoxifier.

Your brain needs plenty of B vitamins to function properly. It also needs amino acids, stable blood sugar, and plenty of oxygen. The brain also needs glucose in abundance. Glucose is a sugar that the body makes from the food we eat. It is the primary source of energy for the brain. Your brain literally cannot function without it. If your glucose or blood sugar levels remain relatively stable, your brain will work better. That means keeping your weight down, avoiding sweets and other refined foods, and getting some exercise.

Exercise improves circulation, increasing your oxygen supply to the brain via better blood flow. Glucose and oxygen work together in the brain. If your blood isn't getting enough oxygen, your brain won't work as well. Exercise is one of the best ways to increase blood flow to the brain.

Preventing Memory Loss and Brain Fog

If glucose is the energy source for the brain, a substance called glutamate is the mainstay of the communications system of the brain. Glutamate is a brain "excitor," meaning it excites brain cells into action. With the proper balance of glutamate, your brain functions well. Too little glutamate is rarely a problem. However, if the brain gets too much glutamate, the brain cells excite themselves to death. And if this continues, you lose brain function, starting with memory.

Glutamate is probably a familiar word to you because you've heard of monosodium glutamate, or MSG. Millions of pounds of MSG are dumped in our food every year, much to the detriment of our brain health. Since MSG has gotten a bad reputation, food manufacturers, ever alert to increasing profits at the expense of your health, have learned to disguise MSG on labels by calling it natural flavoring, hydrolyzed vegetable protein, vegetable protein, and spices (while the FDA looks the other way). New labeling laws were supposed to mandate that all MSG-type products be labeled as glutamate, but somehow they got lost in the political maze of the FDA. The best way to avoid glutamate is to avoid processed foods and be discriminating about eating in restaurants.

Glutamate has a close cousin called aspartate, another brain excitor that also has important functions in brain communications. Aspartate should be familiar to you as a part of the artificial sweetener aspartame, otherwise known as Nutra-Sweet. Test animals fed MSG and aspartate, even in low doses over a long period of time, end up with symptoms identical to Alzheimer's. If you want to keep your memory powered up for life, I urge you to avoid these substances. This means avoiding refined foods, diet sodas, and other artificially sweetened foods and drinks. There's no doubt that MSG and all its relatives make food tastier, but who wants to sacrifice brain cells and memory?

The amino acid glutamine is closely related to glutamate, but when you take it as a supplement, your body can either turn it into glutamine, as needed, or into other related amino acids.

Brain fog can have many causes or a combination of causes. Some of the most common are unstable blood sugar, excess estrogen, low thyroid, exhausted adrenal glands, and lack of sleep. Other common causes of brain fog are pollen allergies and food allergies and sensitivities (see page 226).

If you are sensitive to environmental toxins and irritants such as car exhaust, pesticides, fumes from newly painted rooms or new carpets, solvents, scented laundry soaps, fabric softeners, and perfumes, your brain can "crash" just from exposure to these substances. If this describes you, your best approach is to make every effort to avoid exposure to such substances while building up your immune system as much as possible. I recommend working with a health care professional knowledgeable in alternative medicine if you have environmental sensitivities.

Is Your Prescription Fogging Your Brain?

If you're taking prescription drugs, keep in mind that many of them can cause memory loss and brain fog. The most common types of drugs that can cause memory loss are the ulcer drugs, such as Tagamet and Zantac; the high blood pressure drugs, such as beta-blockers and diuretics; and the antidepressants, antipsychotics, barbiturates, sleeping pills, and tranquilizers, such as Prozac, Nembutal, Atarax, Dalmane, and Valium.

Remember, keeping your memory powered up for life is mainly a matter of a healthy lifestyle. If you supply your brain with a good environment, it will supply you with a good memory.

Sometimes during times of stress or illness, or as we age, we need some help powering up the brain. Here are some natural ways to boost your brain power while also boosting your energy.

Memory and Energy Boosters

Ginkgo Biloba

This is one of my favorite memory boosters because it's very effective, very safe, and not expensive. It's been extensively researched and is sold in standardized amounts, so you know what you're getting.

The ginkgo biloba tree has been on this planet longer than any other species of tree. It has been around for at least three hundred million years! The Chinese have been using ginkgo medicinally for at least five thousand years.

Ginkgo has been shown over and over again in European research studies to be very effective in treating what is called in medical circles "cerebral insufficiency," or impaired blood flow to the brain. It can improve the ability to remember, the speed of memory, and mental performance, as well as relieving other symptoms of cerebral insufficiency, such as headaches, dizziness, ringing in the ears, clumsiness, and hearing impairment.

Ginkgo may be one of our most important anti-aging medicines. If you're over the age of sixty, I recommend you take it daily as health insurance. It may be a few weeks before you notice results.

The best way to take ginkgo is in a liquid extract, capsules, or tablets that are at least 24 percent ginkgo flavoglycosides.

Acetylcholine

Acetylcholine is a neurotransmitter, a chemical that transfers messages from one brain cell to another. When those messages are disrupted by a lack of acetylcholine or less effective acetylcholine receptors in the brain cells, symptoms such as memory loss and confused thinking can result. Researchers at the University of California have theorized that one of the causes of Alzheimer's disease is a destruction of the cells that supply acetylcholine to the parts of the brain involved in memory and cognitive thinking. When they increased acetylcholine levels in the brains of rats with brain damage equivalent to Alzheimer's, they found they could restore their memory.

In another study done at Hebrew University, a research team discovered that memory loss could be caused simply by an excess of a brain enzyme called acetylcholinesterase, which breaks down acetylcholine.

Increasing your brain's supply of acetylcholine is a safe, natural way to give your brain what it needs to do the job. One of the other jobs acetylcholine has in the body is to make your muscles contract. If you are taking anticholinergic drugs to treat Parkinson's disease, you won't want to use supplements that boost acetylcholine. Anticholinergic drugs are used in Parkinson's and in some digestive tract diseases to reduce muscle contraction. The next four supplements listed will help you build your acetylcholine levels.

Pantothenic acid. Also known as vitamin B_5 or pantothenate, pantothenic acid acts as an enzyme that builds the acteylcholine molecule. Take 200–500 mg daily.

Phosphatidylcholine. The active ingredient in lecithin, phosphatidylcholine is a building block for acetylcholine. You can take it as a liquid, as a capsule, or as 1 tablespoon daily of lecithin granules that can be sprinkled on cereal or other foods or just eaten plain. Be sure the lecithin is at least 55 percent phosphatidylcholine, and be sure that it is fresh, not rancid. It should have a pleasant, nutty smell and taste. Since choline increases the secretion of stomach acid, this may be helpful if your digestion is poor; but if you have ulcers, wait until they're healed before using choline. Take 1,500–2,500 mg daily.

Niacin. Also called niacinamide or vitamin B_3, niacin is a cofactor in building acetylcholine. Take 50–100 mg of niacin in the form of niacinamide daily. If you are experiencing flushing, take it with a meal. With this small a dose, flushing usually goes away after a week or two.

Glutamic acid. Glutamic acid is a brain-stimulating amino acid that may increase the number of acetylcholine receptor sites in your brain cells. It is the amino acid found in the highest concentration in the brain after aspartate, and the brain spends a great deal of energy keeping it balanced with its close relatives glutamine and gamma-aminobutyric acid (GABA). It can also be made into glutamate, which may sound familiar from the flavor enhancer monosodium glutamate (MSG), a highly absorbable and easily toxic form of glutamic acid. Because glutamate in excess can become a brain toxin, you should take this amino acid in the form of glutamine, which the body will easily convert to whichever form it needs in the brain without toxicity. If you have cancer, do not take glutamine, as it can act as a food for cancerous tumors. Take 500–1,000 mg daily.

Carnitine

Carnitine is a nonessential amino acid that can become essential if your brain isn't functioning as well as it could. Although carnitine is not an essential amino acid, meaning that our bodies can synthesize it, a deficiency can cause fatigue, muscle weakness, heart disease, acidic blood, high triglyceride levels, and brain degeneration. Taking carnitine as a supplement can enhance the body's ability to burn fat, prevent heart disease, and improve brain deterioration as we age.

We get carnitine in meat, and we make it from lysine, which is found in whole grains, legumes such as soy, and meats. To manufacture carnitine, the body also needs vitamin B_6, niacin, iron, and vitamin C.

It's only been recently that researchers have made advances in understanding how carnitine affects the brain. Current theory is that carnitine enhances brain function by improving the energy levels of brain cells, transporting fats across cell membranes into the mitochondria. In one double-blind, placebo-controlled study of carnitine, thirty mildly to moderately demented patients with probable Alzheimer's disease were randomly assigned to receive either carnitine or a placebo. After six months, the treated group showed significantly less brain deterioration. This is just one of several recently published studies showing similar results. No pharmaceutical drug has shown these kinds of results. Carnitine is already being used extensively in Italy to treat brain deterioration.

And you don't need to have a failing memory to benefit from carnitine. A study done in Italy of healthy people showed that after thirty days of carnitine supplementation, they were better able to pay attention and had faster reflexes and better eye-hand coordination. Other studies have shown that carnitine supplementation improves long-term memory, increases alertness, and improves learning ability. In every study, a certain percentage of people also reported improved mood. Carnitine's ability to protect brain neurons and enhance their responsiveness also makes it one of our most important antiaging supplements.

Carnitine comes in several forms at your health food store. The forms I recommend are either L-carnitine, acetyl-L-carnitine, or L-acetylcarnitine. The acetylated forms may help absorption, but they also tend to be more expensive. Please do not take the synthetic D or DL forms of carnitine, as they can have negative side effects.

Carnitine comes in tablets or capsules, usually in 250 or 500 mg amounts. For fat burning and improved brain function, I recommend 1,000–2,000 mg daily on an empty stomach, in divided doses. In other words, take 500 mg three or four times a day. As a maintenance and prevention supplement, you can take 250–500 mg daily.

Carnitine's ability to improve alertness and attention can also cause insomnia in some people. If this happens to you, try taking the last supplement half an hour before dinner.

Vitamin C

Vitamin C will greatly enhance your body's ability to use carnitine, so be sure you're getting at least 1,000 mg of vitamin C daily (which I recommend everyone take anyway) when you're taking carnitine.

Vitamin B_{12}

Many elderly people diagnosed with senility or Alzheimer's disease simply have a vitamin B_{12} deficiency. Vitamin B_{12}, also called cyanocobalamin, plays a pivotal role in proper brain function.

The symptoms of B_{12} deficiency, such as unsteady gait, fatigue, and memory loss, can begin showing up long before a blood test will show a deficiency. However, since the neurological damage done by a true B_{12} deficiency seems to be largely irreversible, it's not worth waiting around for it to show up that way. If you or a loved one is showing symptoms of a B_{12} deficiency, find a health care practitioner who will give four to eight weeks of B_{12} injections to see if the symptoms improve. In the meantime, start using betain hydrochloride and digestive enzyme supplements to improve digestion and absorption of nutrients. If a B_{12} deficiency is the cause of the symptoms, they usually clear up dramatically within a few weeks of B_{12} injections.

Some people may need to continue getting regular B_{12} injections, and others may do fine maintaining with B_{12} supplements. It can be taken in supplement form as a nasal gel or sublingually (under the tongue). Vitamin B_{12} is not well absorbed when taken in pill form.

Magnesium

Magnesium is one of the magic minerals, and it is essential to a high-energy lifestyle and brainpower. The oxygen deficiency and muscle spasms caused by magnesium deficiency narrow the coronary arteries, interfering with heart function and impairing blood flow to the brain. A deficiency also makes the blood "sticky," which can contribute to causing stroke.

Nearly every important biological process in the body relies on magnesium. Among its more important jobs are maintaining fluid and electrical balance in our cells, sending messages through the nerves, maintaining blood vessel strength, relaxing smooth muscles, and keeping blood flowing smoothly, cholesterol balanced, and the heart beating smoothly. It regulates how we absorb and use calcium and other minerals and helps regulate how we use proteins and carbohydrates.

This magic mineral is also a key to energy production in the body, taking part in more than three hundred enzyme reactions. The enzyme reactions regulate how the body uses nutrients and other substances, such as hormones. For example, vitamin B_6, vitamin E, and vitamin C all need magnesium in order to work properly.

Magnesium can be depleted by stress, excessive alcohol, sugar, diabetes, kidney disease, chronic diarrhea, not enough protein in the diet, too much protein in the diet, and thyroid disorders. Drugs that can deplete magnesium include corticosteroids (prednisone), loop and thiazide diuretics used to lower blood pressure (Diuril, Chlorothiazide, Oretic, Esidrix, Furosemide, Lasix, Bumex), aminoglycosides (antibiotics such as streptomycin, gentamicin, and amikacin), and cisplatin (in some chemotherapy drugs).

Magnesium by itself can cause diarrhea, so unless you are constipated, be sure to take it in a multivitamin, in combination with calcium, or in the form of magnesium glycinate or magnesium citrate. I recommend that you take 300–400 mg of magnesium daily as a supplement.

Coenzyme Q10

As an energy and memory booster, coenzyme Q10 is one of the best-kept secrets around. It is a vital enzyme, or catalyst, to the production of energy in our cells. Without it, our cells simply won't work. Its chemical name is *ubiquinone*—it is ubiquitous, or everywhere, where there is life. Its levels in the human body are highest in the heart and liver. When we are ill or stressed, and as we age, our bodies are less able to produce CoQ10. Many older people who try CoQ10 report an almost immediate boost in their energy levels.

CoQ10 should come as a powder in a capsule and be a deep yellow color. Also be sure that the product says "coenzyme Q10" or "CoQ10." Variations of it will not be as effective. The purity and quality of CoQ10 does vary, and since it's not a cheap supplement, it pays to get a high-quality brand. Most CoQ10 comes in 30 mg capsules. You can take one 30 mg capsule three times a day with meals, and up to 200 mg daily if your energy is low.

If you want to know more about CoQ10, read *The Miracle Nutrient: Coenzyme Q10* by Emile G. Bliznakov, MD, and Gerald L. Hunt (Bantam Books, 1987).

BEATING DEPRESSION NATURALLY

With very few exceptions, we all have periods in our lives when we're down, periods when we're up, and periods when we're somewhere in between. It's quite normal to feel some level of depression before, during, or after a major life change, such as the death of someone close, illness or injury, birth, marriage, divorce, job change, or a move. When we're very "high," or excited about something, we'll eventually have a corresponding dip in our emotions. These emotional ups and downs are all part of being human, and most of us learn to cope with them pretty well by the time we're middle-aged. Debilitating depression that makes a person nonfunctional for weeks or months at a time is another story and should be treated by a competent health care professional.

Minor depression can be a form of time-out for adults. Sometimes it's nature's way of giving us a rest.

Or perhaps we need to go within ourselves and be reflective. Maybe it's a message from the psyche telling us we need to reevaluate our lives. This reevaluation is most often an inner call to align ourselves with a sense of purpose, or a mission in life—to go for what we *really* want, to reach for our dreams, even if they seem completely out of reach.

Unfortunately, thanks to a massive, multimillion-dollar public relations campaign on the part of the giant pharmaceutical companies who sell drugs such as Prozac, millions of people are suffering under the illusion that if they aren't feeling wonderful all the time, something must be wrong with them and they need to fix it by taking a pill. Never mind that the pills are expensive, addictive, and have serious side effects!

Once you've had your time-out or your grieving time, the first step toward healing depression is to get up out of bed, up out of the armchair, or off the couch, and *do* something—*anything*. Sweep the floor, go for a walk in the park, get a haircut, call a friend. Getting up and moving is one of the great cures for depression. Giving to others, forgiving others, and remembering what you're grateful for helps, too. I realize that this is easier said than done when you're actually *in* a depression, but go ahead and do it anyway!

If you're depressed to the point of being nonfunctional for weeks or months at a time and haven't had any luck with conventional medicine, try to find a reputable alternative health care professional. Very often, the skillful use of nutrition and supplements can help people with mild to moderate depression.

The most common physical causes of depression tend to be the same as those that cause a lack of energy: chronic stress, poor nutrition, lack of exercise. Some of us may also be more genetically predisposed to have biochemical imbalances in the brain that contribute to depression.

Amino Acids

Many alternative health care practitioners have had great success treating depression with amino acids. Amino acids are the building blocks of protein and play a vital role in the production and regulation of brain chemicals. Most of the new "personality" drugs have much the same effects on brain chemistry as the amino acids tryptophan, L-tyrosine, and L-phenylalanine. These substances affect the brain's production of serotonin, a neurotransmitter that influences our moods. However, first try the simpler solutions, such as nutrition and exercise, for treating depression. It's always preferable to begin with the most simple, down-to-earth solutions.

Although amino acids are safe, especially when compared to the prescription drugs, I strongly recommend that you not take more than the recommended dose, unless so advised by a health care professional, and that you monitor yourself carefully to track how the amino acids affect you. (Keeping a daily diary of how you're feeling works well.) The stimulating amino acids, such as tyrosine and phenylalanine, can cause irritability in some people.

If you have chronic, recurring depression, I would advise that you work with a health care professional. And do *not* take amino acids for depression without consulting your physician if you are already taking a prescription drug for it.

If you or your physician or health care professional want to know more about amino acids in detail, I recommend the book *The Healing Nutrients Within* by Eric R. Braverman, MD, and Carl C. Pfeiffer, MD (Keats Publishing, 1987). Your physician may want to check out some of the 120 pages of references cited. Very few prescription drugs have been so thoroughly tested.

Tryptophan

As I mentioned in our discussion on sleep, the amino acid tryptophan has, for all practical purposes, been banned by the FDA, even though uncontaminated tryptophan is perfectly safe and makes a wonderful antidepressant and sleep aid. Ironically, tryptophan is still included in baby formulas and nutritional powders for senior citizens because it is an essential amino acid, but you can't get it by itself as a supplement in this country, even with a prescription. Tryptophan is often quite effective for treating depression, especially if there is an anxiety component to it, and if you have a reputable source outside the United States, it may be worth trying.

Tyrosine

Tyrosine is fairly well established through research and the experience of hundreds of alternative health care practitioners as a safe and effective remedy for depression. Tyrosine is the precursor to some of our most important neurotransmitters, so it is an important part of our brain's nutrition. It is also a precursor to adrenaline, thyroid hormones, and some types of estrogen. It has been shown to lower blood pressure, increase sex drive, and suppress appetite. L-dopa, which is used to treat Parkinson's disease, is made from tyrosine.

Start with 500 mg of tyrosine three times a day with meals. If that doesn't work, try 1,000 mg. The most you should take without consulting a health professional is 1,500 mg. Although tyrosine is considered one of the safest amino acids, it can trigger a migraine headache in some people and shouldn't be used in conjunction with MAO inhibitors.

Phenylalanine

Phenylalanine is the precursor to tyrosine and has been used in numerous studies to successfully treat depression. Many supplement manufacturers will combine tyrosine and phenylalanine, but vitamin B_6 should be added to this combination for better utilization.

This amino acid should be avoided by people who have PKU (phenylketonuria), a genetic defect in the body's ability to process and use phenylalanine. This defect can cause severe retardation. If it is caught early enough, retardation can be avoided with a phenylalanine-free diet. Some researchers believe that many children who are hyperactive or have learning disabilities are suffering from a mild form of PKU. Because there are a small number of women whose phenylalanine levels fluctuate when they are pregnant, this amino acid should be avoided if you are pregnant, just to be on the safe side.

The most common source of phenylalanine these days is the artificial sweetener aspartame (Nutra-Sweet). Every time you use aspartame, you get some phenylalanine and aspartic acid. However, I recommend that you take phenylalanine in a supplement because we don't know enough about aspartic acid and its side effects or what it does in combination with phenylalanine.

Phenylalanine has been reported to raise blood pressure, so if you have high blood pressure, monitor it carefully or consult your physician. Phenylalanine also gives some people headaches. A few studies suggest that L-phenylalanine may promote the growth of cancerous tumors, so if you have cancer, this would not be your antidepressant of choice, and please avoid the aspartame! You can take up to 500 mg of L-phenylalanine three times a day.

The B Vitamins

The B vitamins play an essential role in our neurological health, and yet most adult Americans are deficient in them. Although each of the B vitamins plays some role in brain function, vitamin B_{12} is best known for its ability to combat depression. For years, alternative health professionals have given vitamin B_{12} shots as part of an overall treatment program for people who are extremely stressed out or depressed. Until recently, this practice has been pooh-poohed, but now more and more MDs are jumping on the B_{12} bandwagon.

If you want to try B_{12} as an antidote for stress or depression, it's important to know that it's not well absorbed when you take it orally (by mouth), which is why it is given in the form of injections. However, there are B_{12} supplements you can buy at your local health food store that are sublingual (dissolve under the tongue) and intranasal (in the nose). You'll want to take about 1,000 mcg (1 mg) at least every other day for treating depression.

WORKING WITH YOUR MIND AND BODY TO BEAT STRESS

While this is primarily a chapter about using nutrition to maintain an active lifestyle and handle stress effectively, exercise and the mind/body connection are such important factors in maintaining physical, mental, and emotional balance that I feel compelled to address these issues here.

The word *stress* has its roots in the Latin for "narrow" or "tight." Have you ever felt the pressure

---

Prescription Drugs That Can Cause Depression

One of the most common caus is prescription drugs. Here is a the most common prescription drugs that can cause depression:

- Amphetamines
- Antibiotics
- Anticonvulsants
- Antidepressants (I kid you not!)
- Barbiturates
- High blood pressure drugs (beta-blockers, diuretics)
- Hormones (estrogen, including Premarin, and synthetic progestins, such as Provera)
- Narcotics
- Painkillers
- Sleeping pills
- Systemic corticosteroids (prednisone, cortisone)
- Tagamet and Zantac
- Tranquilizers (Halcion, Librium, Restoril, Xanax)

---

of anxiety? Does your schedule keep getting tighter and tighter? Mental constriction is a familiar form of stress. We all know the physical expressions, too, revealed most obviously in the tightening of muscles. Bodily signs are easy to identify and offer an excellent opportunity to beat stress through relaxation. A physical approach, such as massage or exercise, will help relieve the adverse effects of stress in the body, including the buildup of toxic substances, sluggish circulation, and shallow breathing. Any habit of physical activity also establishes a healthy substitute for time spent worrying. The best approach to relaxation, however, is a combination of mind and body work.

Working with the body redirects energy that has been channeled by emotional reactions that are stuck in a negative groove. Even mild resistance as you grit your teeth in heavy commuter traffic or do daily mundane chores after a long day manifests itself in tenseness somewhere in your body. Build in some form of physical exertion to your daily schedule, and you will help undo the symptoms of stress.

The real key, however, is also to address the *causes* of stress. External pressures from career, relationships, and money, for example, are often considered causes. But the true origins of stress lie in our personal *reactions* to external factors. The mind has a tremendous capacity for retraining. People do lose the urge to smoke, drivers do stay calm in the face of road hogs, and even the boss has a lighter side to appreciate. Learn to focus your mind as well as your body, and you will release the habitual thought patterns and responses that actually create stress.

Exercise

Exercise is a depression lifter. It stimulates the release of mood-enhancing chemicals in the brain and bloodstream. An aerobic workout is a much better immediate stress tonic than a cocktail or dose of caffeine. We instinctively recognize this when we take that walk around the block to "cool off." The pent-up energy is channeled in a healthy way. Establish a sensible exercise routine and you'll discover long-term benefits as your mood lifts and stabilizes.

Exercise also counters the draining effects of stress. Using physical energy actually trains the body to generate more. Get physically fit, and your ability to meet stress increases. You will also build your resistance to illness, as moderate exercise has been shown to boost the immune system.

Stress leads to bad posture, poor breathing, and harmful substances in the bloodstream. These physical signs are part of the tightening, clogging effects that come from feeling mentally strained. Exercise counters them all, and in a cyclical manner; improve one and the others tend to follow. Training the muscles of the body to overcome moderate resistance keeps them strong and toned. As tension relaxes, posture improves. Improved posture brings better breathing habits. Improve breathing, and circulation becomes more efficient. Blood vessel networks expand, blood pressure improves, and the heart grows stronger. Muscle tone increases with a better blood

supply, and toxins are flushed out of the system, contributing to general well-being.

Exercise can help with specific forms of stress, such as premenstrual syndrome (PMS) and insomnia. Improvements in digestion, metabolism, and circulation that come with a regular physical workout result in better uptake of nutrients essential for trouble-free menstrual cycles and menopause, sleep, and other bodily functions. The body's natural mood elevators and painkillers, called endorphins, circulate more freely with exercise. Research even shows that exercise can improve short-term memory.

The only downside for some people is the tendency to become exercise dependent, creating an inability to function normally without a workout "fix." If you find this happening, it's a sign that you need to work more with your mind. Relish your fitness, but expand your choice to include an Eastern approach, such as yoga, chi gong, or some form of meditation.

Your Exercise Choice

How do you include yet another activity in an already active life? Make it fun. Keep competition to a minimum, especially if it gets you worked up. Unless your exercise choice is pleasurable, you'll find that it becomes another source of stress. Choose a sport to suit your character. Are you a sociable, team sports personality type or more of a loner, happy to squeeze in a daily workout? Are you an indoor, rowing machine sort or an outdoor jogger? Make your choice from the wide range of aerobic exercises to bring the cardiovascular benefits that will refresh and boost your system. Or take up a nonaerobic form, such as yoga, to condition your body and mind.

Walking, running, swimming, cycling, skating, racquetball, tennis, squash, jump rope, stair climbing, rowing, and cross-country skiing are all excellent aerobic activities. Many of these adapt to intense, indoor aerobic exercise using equipment, which for some creates a more predictable and sustainable workout often better suited to city lifestyles. Don't ignore ordinary activities, either, from vigorous house cleaning and raking the leaves to painting the house and pulling the weeds.

For standard exercise, aim at a minimum of twenty minutes a day. Build in a routine for five to six days a week, as this allows for necessary recovery time and lessens the tendency for addictive types to overdo it.

Take the time you need to select a suitable exercise, and remember that about three months are needed to establish a new habit of any kind. Make sensible exercise a part of your routine, and you automatically bring stress relief to your life.

Biofeedback

If you like hands-on technology, you'll enjoy biofeedback. Biofeedback is a form of body training that brings under conscious control certain body functions that were previously subconscious. This type of training is ideal if you manifest stress in mainly physical ways. Biofeedback can be used to treat headaches, migraines, hypertension (high blood pressure), ulcers, and digestive problems, for example. Biofeedback is also an aid in relaxation and meditation, as it can be applied to brain wave monitoring.

Our nervous system works on two levels—sympathetic and parasympathetic. The sympathetic system narrows blood vessels, raises blood pressure, and speeds up heart rate. Under the parasympathetic system, heart rate is slowed, intestinal and gland activity increases, and sphincter (passage-closing) muscles relax. Biofeedback normally increases the parasympathetic influence with the effect of slower heart rate, for example.

In most biofeedback systems, your hand or some other part of your body is hooked up to a machine sensitive to brain waves, body temperature, or some other body function. The machine beeps or gives you some other cue when you have achieved your goal: slower heart rate, lower body temperature, or more relaxed brain waves, for example. The idea is to use a "soft" form of concentration to control the body, and this can be surprisingly easy to achieve once you know how. The beeps are the feedback that lets you know that your focused thoughts and relaxation are having an effect.

There is a good reason for using skin temperature in biofeedback intended to beat stress reactions. Skin temperature increases when blood vessels are dilated, allowing blood to flow to the skin. Constriction of blood vessels is one effect of stress. This is an involuntary sympathetic nervous system response geared to conserve energy when it appears that the body is under threat. If you were asked to reverse this reaction and relax your body systems, it would be difficult to know where to start. Biofeedback shows you exactly what mind-set and relaxation is needed to achieve control of this involuntary response.

Biofeedback tends to be very rewarding as you get better and better at producing the desired effects. Physical benefits can include the warming of hands and feet that have previously been permanent cold zones, relief from muscle tension, improved digestion, and lowered blood pressure and heart rate. Gaining practice at bringing the nervous system into balance is also practice for bringing the mind into focus.

Biofeedback Programs

It is not advisable to simply buy and use biofeedback equipment without formal training. Seek out an experienced therapist with an excellent reputation, getting recommendations if you can. Listings are found at hospitals and spas as well as in telephone directories. If your doctor refers you, you may find that you are covered by your medical insurance. A good practitioner will offer a personalized program of about ten sessions, each about an hour long. A well-designed program will take you to the point where you are sure enough of the "bio" that you no longer need the feedback.

Meditation

Have you ever tried to "empty your mind" or obey a command *not* to think of a pink elephant? Meditation is not about banishing thoughts or blanking your mind. Meditation comes from the Latin "to think over." It means focused thinking. Some forms of meditation are used much like biofeedback. As with biofeedback, the physical results stem from a nervous system brought back into balance. Benefits are similar, including lowered heart rate and blood pressure, improved digestion, and improved blood flow. Apparently, Tibetan monks are even asked to demonstrate their meditative powers under extreme physical stress. The robes of the meditating monks are soaked with ice-cold water. The monks are said to have achieved the desired state when they have, by thought alone, increased their body temperature to the point where the robes are dried—not just once but six times in one long session!

The simplest meditation techniques are breathing exercises. A few minutes' concentration on deep, controlled breathing alone is a powerful tool, useful in everyday stressful situations. Cardiovascular benefits result as the body responds to the improved flow of oxygen. Calmness is felt as relaxation is induced.

Calmness and higher states of consciousness are often sought as aims of meditation. Many approaches are rooted in spiritual teachings from the East, such as Zen Buddhism, although no religious beliefs are necessary to take up most forms of meditation. Some techniques require the repetition of a word or phrase. Others advise certain postures, while some methods require only a relaxed sitting or lying position. Taking a course of instruction can make meditation a part of your social life, or a book can lead to a solo path. There are numerous books and classes to provide you with an introduction to a wide range of techniques. As your mind is your own, the choice is yours.

Chi Gong

Starting with either mind or body, stress is ultimately only fully addressed with a balanced approach to both. This seems to have been understood for centuries in the East. Many Eastern practices, from martial arts and tai chi to acupuncture and meditation, have been exported to the West. Part of the appeal of such techniques lies in the fact that they tend to involve the whole person, rather than isolating mind and emotion from physical expression. As such,

Eastern disciplines make effective stress relievers. What is not well known is that chi gong lies at the root of such practices. The significant element in chi gong practice is becoming aware of and moving your energy, the very thing that is depleted or stretched to the breaking point with stress.

Also known as qi gong and chi kung, chi gong is the cultivation of energy. *Chi*, or *ki*, is the Chinese term for vital energy. *Kung*, or *gong*, means cultivation. By nurturing chi, the aim is to increase general health and well-being. Many variations of its practice exist, but books such as *Chi Kung: Cultivating Personal Energy* by James MacRitchie (Element, 1997) are useful starting points. Seek out a reputable teacher for initial instruction when you are ready to integrate this ancient practice into your own life.

Simply explained, chi gong is a progressive series of calm, slow exercises, often in sets and involving concentration on breathing as well as movement. The aims of chi gong are fourfold: that energy be balanced, free flowing, of good quality, and of good volume. The exercises are meditative in that they ask for focus on specific chi points in the body, based on Eastern theories of anatomy and physiology as practiced, for example, in acupuncture.

We instinctively adopt chi gong postures as we naturally stretch and relax. Lying with our hands behind the head as people do all over the world, for example, directs energy to a point at the base of the skull, helping to relax vessels in the lower brain, from where functions such as temperature and heart rate are regulated. As with meditation and ordinary exercise, you will get the most out of chi gong when you have regular practice. Benefits can include clearheadedness, body toning, a boost to the immune system, and improved lymph circulation, as well as improved blood flow, blood pressure, and heart rate.

10 STAYING FIT ~

THE BENEFITS OF STAYING FIT

Fitness is feeling up to the task. Climb a mountain or walk two blocks—the task is up to you. Whatever activity you choose, do you feel enthusiastic and confident? Does your body respond well to the exertion? Do you feel energized and ready for more?

Fitness is much more than the absence of disease. It is both emotional and physical. Tune up the body and feel your mind tune in. An enjoyable sense of general well-being comes from good muscle tone, a healthy heart and lungs, and strong, flexible joints.

How are these achieved? Athletes know that diet and supplements alone will never produce overall fitness. Our bodies are designed to move! Muscles need stretching; bones get stronger with stress; and lungs and heart are more efficient with exercise. Research shows that you're prolonging your life with just half an hour of exercise a day. Since 1962, a study of over ten thousand Harvard alumni has shown that a sedentary lifestyle leads to a 44 percent higher risk of death compared to men of the same age who engage moderately in sports like running, swimming, and racquetball.

Harking back to distant ancestors, your choice of exercise or sport makes up for the loss of a hunter-gatherer culture. Hunting mammoths or trekking miles for water may no longer be necessary, but the human body is still equipped to do both; it isn't truly suited to modern, desk-bound, car-driving lives. We get the best out of the body by using it, just as we get the best out of a musical instrument when it is played.

Exercise combined with good nutrition and the right supplements produces real fitness. How much exercise and food, and which supplements? The answer lies in the level of activity that gives you the most pleasure. There's no sense in striving for ironman standards and appetites if a round of golf is more your style. Beyond basic health, your level of fitness is your choice. Simply speaking, aiming to be fit for the sports or activities you find fun produces the maximum benefits.

Fitness Promotes Energy

Anyone who exercises regularly knows that you use energy or lose it. Working the body keeps its fuel systems active. Exercise brings in the oxygen used by every cell of our bodies as fuel to burn the calories taken in from food. Burning the calories produces energy. Just as a neglected machine works slowly, gathering dust and rust, the sedentary, low-oxygen body suffers low energy levels and disease symptoms such as high cholesterol and wasted muscles.

There is not a point in our lives when fitness doesn't matter. Energy is needed for every activity, even sleeping. When you have optimum fitness, you'll have optimum energy. The greater the energy, the more active you can be, not only in your chosen sport or exercise, but in every area of your life.

Exercise can also free up energy by relieving pain. Believe it or not, one of the best ways to handle arthritis is exercise. I'm not talking about running a marathon—just moving the body, even if gently and slowly. The same applies to back pain.

Contrary to the advice that used to be given for back pain, most of the time it's best to keep on moving—with care. Going to bed for days on end can actually make back pain worse in the long run.

Ten Major Exercise Benefits

In case you had any doubt about the value of exercise, check out the following ways that exercise improves your overall health—and this is just a small sample.

1. *Boosts energy.* Using energy helps you keep it!
2. *Boosts the immune system.* Exercise in moderation increases disease-fighting white blood cells.
3. *Reduces the risk of heart disease and stroke.* Fitness strengthens the heart and circulatory system.
4. *Relieves depression.* Exercise stimulates the release of mood-enhancing chemicals in the brain and bloodstream.
5. *Improves cholesterol profile.* Exercise raises levels of "good" heart-protective HDL cholesterol and lowers "bad" LDL cholesterol levels.
6. *Controls weight.* Exercise helps keep weight off—or on!
7. *Relieves PMS.* Exercise helps balance hormones.
8. *Strengthens bones and reduces the risk of osteoporosis.* Regular exercise actually strengthens bones, reducing the risk of brittle bones caused by calcium loss, especially in old age.
9. *Relieves insomnia.* Exercise is one of the best sleeping remedies I know. Just a brisk half-hour walk in the late afternoon can set you up for a sound night's sleep.
10. *Improves your sex life.* Keeping hormones balanced and blood circulating leads to a healthier sex life at any age.

HOW THE BODY PRODUCES ENERGY

Take an in-depth look at energy in the human body, and you'll find that humans are actually solar powered. People are part of the food webs and food chains that rely on the great power of sunlight. Plants and their leaves, fruits, and seeds absorb the sun's energy and use carbon dioxide and water to create sugars and starches. The sugars and starches come with a natural taste-good factor, so the plants are soon snapped up by foraging animals. The energy stored in the plant chemicals is released inside the foragers' bodies. There it is used for all activities, including the formation of body tissues. Eat a chicken, and you, the human, are absorbing energy originally taken in by the plants. The energy has been converted once again and bound up in a drumstick on your plate. There is a more direct link when we eat vegetables.

Metabolism Is Your Key to Optimal Fitness

Metabolism is the name for the bodily processes that extract energy from foods and synthesize different compounds for use in the body. Digestion reduces food to manageable parts. Specialized proteins called enzymes trigger and speed up the metabolic processes, including digestion. Blood absorbs the results of digestion and transports them to cells all over the body. The cells take up the nutrients in the form of carbohydrates, fats, and proteins.

Cells also receive oxygen and use it to break the chemical bonds of the nutrients. This process releases the energy. Cells would be damaged by the release of a great amount of energy at one time. Instead, new molecules of a substance called ATP (adenosine triphosphate) are formed, which store the energy. ATP molecules are broken down by cells when energy is needed.

When nutrients are broken down, part of the energy released is heat. In fact, 75 percent of the energy produced by the body is heat. Heat production is important for keeping body temperature in the narrow range required for full functioning. The heat produced is measured in calories. Different foods store different amounts of energy and so contain varying amounts of calories. Take in excess calories, and the body metabolizes the nutrients into forms it can store. Storage of excess is mainly in that very familiar form—fat.

A measure of metabolism is the rate at which the body uses energy. An efficient metabolism is part of fitness. A regular exercise program can increase underlying, *basal* metabolism by as much as 10 percent. Increasing basal metabolism means that the body burns more calories when at rest. A state of fitness also creates a metabolism able to adjust more smoothly to the demands of the body and ensures that the body always has the energy it needs. Establish an exercise habit, and you naturally improve your energy levels.

Metabolism and Weight

We all know that the more excess fat we're carrying, the less healthy we are, right? If we know that, then why do we continue to put on the pounds? A recent article in the *Journal of the American Medical Association* published the results of a nationwide survey of weight gain among Americans age twenty and older. The study found that for the past few decades, Americans have been carrying an average of 8 percent more weight on their bodies. That's a big gain! If you weigh 140 pounds, 8 percent of that is just over 11 pounds. Furthermore, the survey shows that we keep gaining weight until we're about sixty years old, when it begins to decline.

So what's a body to do? We know that dieting doesn't work. In fact, I recommend that you throw away your scale. We also know that keeping the weight off may not be as simple as eating less and exercising more, although it will make a big difference for most people. However, if your metabolism is slow or your hormones are out of balance, you still won't be burning calories efficiently.

Whether you have a "fast" or "slow" metabolism depends on how much energy is required to maintain your body. The "faster" the metabolism, the more efficiently your body burns calories and the more you can eat without adding fat to your body. If your body gets the message that it's well nourished and healthy, metabolism stays fast. If your body gets the message that it's going to starve (as in dieting) or that it's malnourished, diseased, or

stressed, metabolism usually slows down as a way of conserving energy.

Metabolism varies widely and depends on a complex interplay of factors:

- Men generally have a faster metabolism than women; this is related to their testosterone levels. (Women make testosterone, too; they just make less.)
- Women's slower metabolism is related to estrogen. High estrogen levels slow metabolism.
- As we age, our metabolism tends to slow down.
- The colder the climate, the faster the metabolism.
- The higher the percentage of fat on the body, the slower the metabolism, and conversely, the more muscular (not thin, muscular!) the body, the faster the metabolism.
- Some drugs slow the metabolism—for example, alcohol, barbiturates, meprobamate, narcotics, hypnotics, and antidepressants.
- Low-calorie diets and malnutrition slow metabolism.
- Stress slows metabolism in some people and speeds it up in others.
- An infection can slow metabolism.
- Regular moderate exercise will speed up metabolism. Extreme exercise will slow metabolism if the body is stressed.
- An underactive thyroid (hypothyroidism) slows metabolism.
- Genetic factors can predispose us to a fast or slow metabolism.

Here's a metabolic formula that will clarify how metabolism works:

Exercise + testosterone + protein = muscle
More muscle = faster metabolism
Faster metabolism = more calories burned

Exercise is one of the best ways to get your metabolism moving again. As we all know, exercise burns calories. But more importantly over the long haul, regular moderate exercise replaces fat with muscle, and we burn most of our calories in muscle. The more muscle we have on our bodies, the faster our metabolism will be. A combination of exercise plus testosterone plus protein builds muscle. Thanks to their higher levels of testosterone, men have an edge over women in building muscle.

A very low-calorie, low-fat diet causes a loss of muscle and slows the metabolism. As our metabolism decreases, we tend to convert our energy to fat instead of muscle. It's a vicious cycle—we eat less and we get fatter!

If you try to burn off your fat too quickly, you'll start burning off muscle, too, and your metabolism will slow down. Approach losing your fat as a gradual process that's related to a gradual change in your lifestyle. Since most people gain at least a pound a year from ages thirty to sixty, if you start out trim and then maintain a healthy lifestyle, you'll stay in good shape. You don't have to look like a thirty-year-old when you're fifty. It's natural to gain a little weight as you age. But most Americans are overdoing it by at *least* 10 pounds!

As you exercise more and gain more muscle, your weight may stay the same or increase. That's because muscle weighs more than fat. The scale may stay the same, but you'll notice that your clothes fit better or are becoming looser. If the truth be told, we all know when we're fat and when we're trim, regardless of what the scale says.

The very best way to shift your metabolism into a higher gear is to exercise. If you're working to change to a healthier lifestyle and want to give yourself a little extra boost, there are some supplements that can help you change your metabolism. However, these are not magic pills that will work without exercise and good nutrition, and they are only meant to be used for a couple of weeks to a few months. Do not use any of these products long-term. If your own metabolism doesn't kick in and do its job, you need to find out why.

Garcinia cambogia

Garcinia cambogia is a citruslike fruit from Asia, where the fruit or its dried rind is used as a food, spice, or condiment. It is also called Malabar tamarind, even though it is not a tamarind. Studies done on rats by Hoffman-La Roche, which is distributing the product in the United States, have shown that a substance in *Garcinia* called hydroxycitric acid (HCA) suppresses appetite, improves the body's ability to use fatty acids, and reduces the conversion of carbohydrates to fat. It has produced significant weight loss in rats with no side effects. Because it is eaten in Asia as a food, I feel that it is safe to use to assist with weight loss and change in metabolism, for up to six months.

Chromium Picolinate

Chromium is an essential mineral that plays a role in regulating insulin, which in turn regulates blood sugar levels. Studies have show that it makes insulin more efficient and thus better able to metabolize sugar and fats. Chromium can increase lean muscle mass when used in conjunction with exercise. Chromium picolinate is a better-absorbed form of this mineral. Some supplement formulas combine *Garcinia* and chromium picolinate.

L-Carnitine

Carnitine is an interesting amino acid because one of its primary roles in the body is to carry fat across cell membranes into the mitochondria, our cells' power plants. The fat is then turned into the ATP I mentioned earlier, which supplies energy for many bodily functions, especially muscle contraction. The more carnitine available in the body, the more fat can be transported into the mitochondria and burned for energy. Some researchers suggest that carnitine also allows the body to exercise longer without becoming fatigued.

Carnitine is an especially important supplement to take when you're losing weight because it cleans up substances in the blood called ketones, formed when the body is breaking down fat. There is also evidence that it speeds up the liver's ability to break down fats for excretion.

Carnitine comes in several forms at your health food store. The forms I recommend are either L-carnitine, acetyl-L-carnitine, or L-acetylcarnitine. The acetylated forms may help absorption, but they also tend to be more expensive. Please *do not* take the synthetic D or DL forms of carnitine, as they can have negative side effects.

Carnitine comes in tablets or capsules, usually in 250 or 500 mg amounts. For fat burning and improved brain function, I recommend 1,000–2,000 mg daily on an empty stomach, in divided doses. In other words, take 500 mg two to four times a day. As a maintenance and prevention supplement, you can take 250–500 mg daily. Vitamin C will greatly enhance your body's ability to use carnitine, so be sure you're getting at least 1,000 mg of vitamin C daily (which I recommend everyone take anyway) when you're taking carnitine. Carnitine's ability to improve alertness and attention can also cause insomnia in some people. If this happens to you, try taking the last supplement half an hour before dinner.

THE TWO ENERGY PATHWAYS

Everyone who exercises knows that it doesn't take long to get over the beginner's huffing, puffing, and next-day aches. But why do people have to go through this? The unfit body has to call on energy pathways weak from underuse and a backup system forced into overdrive. Getting fit brings the pathways back into balance, and exercise soon becomes a pleasure.

A basic understanding of the main energy routes your body uses to fuel itself will help explain how exercise becomes easier and how different forms of exercise affect the body.

Many of the processes that produce energy in cells use up one gas, oxygen, and produce another gas, carbon dioxide. This exchange of gases is called *respiration*, the same term we use for the exchange of gases when we breathe.

Burning up calories using oxygen as a fuel is known as *aerobic* respiration. Aerobic respiration burns calories at a high rate for a short period of time and occurs when the blood and tissues are kept topped up with oxygen. The need to breathe more quickly during exercise is the response to the need for more oxygen.

Aerobic exercise happens when the heart rate is high. Other things are happening in the body at the same time: The levels of insulin, the hormone that pulls glucose, or sugar, out of the blood and stores it as fat, is reduced. At the same time, the supply of glucagon, a substance that releases stored glucose from the liver, is increased. When this happens for more than a few minutes, the body shifts into a mode of burning stored fat, which is what you want to happen when you're on a weight loss program. Aerobic exercise doesn't tend to build muscle. Examples of aerobic exercise are given later in this chapter.

Anaerobic respiration is the term used when cells produce energy with limited oxygen; instead, energy is taken from stored carbohydrates once the supply of ATP stored in the muscles is used up (which is almost immediately). Anaerobic respiration is not very efficient, and it produces *lactic acid*. A buildup of lactic acid causes that notorious muscle soreness as well as limiting the normal functioning of the body. Fortunately, lactic acid is easily recycled once oxygen is available again. According to Barry Sears, author of the book *Entering the Zone*, anaerobic exercise is an important part of an exercise program because it releases growth hormone, which in turn burns fat and builds muscle. Injections of growth hormone have become something of an antiaging fad, but I don't recommend it, as we have virtually no research on its side effects and it may increase the risk of diabetes. Some examples of anaerobic exercise are given later in the book.

A sensible exercise program will include both aerobic and anaerobic conditioning, building up both the aerobic and anaerobic pathways.

Why Exercise Leads to Energy Efficiency

Short-burst exercise allows the body to rebuild stores of energy in rest periods. This was useful to cave dwellers who needed a source of instant energy to flee from predators. A continuous fast run depletes stored energy rapidly, but a moderate run will force the body to burn stored fat in other areas than the muscles being used. Once the body reaches its optimum weight—not too heavy and not too light—it will use energy most efficiently.

The wise athlete knows his or her body and its tolerance levels well. Warm-ups, workouts, and training routines are designed to exercise the body's systems in a way that improves them rather than straining them. Energy efficiency increases in athletes because the body responds to exercise in the following ways:

- Increased number of capillaries to muscle tissue
- Increased efficiency of heart contractions
- Increased ability of blood to take up oxygen
- Increased lung efficiency
- Better energy storage
- Better resistance to the effects of lactic acid

HOW MUSCLES STORE AND USE ENERGY

The main product of carbohydrate digestion is sugar, particularly glucose. When blood sugar levels are referred to, they are a measure mostly of the amount of glucose being transported by the blood. When blood sugar levels are too high for the body's energy needs, storage mechanisms kick in. Glucose is converted to a substance called glycogen, which means "sugar former." The largest site of glycogen in the body is the liver, which stores about 320 calories' worth. The muscles, however, also store glycogen and at a higher level of around 1,400 calories in total.

Low blood sugar levels trigger the breakdown of glycogen, which makes the stored energy available again. Glycogen in the liver breaks back down to glucose, leading to high energy release. Muscle glycogen is broken down to lactic acid by anaerobic respiration, which results in lower energy production rates. Used either way, glycogen can be regarded as fuel for the athlete. Muscles also store a source of energy derived from fats (a topic covered shortly).

The responses of the body to store or release sugar are a marvelous balancing feat. Adjustments are automatic, answering a built-in aim to keep all systems at optimum levels. That state of synchronized regulation is known as *homeostasis*. As an athlete, you are testing your body systems regularly, keeping them operational and finely tuned. It's a completely different story for those who indulge in high-sugar snacks and long hours of TV watching. Blood sugar regulation in couch potatoes is tested beyond exertion to exhaustion!

Athletes probably look more positively on fat than anyone else, partly because they don't have too much of it. They appreciate its protective cushioning of internal organs and its insulation as they put the body through its paces. They also realize its potential— literally. A conditioned athlete stores about 50,000 calories of fat. That's roughly twenty times more than the energy stores of carbohydrates. Fats contain twice as much energy per unit weight as carbohydrates. They also take up much less room, because water is needed for the storage of carbohydrates.

Just as the body triggers the storage of excess carbohydrate/sugar calories as glycogen in the liver and muscles, so it also stimulates other areas to store them as fat. Fat, just like glucose, is used to make ATP, although the body's first call is always on sugar as the fastest way to create these molecules.

At the right signal, fats are first deconstructed, releasing *free fatty acids* (FFAs) into the bloodstream, where they are then carried to the muscles. As with glycogen, the breakdown of FFAs in the muscle fibers leads to energy by producing ATP.

One drawback to fats is that they use up more oxygen per unit than carbohydrates to make the ATP. Although the need for oxygen is greater, fat reserves are extensive and very useful for distance work. The trained athlete sees the most energy benefit from burning fat because his or her oxygen uptake and delivery mechanisms will be in good shape.

Expert marathon runners burn more than twice as much fat as carbohydrates during their races. It's slow, long distance running triggering the burning of fat stores that makes it the most efficient way to lose fat. "Hitting the wall" describes the experience of the runner whose body isn't yet trained to move smoothly into the burning of fat when his or her carbohydrate stores are depleted.

Distance training sees the body adapt to "burn leaner" with a lower body fat ratio because the rate of calorie burning increases. Normal benefits of all exercise also apply, including improved blood supply and heart and lung function. In addition, if you train for long distance, your muscles will increase their ability to process FFAs, and you'll have a better supply of FFAs in your bloodstream. And by the way, you can get your distance training by running, but you can also get it by swimming and walking.

CARDIAC FITNESS FIRST

Unless people exercise regularly or practice deep breathing techniques, much of the oxygen they breathe in is wasted, since it goes unabsorbed. Lungs may take in oxygen, but the network of tiny blood vessels called capillaries must be extensive enough to make use of lung capacity. In addition, the blood supply needs to be ample, with enough factors like hemoglobin, the red pigment that binds with oxygen and transports it.

The strength of the heart is of great importance in creating an effective blood supply and ensuring that cells get the oxygen they need. Daily sessions of sensible exercise produce these extremely worthwhile cardiac results:

- Heart muscle becomes larger.
- Each contraction pumps more blood.
- The overall quantity of blood pumped increases.

An increase in the amount of blood pumped per minute is an improvement in *minute volume*. The other main measure of heart capacity, the amount of blood pumped by each contraction, is known as *stroke volume*. At rest, the heart can pump about 4 L of blood per minute. Exercise regularly, and your heart's capacity will increase by about eight to ten times. This ensures a sufficient oxygen supply and therefore sufficient energy to meet every need.

Greater heart fitness doesn't happen in isolation. Training puts a load on the cardiovascular and pulmonary systems as a whole. Besides better heart function, blood flows faster under improved pressure and carries greater amounts of oxygen. The lungs gain from these changes as their arteries and networks of capillaries become more effective and more oxygen is absorbed at a faster rate.

The blood vessel improvements extend to the muscles of the body as new webs of capillaries grow and old ones expand. Where athletes experience such effects, scientists see greater muscular endurance. Another effect of cardiac fitness is a steady drop in pulse rate at rest, an indication of more efficient underlying, or basal, metabolism.

Aerobic conditioning, daily exercise that uses the aerobic energy pathways, is wonderful for the heart. Persist with training that increases the time you can steadily use your large muscles, especially thighs, to beat the force of gravity, and cardiac fitness will be a sure result.

BUILDING MUSCLE FIBER

Muscles are made up of long fibers bound together. Muscle power comes from fiber contractions strong enough to lift bones and beat the pull of gravity. Muscle fibers come in two types, red and white. The difference lies in the speed of contraction: White fibers contract much more quickly than red ones. For this reason, white fibers have come to be known as *fast twitch* and red ones as *slow twitch*. Each individual inherits his or her own particular proportion of fast- and slow-twitch fibers. Different training styles are used to bring about changes in each type, but the original proportion cannot be changed.

A greater number of red, slow-twitch fibers is typical for the muscles of distance runners. Slow-twitch fibers are adapted mainly for aerobic respiration, which is suited to less intense, long-duration work. White, fast-twitch fibers are primarily designed for anaerobic respiration. Fast-twitch fibers lend themselves to fast, intense activity and are the source of an athlete's "explosive" power, characteristic of sprinters.

Athletes tend to respect their natural muscular limitations, choosing suitable sports and exercises. Many top distance runners, for example, show proportions of about 80 percent red, slow-twitch fibers to 20 percent white, fast-twitch fibers. No matter the choice of activity, however, exercise strengthens all muscle fibers. Muscular payoffs include greater storage of energy as well as improved fatigue tolerance and endurance characteristics.

A quick way to assess which fibers dominate your muscles is the vertical jump. Stand sideways next to a wall against a yardstick. Raise the hand you use the most as high as you can, noting the height reached. Step about 6 inches to a foot away from the wall and jump upward, without taking a step, reaching as high as you can with your hand. Record the difference between the reach from standing and the reach from jumping. Do this three times, taking your highest measurement as your score.

Studies show correlations between vertical jump scores and types of events. Many champion sprint swimmers like Mark Spitz, for example, are seen to have higher scores than several top distance swimmers. This kind of correlation shows how fast-twitch fibers are suited to shorter, faster events.

Knowing your fiber type can help if you are making serious training choices. For all-around fitness training, muscle fiber type is not too important, but it may guide you in terms of your body's natural tolerance limits. The characteristics of both fiber types can be altered to a degree, but it should be remembered that general exercise increases all muscle fiber strength because it involves movements of all kinds. Keep in mind that intense, anaerobic movements do not affect red, slow-twitch fibers and that white, fast-twitch fibers are unaffected by long, slow exercise.

Your choice of training will be affected by your need to build or shape your muscles a particular way to suit your chosen activity. The focus can be general—for instance, concentrating on sprints to improve explosive power. Exercise can also be very refined, with specific styles used to deliberately influence the makeup of your muscles.

Changing White Fibers

Speed potential is enhanced by increasing the size and strength of white, fast-twitch fibers. This is done by exercising fast against high resistance, which produces a greater volume of white, fast-twitch fibers than red, slow-twitch fibers. The proportion doesn't change, but the relative bulk does. Sprint swimming can produce the desired result more easily than working with weights.

To improve distance performance, work at exercises that increase the endurance characteristics of white fibers. Guess what? This calls for a lot of distance work! You have to sacrifice some of the speed potential of white fiber, so sprinters—be careful how you go about this type of muscle work.

Changing Red Fibers

Exercising moderately or slowly with heavy resistance will make red fibers grow and strengthen. If your emphasis is on this kind of exercise, the result will be an increase in the mass of red, slow-twitch muscle relative to the mass of white, fast-twitch fibers. The muscle will be big and strong and appear bulked up, which is why heavy resistance exercises are used by bodybuilders.

The endurance characteristics of red fibers can be enhanced by many repetitions of exercise against medium resistance. This results in a greater ability of the muscle to use oxygen because it produces a more efficient enzyme action. Resistance trainers adapt their workouts to suit their training aims, adding more weight as resistance, for example, or changing the number of exercise repetitions they perform.

FITNESS AND WEIGHT

While being extremely heavy or extremely thin may be a requirement of particular sports, the healthiest weight lies between these extremes. Weight as a fitness issue is nowadays guided by measuring the percentage of body fat. This is more useful than judging the weight of an individual in relation only to height, frame, and age. Body fat measurements make it easier to see how weight comes from useful bone, muscle, and essential fat, not just flab. This can lessen the anxiety of gymnasts and bring flabby football players, mistakenly proud of their bulk, down to earth.

Body fat varies with age and sex. Average figures for college-age adults are about 18 percent body fat for men and 25 percent for women. The norm for nonathletic American adults between thirty and fifty years of age is about 30 percent for men and 35 percent for women.

Body fat varies from sport to sport. As might be expected, however, athletes generally have a smaller percentage of fat than nonathletes. Exceptions occur, as with long-distance swimmers, who often exceed the average by about 5 to 7 percent because they build up fat insulation as protection during long spells in cold water. Only about 3 to 5 percent body fat in men is truly essential and 13 percent in women. Some research suggests that it is dangerous for men to drop below 5 percent body fat. Low body fat in premenopausal women may be a contributory factor when menstrual cycles are absent (amenorrhea).

Essential fat is found in the spleen, liver, kidneys, heart, nervous tissue, muscles, and cell membranes. Most of this fat, around 70 to 80 percent, is stored under the skin. This is subcutaneous fat, and it is measured using calipers on specific skin fold points on the body. Calipers are the most common and easiest tool for the calculation of body fat percentage. There is underwater weighing, too, and a hi-tech method called electrical impedance. Unfortunately, inaccurate body fat measurements are all too common. Always use a health professional who is experienced in the chosen measuring technique.

HEALTHY WEIGHT LOSS

No one should lose weight if doing so brings ill health. Many athletes achieve low body fat percentages naturally through exercise. Weight loss does become an issue for competitive athletes toward the season start or after any long period of rest. Here's why:

- Extra weight means excess stress on body parts such as ankles and knees and therefore greater risk of injury.
- Excess fat means greater storage of heat produced internally and therefore increased risk of heat stroke and heat exhaustion.
- Heavier bodies take more effort to get across the finish line.

For many people, losing a few pounds is rightly seen as an essential part of getting fit. Diet and supplements alone will not achieve fitness, so it follows that they are also not the path to permanent weight loss. Unfortunately, this doesn't deter millions of Americans from ignoring their general physical condition and relying on diets alone. The result is that most people regain those lost pounds sooner or later. The message is: Keep moving to keep weight off. Still, diet and supplements are useful tools to make weight loss easier, and I'll cover them later.

Excess pounds accumulate because not enough movement occurs to burn them off. Although to lose weight you will have to eat less (but no fewer than 1,200 to 1,500 calories per day), shortcuts don't work. Sooner or later, the movement that didn't occur while weight went up will have to happen if weight loss and fitness are going to stick. Body systems won't be tricked for long. Once geared to gain weight, they have to be regeared to stay at a lower weight. Basal metabolism will adjust upward and the pounds will stay off if lower calorie intake is combined with increased calorie burning. Persistence is

important, as it can take up to six months to make this kind of major change in body chemistry.

It may seem strange, but drastically lowering food intake is not an efficient way to lose weight. The body's response to starving is to slow down the processes of metabolism and conserve energy stores, including fat. An extremely low-carbohydrate, high-protein regimen will produce initial weight loss, but only through the diuretic effect of shedding water. Any program of weight loss and fitness should involve a sensible reduction in calories as well as an adjustment to a healthy diet. An improved supply of nutrients is a helpful backup to a body asked to meet new stresses. An undersupply of food leads only to quick fatigue during exercise.

The High-Protein Diet

It used to be gospel in the sports world that the way to be most competitive and get the nutritional edge was to do "carbohydrate loading" to supply the muscles with plenty of glycogen. However, what we now know is that for most athletes, too many carbohydrates and not enough protein make it hard to lose weight and gain muscle and can contribute to sluggish performance. As always, the key is balance.

Protein is made up of strings of amino acids and is not only important to good health but essential. Protein is used by the body for repairing tissue, for growth, and specifically for building muscle. It's also a factor in synthesizing enzymes, neurotransmitters, and the hormone insulin.

Protein is not converted to fat in the body, and it is used to make muscle. More muscle means higher metabolism, which means burning off calories faster. It is important for athletes to get enough protein in the diet, but too much can cause fatigue and irritability, stress the kidneys, throw off the mineral balance in the cells, cause a calcium deficiency (increasing the chance of getting osteoporosis), and increase the risk of certain types of cancer.

You can encourage your body to burn fat through diet by making sure that you always combine protein with carbohydrate. When you eat carbohydrates alone, your body immediately stores them as fat if they aren't burned off, but eating them with protein slows carbohydrate breakdown, giving your body greater opportunities for burning these calories.

Keep your carbohydrate portions small and in the form of complex carbohydrates, such as whole grains, vegetables, and fruits. Remember, carbohydrates are abundant in grains, legumes, and many vegetables. Getting enough carbohydrates is rarely a problem. Because fruit is high in sugar, a form of carbohydrate, keep your fruit consumption to a maximum of two pieces daily, eaten alone, and while you're in weight loss mode, skip the fruit juice.

Some weight lifters recommend a diet that is 40 percent protein, 40 percent carbohydrates, and 20 percent fat, with 250–300 g of protein a day, but you have to be very large and a very intense athlete to consume that much protein.

You have to find the balance that works best for you through experience. Some people have a difficult time digesting grains, while others have trouble with fats. For some people, refined sugar is a recipe for fatigue and illness, while others can tolerate it. I recommend that you experiment and find out what combinations and types of food make you feel most energetic and clearheaded. Many people have increased their energy, lost weight, and increased athletic performance by using the principles in Barry Sears's book *Entering the Zone*.

Training for Weight Loss

Remember, body fat measurements are a more accurate guide to over- or underweight than the scale. Cultural images are unimportant. What counts is your ability to meet enjoyable physical challenges without too much stress or discomfort. Exercise is also more fruitful without one eye always on the scale. Concentrate on exercise instead of your weight. Don't be distracted by sudden weight fluctuations, as these have more to do with water loss or retention than true weight loss or gain. To lose weight, adjust your diet and be prepared to stay with your training regimen. Take heart if you're heavier than most, since you will burn more calories. The bulkier the body, the more energy it takes to move it.

Exercise has to go on to the point where fat begins to be burned. The metabolism switches to fat burning after about 40 minutes of exercise. Losing 1 pound of fat means burning 3,500 calories. Running 1 mile burns at least 100 calories. This all translates into the need for consistent training. Doing only short, intensive workouts is out. Slow, long distance sports are in, although sustained increases in the rate at which you work will burn calories faster. For example, cycling at 5.5 miles per hour burns 2.5 calories per minute, whereas 11.6 calories are burned per minute at 13.1 miles per hour. The major point is that slow, long distance work turns on the fat-burning processes. A big bonus is that fat burning continues for several hours after this kind of exercise.

It might be thought that the higher body fat stores of women would make them better distance runners. Greater natural fat reserves, however, are not an advantage. The significant factor is the ability to burn fat, which is regulated by metabolism and dependent on heart and lungs.

Inherited body type, gender, and even prebirth nutrition all affect fat distribution. These lead to certain recognizable body types, from pear-shaped to boxy to hourglass figures. The tendency in men is for excess fat concentration around the waist. In women, fat buildup more often begins around the hips and thighs.

The distribution of weight on the body affects running power. Whether your weight is high on your body or low on your body will make a difference. It takes four times as much energy to carry 1 pound on a foot than to carry 1 pound on the back. This sets runners with big legs at some disadvantage. It is also the reason why ankle weights don't work, since they frequently create enough excess stress to cause injury. Include leg workouts, without weights, to help strengthen leg muscles and chase flab off thighs.

Experts agree that no more than 15 percent of total body weight should be lost during any one period. A realistic and healthy aim is 5 to 10 percent. The goal can be revised as you meet your targets.

A firm rule for all athletes is to stabilize your weight well before an event. Make your target weight at least three to four days before short, intensive competition and as far ahead as six weeks before a triathlon. Dieting is stressful for the body and can involve fatigue and weakness. Stay with your weight loss program, but go easy, heeding any negative signs.

Fat Burners

If you're working off some excess weight, your most important job is to get plenty of exercise and keep your calorie intake moderate. If you need some extra help burning off that fat, there are supplements that can help you do the job.

GLA Oils

My favorite fat burner is gamma-linolenic acid (GLA) supplements, because they are entirely safe, can be taken long-term, and can be taken by anyone. You can give yourself the same benefits as aspirin by making sure your GLA levels are high. GLA is an omega-6 fatty acid normally made in the body from the essential fatty acid linoleic acid, which is found in some unprocessed vegetable oils and nuts. GLA plays an essential role in the body's formation of "good" prostaglandins, which are hormonelike substances that, among other things (such as inhibiting inflammation), help the body burn fat more easily. You can take GLA in the form of a supplement of evening primrose oil or borage oil. Follow the directions on the container.

The Pep Pills

Please be very cautious in using the so-called "diet pills" or "pep pills." The FDA has received more than one hundred reports of adverse effects from taking a weight loss product containing ma huang and kola nut and in response has issued a public warning. For once, I am in agreement with them. Ma huang is a source of ephedrine, a stimulant, and kola nut is a source of caffeine. The combination is popular because it helps burn fat. However, taken in high doses or over a long period of time or in combination with other drugs, such as alcohol, these products are most definitely dangerous, especially if you have high blood pressure or heart disease.

Taken for short periods of time, in recommended doses, they can be helpful in weight loss programs.

But overdoing it with these drugs is extremely dangerous. I also want to point out that if you take an over-the-counter antihistamine, such as Sudafed, and drink a couple of cups of coffee, you're getting essentially the same thing, so it is a bit hypocritical of the FDA to pounce on one company for pushing this type of product.

Here are some supplements you can take, for a few weeks at a time, to help you get going on your weight loss program. Please don't take them long-term, and notice if you are experiencing any adverse effects, such as rapid heartbeat, irritability, and insomnia. If you have any type of heart disease, high blood pressure, diabetes, or liver disease, do not take these supplements. If you're stressed out and need an energy boost, try a cup of ginseng tea, which has a tonic effect rather than a stimulating effect.

Ephedra/Ma huang. The major ingredient in most diet pills is *Ephedra sineica*, also called Mormon tea, desert tea, or the Chinese version, ma huang. The key substance in ephedra is a stimulant called ephedrine. If you're thinking that this name sounds familiar, you're right. Pseudoephedrine, a synthetic version of ephedrine, is the active ingredient in most over-the-counter allergy and decongestant medicines. While it decreases appetite and increases energy, the side effects can be the same as if you were taking an allergy medicine: irritability, anxiety, restlessness, and insomnia. This ingredient is closely related to amphetamines or, in street drug parlance, "speed."

Some products combine ephedra with caffeine and aspirin. This combination does seem to increase the body's ability to burn fat, but it's a potent combination and I recommend you use it with care.

Yohimbine. Another popular diet pill ingredient comes from a plant called *Corynanthe yohimbe*. This herb is a fat burner, essentially increasing energy by speeding things up. This can be the good news if it improves your mood—or the bad news if you suffer from its side effects, which can include panic attacks, high blood pressure, and heart palpitations. Yohimbine also has a reputation as an aphrodisiac for men, which seems to have some scientific basis in fact. It should not be used if you have ulcers, kidney disease, or heart disease, nor should it be used if you're taking high blood pressure medication, tranquilizers, antidepressants, or any other mood-altering drug.

Guarana. This Brazilian plant (*Paulina cupana*) contains caffeine, so it can be quite stimulating. As you know, I'm not a big fan of ongoing caffeine use, but it can be used if you need a mental pick-me-up or a temporary energy boost. I do not recommend you use it long-term.

Chromium picolinate. We talked about chromium as a metabolism booster. Now let's talk about its other primary effect, which is to burn fat. Chromium is an important mineral involved in food digestion and metabolism, as well as the regulation of insulin and cholesterol. Taken as a supplement, it can lower cholesterol, especially when combined with niacin (chromium nicotinate). There is some evidence that it stimulates the body to store calories as muscle rather than fat. You can also increase your chromium levels by taking a brisk walk!

A chromium deficiency, which I suspect most Americans have, can disrupt the way the body handles glucose, or sugar. Eating refined sugar depletes the body of chromium.

Gotu kola. Gotu kola (*Centella asiatica*) is used in India in Ayurvedic medicine and in China, where it is called fo ti tieng. When gotu kola first came on the market, it was often billed as an "upper." However, many people had it confused with the South American plant *Cola nitida*, which contains caffeine. In reality, gotu kola tends to have a sedating and tonic effect. The Chinese use it to improve memory, for exhaustion, and for a variety of "nervous" disorders. It may actually have the effect of countering some of the side effects of ephedra and yohimbine. Research has shown that gotu kola does improve circulation by strengthening the veins and capillaries, which may account for its role as a memory enhancer.

Do Not Dehydrate

Dehydration plays no positive role in fitness or weight loss. Fluid deprivation and fluid loss through sweating can take off the extra weight, but the body will be highly stressed and the loss will be temporary. Dehydration is also bad for athletic performance in the following ways:

- Glycogen stores decrease
- Oxygen uptake decreases
- Heart function decreases
- Blood volume decreases
- Muscular endurance decreases
- Muscular strength decreases

If you are working to make a strict weight class in a sport like wrestling, do it well ahead of time with a sensible reduction in calorie intake, long slow workouts, and a distance training program.

Recent research has shown that dehydrated weight lifters had higher cortisol levels, implying that dehydration created a stress response by the adrenal glands. Some researchers theorize that chronically increased cortisol could lead to reduced levels of testosterone.

Your first choice of fluids before, during, and after exercise should be water, water, and water. Once you've had some water, you can move on to sports drinks or fruit juices to replace minerals. Orange juice and apple juice have as much as 200–400 mg of potassium per cup, significantly more than most sports drinks unless they are fortified. (Yet another good reason to read labels carefully!)

Most adults need six to eight glasses of water a day, but when you are exercising, that need goes up. How do you know if you're drinking enough water? If your urine is dark, it means that it's too concentrated, and you probably need more water. Some vitamins can darken urine, but in general urine should be nearly clear.

Caffeine and alcohol will actually contribute to dehydration, so choose your fluids wisely. If you are running a marathon or doing some other type of extended intensive exercise, you may need a sugary drink to refuel the glucose in your muscles and liver, but it's ideal if you can get some vitamins and minerals with your sugar. In other words, choose a sports drink that is fortified with vitamins and minerals, or choose fruit juices. I strongly recommend that you avoid diet sodas sweetened with artificial sweeteners such as aspartame.

Although it's fine to drink water up to 30 to 40 minutes before exercise, be very cautious about sugary drinks before exercise, as they can cause hypoglycemia. These types of drinks are best consumed during exercise, when your body can burn them off immediately.

Replacing Electrolytes and Key Minerals

When you sweat during exercise, your body loses minerals (called electrolytes in this context), especially sodium (salt) and potassium, which regulate fluid balance in your cells. Intensive exercise in very hot weather can cause an athlete to lose as many as 5 pounds of water weight, but it is very important that this be replaced with high-quality fluids over the next few days.

Potassium

Potassium not only balances sodium in the cells but, along with calcium and magnesium, plays a role in regulating heart rhythm. A potassium deficiency can cause the nerves and muscles to malfunction, as well as causing water retention, ringing in the ears, and insomnia.

This important mineral is found naturally in citrus fruits, apricots, bananas, apples, cantaloupe, tomatoes, watercress, all green leafy vegetables, the mints, sunflower seeds, and potatoes. Most people can easily get enough potassium in their daily diet, and many multivitamins contain potassium.

It may benefit you to get some potassium from a sports drink after or during intensive exercise, but since potassium is so plentiful in most foods, you can get most of it through diet. Athletes doing intensive exercise may want to take a potassium supplement of 100–500 mg daily with food.

Sodium

Sodium has a bad name in nutrition because in excess it can contribute to high blood pressure. But in fact, it is an essential mineral and is especially important to athletes who are losing it through sweating. However, most people get more than enough salt in

to conserve it, even ere is no need to sup-

Magnesium

Magnesium is one of the superstars of the mineral world, and it is especially important for athletes because it plays a key role in regulating fluid balance in the cells and in energy metabolism and muscle contraction. Fatigue and muscle weakness can be signs of magnesium deficiency. Magnesium is necessary for calcium and vitamin C metabolism and literally hundreds of enzyme reactions in the body. Athletes should be getting 300–400 mg of magnesium daily in supplement form. Magnesium is found naturally in whole grains, figs, nuts and seeds, bananas and other fruits, and green vegetables.

Calcium

Calcium is the most abundant mineral in the body and is essential for strong bones. For athletes, adequate calcium and magnesium help prevent muscle cramps, help blood to clot, and can improve endurance. Calcium by itself won't do you a bit of good. To be absorbed, it needs other minerals, especially magnesium and phosphorus.

Athletes should be taking 400–1,600 mg of extra calcium in supplement form, with magnesium. You should be getting the other minerals that help calcium build bone in your multivitamin. These include boron, manganese, zinc, and copper. For more on calcium, refer back to chapter 1.

HEALTHY WEIGHT GAIN

Calories should go up for weight gain, but exercise should not go down if you want to stay fit. The trick is to consume more calories than you burn without adding too much body fat.

Sports like weight lifting and discus call for a larger body mass for the power it brings. Greater-than-average body fat may benefit long-distance athletes in the form of extra fuel reserves and insulation, but never at the expense of oxygen uptake and delivery systems. This is why increasing body mass does not have to mean increasing body fat. Aerobic conditioning, as in long workouts and distance training, incorporated in every weight gain program, will ensure that not all weight gained is fat. Heavy weight lifting, always with expert instruction and supervision, is also essential. Slow use of heavy weights builds bulk as muscle, thickening red, slow-twitch fibers.

Weight is gained easily at the rate of about 1.5 pounds per week until it reaches the body's *set point*. The body works against any increase in weight once it hits this plateau. After this point, weight will only increase at about 0.5 to 2 pounds a month unless you adjust your diet and take supplements to overcome that process.

You can shift the set point up to a new level by keeping your weight a few pounds above the original plateau for two to three months. This period of stability gives your body time to adapt. Expect a slower rate of weight gain once you start to work toward increasing weight again. Keep up both weights and aerobic conditioning throughout all stages of a weight gain program to ensure that fat increase is kept to a minimum.

Supplements for Gaining Weight and Muscle

On the shelves of most health food stores and body-building gyms, there are dozens of supplements with labels promising to get you "ripped" and "bulked up." Some will help you and others are just hype. Here are the weight-gain supplements backed up by the research.

DHEA (Dehydroepiandrosterone)

This is a steroid hormone made in the adrenal glands. It is a key factor in synthesizing and repairing protein. Because it is an androgen, or male hormone, it also tends to build muscle and burn fat. DHEA may also increase the effects of insulin and boost thyroid function, which would increase metabolism and thus burn fat. Nearly all the research done with DHEA has been done on men, and because it is an androgen, women should use it with caution. Used in excess, it can cause

hair growth in places women don't want it! Because DHEA production declines with age, if you are under the age of fifty, I don't recommend that you use DHEA long-term, since it could suppress your natural production of it. If you are a man over the age of fifty, you may benefit from taking 50–100 mg of DHEA daily. Your best guide is how you feel. If you are a woman, you should not be taking more than 25 mg daily, and some health care professionals recommend 25 mg every other day for women.

Protein Powders

Most athletes can get all the protein they need from foods, but for those intensively trying to build muscle, protein powders may help. There are dozens of protein powders on the market, with a dizzying array of ingredients. These powders are usually made from eggs, whey, soy, or casein (milk protein). They are high in protein and low in fat and usually also contain a selection of amino acids, herbs, vitamins, and minerals. Each manufacturer will have its list of reasons why it has a superior product. The bottom line is to find what works for your body. If it tastes good, it digests well, and you're seeing results, then it's probably right for you. If you know that you are allergic to milk, avoid powders made with casein and whey. It's also important to know what your weight and muscle-building goals are and then to read the product literature to find out which product will best meet your goals.

Energy Bars

While these easy-to-eat-and-digest bars are great if you're doing intensive exercise and need some carbohydrate energy, be aware that if you're not exercising, these bars will put on the pounds, because they are primarily made of a variety of sugars and carbohydrates designed to be quick fuel and to be burned rapidly. If you are not doing intense exercise, they will go straight to fat! Use them wisely.

Creatine Monohydrate

Creatine monohydrate is a form of creatine, a nitrogen compound that combines with phosphorus to form high-energy phosphate in the ATP energy cycle. This high-energy phosphate is part of the body's immediate fueling system, essential for such activities as weight lifting, the 100-yard dash, and swimming sprints. Taking a creatine monohydrate supplement can supply the body with an extra reservoir of creatine, from which the ATP energy cycle can be fueled. Creatine monohydrate has been well studied. Athletes who use it tend to increase their performance and, over time, their lean body mass. Most studies indicate that a dosage of 5–10 g daily is optimal.

Branched-Chain Amino Acids

Isoleucine, leucine, and valine are essential amino acids known as branched-chain amino acids (BCAAs). They are key ingredients in the body's ability to handle stress and produce energy. They are used by the muscles for energy and are needed in hemoglobin formation. During high-intensity exercise, more leucine is used than any other amino acid. Taking the BCAAs as a supplement can speed healing after surgery and help build muscle. The BCAAs may also be brain transmitters and have some ability to relieve pain.

Anabolic Steroids Have No Place in Fitness

No rational training program includes steroids. The cost to the body of their use is simply not worth it. Synthesized from plants or extracted from human or animal sources, these powerful chemicals function as androgens, or male hormones. *Anabolism* is part of metabolism. It is the synthesis of complex chemicals from simpler ones. One of the results of anabolism is the greater muscle mass desired by athletes because it means increased power, strength, and speed. Using anabolic steroids as a hormonal trigger in the muscles is a completely unnatural intervention, for which athletes pay dearly with many possible side effects, including:

- Permanent liver damage
- Risky cholesterol levels
- Increased growth of undetected or new malignancies
- Shortened bone length in adolescents
- Decreased sex drive
- Bloating

- In women, development of male characteristics, clitoral enlargement, breast atrophy, and irregular or absent menstrual cycles
- In men, acne, baldness, lowered sperm count, prostate enlargement, and genital atrophy

In addition to this horrific list, steroids are usually a black-market purchase produced in unregulated, often makeshift laboratories. This adds the risk of contamination with allergens at best and toxic substances at worst. Steroids have a limited use in medicine and none in sports and fitness. Persist with a healthy weight gain regimen to see safe, long-lasting increase in muscle mass.

There is no competition that is worth doing this type of damage to the body. If you plan to be a professional athlete who lasts in competition over time, the only way to go is the natural way.

GETTING READY TO GET IN SHAPE

Here are some simple guidelines to help you tailor your workout program to your specific needs. Whether you're a seasoned competitor or just starting out, be sure to include all of the elements in this section when getting in shape.

Aerobic and Anaerobic Exercise

The term *aerobic* means requiring oxygen; it comes from the Greek words for air and life. Aerobic exercise develops the oxygen pathways of the body. This increases aerobic respiration, the efficient, oxygen-fueled process of metabolism.

Exercising brings an initial burst of aerobic energy production that only lasts several seconds. The body burns stored energy anaerobically up to about 2 minutes. The aerobic system will then kick in again once it receives more oxygen. If oxygen isn't being delivered in sufficient quantity at high enough speed and to the right places, then energy production suffers.

Aerobic exercise naturally increases the efficiency of the heart, lungs, and circulation. A strong heart provides necessary oxygen with fewer beats per minute than a weaker one, and it is less easily strained. A greater intake of oxygen travels through more and expanded capillary networks to keep energy fueling at high rates for longer periods of time. Athletes show the results in heart rates much lower than the average 70 beats per minute needed to supply the body when resting.

"Aerobics" refers to a series of intense aerobic exercises with slower-paced intervals. Good aerobics classes will not ask students to push too hard, for it is unwise to raise the pulse very high and then let it drop off suddenly. Definitely avoid the plentiful aerobics classes that become unofficially competitive, seeing who can keep up rather than encouraging each individual to find a pace that exerts that individual, but not too much.

In fact, many forms of exercise are aerobic, and several can be tailored to specific types of training. Whichever activity you choose, aim at five or six days a week. This gives the body time to recover but will get better results than a two- or three-day regimen. However, if you're over thirty-five, you need to avoid stressing your joints and should engage in different aerobic activities on different days.

Anaerobic exercise conditions the energy pathway that is not fueled by oxygen. After about 10 seconds of aerobic energy production at the start of exercise, the anaerobic energy pathway is dominant for up to around 2 minutes. Anaerobic conditioning, then, is produced by short, vigorous bursts of activity. Any exertion you have to cut short because of lack of breath is anaerobic, including, for example, the sprint finish of a long run. Any intense activity period during interval training is also anaerobic exercise.

There are three main characteristics of anaerobic exercise:

- *High intensity*—doing a lot of work, pushing the body to maximum limits
- *Short duration*—taking it to the limit and no further, allowing the aerobic pathway to pay back the oxygen debt incurred
- *Repetition*—constantly testing the muscles to build the fibers and strengthen the anaerobic energy pathway

Warm Up and Cool Down

Whatever exercise activity you choose, it makes good physical and mental sense to begin and end with a warm-up in the form of some stretches. A warm-up is so called because it gets blood moving through the muscles. This literally warms them up.

A cool-down really doesn't have to do with cooling but a redistribution of blood circulating in the muscles. A better term is "warm-down." The aim is to speed up the breakdown of any waste products in the bloodstream by ensuring that blood circulates through all parts of the body.

Despite their importance, warm-ups and cool-downs are probably the most neglected parts of fitness routines. This is unfortunate, for they can increase the gains of exercise and help prevent physical damage. Sudden starts and finishes force the body into different gears, creating uneven and overloaded points of stress, increasing your risk of injury. Think of it like a car. It does no engine any good to go from ignition to high gear in one jump.

If your body is young and already flexible, don't dismiss warm-ups and cool-downs. They will help you maintain your body tone in the future, creating a high base level of conditioning that will be hard to lose.

Warm-ups and cool-downs are a mixture of exertion, relaxation, and flexes that increase flexibility and bring your mind into calm focus. They are a form of resistance training, since you are working against the normal patterns of tension that your body holds against gravity.

Begin a warm-up with an exercise that gets blood circulating through all your muscles. This helps prevent tearing caused by stretching cold muscles. Running or walking in place achieves this well.

Another method is the "rock 'n' roll": Sit on the floor, bring your knees up, and tuck your head in. You'll find that you are curled almost in a ball. Next, rock and roll back and forth at a steady pace, keeping as tucked up as you can. Breathe in as you roll backward and out as you bring your weight back up.

Breathing is essential throughout a warm-up or cool-down. Breathe in as you prepare to stretch, and breathe out as you make the stretch itself. As you stretch, try to really feel the flex of muscles involved and the way they bunch or lengthen. Then focus on the way the rest of your body is responding to the stretch. *Relax* as you make the stretch. Use a slow, calm approach and build in meditative techniques if you enjoy them. The overall approach for a warm-up should be to concentrate body and mind in preparation for a period of enjoyable, focused physical exertion free of unwanted stress.

The cool-down is the reverse, stretches taking you down in gear to continue the rest of your day on an even keel.

A full warm-up lasts about 20 minutes to half an hour. Even for just half an hour of exercise, a 10-minute warm-up is needed. A cool-down is usually shorter than a warm-up, but the same rules apply.

Always:

- Ease into warm-ups, especially after inactivity
- Stretch slowly
- Think of your muscles as lengthening
- Hold the stretch as long as recommended
- Remember to breathe
- Go very easy on injured areas
- Be patient, as flexibility increases slowly

Never:

- Cut stretches short
- Overstretch or you will risk injury
- Bounce on a stretch, as this overstresses muscles
- Skip warm-ups and cool-downs—there are no substitutes!

How to Calculate Your Pulse Target Rate

First, a word of warning. Self-calculation is for young and healthy individuals. Anyone middle-aged or older or with a health problem should consult a physician for advice and professional pulse rate setting. Calculation of target pulse or heart rate depends partly on the intensity of the workout you can comfortably endure. Maximum, or 100 percent, intensity would be the level at which your heart is working to full capacity. Obviously, this level is impossible for most people to maintain for longer than a short period of time.

Working at over 80 percent intensity uses the anaerobic systems, while 60 percent is the minimum required for aerobic conditioning. There is more aerobic benefit to working at 80 percent intensity. Any lower, and you'll have to work for longer to achieve the same conditioning.

Subtract your age from the number 220 to give a maximum heart rate. Next, multiply the result by your chosen intensity percentage. For example, for someone aged thirty-two, the target pulse rate is $220 - 32 = 188 \times 70\%$ (or 0.70) = 131.60. Round up to 132 to give you the figure to aim at.

A watch is useful to help you take your pulse during exercise. Feel your pulse with your middle and index fingers placed on the underside of your wrist, below your thumb joint and inside the wrist bone. Another pulse point is right over the heart. You can also feel your pulse in both sides of the neck, outside the windpipe and two or three fingers down from the jaw. Count the number of beats you feel in 10 seconds. Multiply by 6 to get the number of beats per minute.

Exercise with Antioxidant Power

Exercising to exhaustion or without proper nutrition or in a polluted environment can do you more harm than good. Exercise naturally burns up a lot of oxygen, which creates a lot of free radicals with the potential to cause oxidation damage.

What antioxidants do in the body is help neutralize the damage of oxidation. We can think of oxidation as similar to what happens to metal when it rusts, or to an apple when it turns brown. Have you ever prevented a cut-up apple from turning brown by squeezing some lemon juice on it? The vitamin C in the lemon juice is an antioxidant that is stopping the oxidation process. When meat spoils or oil goes rancid, oxidation is at work.

The damage that free radicals do includes cell mutation that can lead to cancer. Other kinds of damage can contribute to cardiovascular disease, cataracts, macular degeneration, arthritis, and diseases affecting the brain, the kidneys, the lungs, the digestive system, and the immune system. Free radicals are involved in the damage done by alcoholism, aging, radiation injury, iron overload, and diseases involving the blood, such as strokes. Once the process of oxidation begins, it can be hard to stop, so your best health plan is to prevent it in the first place.

Many athletes and sports researchers have noticed that some types of professional athletes and long-distance runners die relatively young from heart disease or cancer. This is most likely because their antioxidant status wasn't high enough to protect them from the free radicals produced by the intensive, long-term exercise. Runners face a double whammy because they often exercise outdoors in an environment polluted with car exhaust, factory pollution, and other types of smog. Inhaling these toxins while the body is at peak output puts tremendous stress on the body's detoxifying system.

Recent research shows that intensive exercise also temporarily suppresses the immune system, making many professional athletes more susceptible to infections, colds, and flu viruses.

All these factors make it extremely important that athletes take plenty of antioxidant supplements. Here are some of my favorites.

Vitamin A/Beta-Carotene

This growth-promoting vitamin helps to fight infections, which is especially important for an athlete in intensive training. In fact, if you have any type of lung infection, taking an extra vitamin A supplement for a week or two can help knock it out. Beta-carotene is a precursor to vitamin A, meaning that the body can make vitamin A from beta-carotene. Refer back to chapter 1 for more in-depth information on these vitamins.

Vitamin C

Vitamin C, also called ascorbic acid, is a powerful antioxidant that plays myriad roles in protecting the free-radical-challenged athlete! Here are some of its powers:

- It plays an important role in healing wounds.
- It helps prevent fatigue.
- It helps fight infections.
- It lowers cholesterol.
- It prevents the production of nitrosamines (cancer-causing agents).
- It lowers the incidence of blood clots in the veins.
- It decreases the severity and length of the common cold.
- It increases the absorption of iron.

Vitamin C also works in a team with other vitamins, minerals, and enzymes, strengthening the collagen in connective tissue and promoting capillary integrity, especially important for tissue repair before and after intensive exercise.

I recommend that you include 1,500–2,000 mg of vitamin C in your daily vitamin regimen and double that when you are exercising intensively. In large doses, vitamin C can cause diarrhea. If this happens, simply lower the dose until the diarrhea goes away. Your tolerance for vitamin C is much, much greater when you're fighting infection or under stress.

Vitamin E

One of vitamin E's most important roles as an antioxidant is to prevent heart disease and stroke, but it is also important to hundreds of biochemical processes in the body. It helps prevent cancer, prevents and dissolves blood clots, helps prevent scarring when used externally on the skin, accelerates burn healing, can lower blood pressure, and enhances the immune system.

Today, many cardiologists recommend 400 IU of vitamin E daily. The dry (succinate) form of vitamin E is preferred for people over forty, because it is more easily absorbed by the digestive system. If you are exercising intensively, increase your intake of vitamin E to 800 IU daily.

The Bioflavonoid Antioxidants

Bioflavonoids are organic compounds found in plants. These powerful antioxidants can be an athlete's best friend by reducing inflammation and pain, strengthening blood vessels, improving circulation, and fighting bacteria and viruses.

Vitamin C is found combined with bioflavonoids in nature, and it works much more effectively when combined with bioflavonoids. The following bioflavonoids are two of my favorite antioxidants for athletes.

Quercetin. You should get to know this antioxidant, anticancer, and antiallergy agent. This bioflavonoid may also have antiviral properties. It works wonders for treating allergies.

Proanthocyanidins/PCOs/Grapeseed extract. PCOs improve circulation and the flexibility of connective tissues. They neutralize free radicals more powerfully than vitamin E while reducing inflammation. Vegetables and fruits are our best food sources, but once these foods reach our tables they are largely depleted of this nutrient. Supplements are usually derived from grapeseeds.

Glutathione

Glutathione (GSH) is an amino acid found in nearly every living cell. Its most important job is neutralizing and disposing of excess free radicals, especially those formed from LDL cholesterol particles. Oxidized LDL is damaging to artery walls. GSH protects the body's infection–fighting lymphatic system, stabilizes blood sugar, fights cancer, and helps to repair cells after a stroke.

Intense exercise, illness, and aging cause glutathione levels to drop. If vitamins C and E levels are low, GSH doesn't function as well.

The best way to raise glutathione levels is by taking a cysteine supplement, 500–1,000 mg daily. You can take it in the form of cysteine or *N*-acetylcysteine. For more on this antioxidant amino acid, refer to chapter 2.

FIVE WAYS TO TRAIN

Some natural athletes discover sports and fitness in childhood and keep them in their lives from that time on. Some people begin exercising to speed up recuperation after illness or to get in shape after poor results from a medical checkup. Childbirth, increasing age, increasing weight—whatever the initial motivating events, the underlying reason to take up exercise is to improve fitness. Choosing which exercise path to follow is the next step.

Different exercises do different things for the body. If repair, rebuilding, or reshaping is your primary aim, you may be well enough motivated to get on with only specific workout routines. Unless an activity aligns with your idea of fun, however, it will fade from your life or become a burden, bringing resentment—which is not part of fitness.

Ask yourself these questions: Are you a natural competitor, a team player, or a loner? Are you looking for a recreational activity or a fitness routine to build into your life? How much time are you willing to set aside for exercise or training? Your answers will narrow down the selection.

Strictly speaking, training is preparation for a particular sport or activity. In fitness, training is often an end in itself when the aim is simply a body in shape or a particular shape. Training consists of either a series of exercises or an activity performed in a particular way. Choose your performance strategy according to the results it produces.

Interval Training

Interval training has been a favorite of athletes since the late 1940s. It builds strength and is the basis of a worthwhile aerobics class. Muscles are worked more thoroughly if intense bursts of exercise are spaced with recovery periods. This relates to the mechanism whereby aerobic refueling kicks in after up to 2 minutes of calories are burned from glycogen alone. The fast interval creates an "oxygen debt." The slow interval allows the body's stores of oxygen and other essential substances to be replenished. If there is no slowing in pace, the oxygen uptake never catches up and lactic acid begins to build up. This is why sprinting over very long distances is not possible for the human body. Repeatedly asking the body to respond to an oxygen debt leads to an improvement of all the internal systems and organs involved. Strictly speaking, interval training is both aerobic and anaerobic, for both respiration pathways are exerted.

Whatever your activity, to make it interval based, simply slow or rest after short set periods from seconds to minutes, depending on your condition. A common ratio is 1:3. An example would be running just under maximum pace for 20 seconds, then taking a slow jog for 1 minute. However, many top athletes prefer to use their body as a guide. With experience, it's possible to recognize the point at which the heart rate is at about 160 to 170 beats per minute (the crossover point from anaerobic back to aerobic respiration) and to feel the sensations of lactic acid building up. Typically, muscles begin to feel more solid, and what was comfortable effort begins to feel stressful. It's important, too, not to make too many repetitions, especially in sprinting. This can overtax the heart. Stay within comfortable limits and monitor your pulse rate to see that it doesn't shoot too high.

A limitation of interval training is the lack of stimulating competition. Conditioning is the major focus, rather than the mental stresses and survival tactics associated with an event. Nevertheless, interval training builds up stamina, endurance, and speed, no matter what your choice of sport or general exercise.

Circuit Training

Circuit training is the use of a series of exercises, often involving weights and *calisthenics* (light gymnastic routines). Safe, productive circuit training involves exercises of both high and low intensity and covers all major muscle groups. An example of a circuit training workout might be in five stations: a push-up station; a squat station (where you would squat and rise holding light weights); a bicep curl station; a sit-up station; and a bent-over row station (which works the back muscles). Using a stopwatch, you would spend 1 to 2 minutes at each station, going around the circuit two or three times. You can also circuit train on the machines at the gym, switching between several machines with short or no rests in between stations. Circuit and interval training combined produce maximum benefit.

Continuous Aerobic Training

Continuous aerobic training is not for the absolute beginner. Exercise is best begun gradually to allow the body time to adjust. A good suggestion is to start this kind of training once exercise is an established habit (part of your routine for at least three months). Continuous aerobic conditioning involves working continuously at your chosen sport, such as running or swimming, keeping your pulse at a target level for as long as you desire. The minimum time recommended is 20 minutes. The pace set should be achieved by working at medium effort. At the right rate, you should still be able to carry on a conversation, even if it does sound huffy. If muscles start to pump up, burn, or tremble, cut back your rate and

review your pulse rate calculation. Strength and endurance will both increase with continuous aerobic conditioning for any exercise or sport.

Resistance Training

Weight lifting is the best-known form of resistance training. Why the term *resistance?* Resistance training uses the muscles on the frame of the body, such as the biceps and chest, to work against an object, such as a weight, barbell, or bench press, that resists their effort. Much of the equipment in gyms and health clubs is designed for resistance work. The aim of resistance training is to strengthen muscles.

Resistance training works by testing a muscle beyond its normal limits and then allowing it time to recover. During the recovery phase, the muscle rebounds, not just back to original endurance levels but slightly beyond them. This is a process of adaptation as the body tries to be sure it is ready in case it has to endure the same stress again. A gradual increase in intensity of resistance produces a parallel gain in muscle strength. This is called progressive resistance training and works by making each new level of adaptation become the baseline for further improvement.

There is a great range of resistance exercises, partly because there is a large number of muscles to work for fitness purposes. The number and variety of exercises are also needed because each muscle group has a range of motions to which it contributes, and these all need to be worked in order to maximize performance and avoid muscle stress from repeating the same exercise over and over again.

Resistance exercises begin with a muscle stretch, either pushing against an object or holding a weight. The muscle is contracted, then stretched once more. The action of stretch to contraction and back again is called a repetition. A number of repetitions in a row is called a set. There are three main repetition ranges: low, six to ten repetitions; medium, ten to fifteen; and high, over fifteen. Low, slow repetitions build strength as they bulk up the red, slow-twitch muscle fibers. This level of resistance training is favored by bodybuilders. General muscle fitness results from medium repetitions. High, fast repetitions help increase the speed potential of white, fast-twitch fibers, but working with weights, endurance improvements and a leaner physique will probably be the main result.

Beginners are best advised to seek a supervised course of instruction on resistance training. This will provide an introduction to the variety of exercises and equipment, in addition to supplying crucial instruction on correct techniques.

Here are some basic guidelines for resistance training:

- Use a varied program of exercises, and don't get stuck in a few routines.
- Aim to execute each repetition perfectly, using the muscle, not momentum.
- Resist weights as you move them back into stretch position. Never let them simply drop back into place.
- Do not pause too long in the middle of workouts.
- Build in recovery time between workouts.
- Do not jar muscles to get weights up.
- Pay attention to pain; don't go past it.
- Get expert advice.

Combination Training

As the name suggests, combination training is a mixture of different methods of conditioning. Each approach brings different physical demands. Combining them develops all of the body's biological systems and exposes the athletes to different conditions. It is also beneficial because it avoids physical stress from repetition, brings variety, and beats boredom. Aerobic conditioning is the choice of most people exercising only for fitness. It's the serious athlete who chooses combination training.

TWELVE WAYS TO SHAPE UP AEROBICALLY

Many sports and fitness routines fill the aerobic bill. This selection represents some of the most popular activities, but there are many more. Some sports, like golf, bring aerobic benefits by incorporating basic activities such as brisk walking. Intense practice of one aspect of a sport will often result in more aerobic conditioning than the sport itself. The stops and starts and frequent bench layoffs of American football are an example. Use the following list of activities as a guide once you're sure of your aims and motivations for beginning exercise. If you're already exercising, check out your choice. See if you're toning up any particular muscle groups and if you're on track to get the most aerobic benefits possible from your chosen activity or your training for it.

Walking

Brisk walking will get the pulse rate up fairly easily unless you are a highly conditioned athlete or very young. Beginner's pace should be about 3 miles per hour. For more aerobic benefits, work up to 5 miles per hour over a period of months. Within four to six weeks, work up from 15 minutes daily to 45 minutes every other day. In the next stage, aim at 45 to 75 minutes daily, which will cover 3 to 4 miles. Essential equipment at all levels is a good pair of comfortable shoes that allow ample room for toes and do not rub heels.

Good shoes and the same aerobic guidelines are just as important for treadmill work. Normal hazards and interruptions such as dogs and drivers can make the treadmill the preferred choice for some walkers and runners. Just watch out as you step on and off the machine.

Walk with your head over your body and your feet pointing straight ahead. Keep poised for your next step with weight always slightly forward over your leading foot. It's a sustained fast pace with vigorous strides and arm actions that provides the necessary exertion. The result is low- to medium-intensity exercise that can be kept up for a long time. You can increase the intensity without increasing speed by using weights. This can come in the form of actual hand or belt weights (never ankle weights) or a weighted backpack.

Walking is often underrated. It actually involves more muscular activity than running. For extra motivation, remember that walking tones legs and buttocks and has even been shown to improve short-term memory and reasoning faculties, especially in people over the age of fifty-five.

Running

Running can vary from a slow jog to an all-out sprint. Running in place counts, too, with or without a treadmill, and is useful for anyone stuck indoors or for TV addicts! It's an exercise for the conditioned exerciser, something to move up to from walking or regular workouts if you're looking for more.

The stresses of running can be grueling, as legs and feet take a hard pounding. The benefits are worth it in all-over toning, but the usual cautions apply, such as the need for gradual progress and avoiding too much too soon. Running in particular can bring stress injuries through too much repetition. Vary your route, take time off, and, if you're past age thirty-five, interchange running with another aerobic exercise.

Indulge yourself with a really good pair of running shoes. Considering the risk of foot injuries, it's not worth cutting costs. If you're running specifically to lose fat or strengthen your heart, monitor your pulse rate as well.

Stair Climbing

This is your chance to join those dedicated bleachers runners down at the track. Stair climbing is actually a useful travel exercise, ideal if you're stuck in a hotel. Three flights are preferable to give a sustained upward climb. Take one or two steps at a time, building up to a speed that takes you to your target pulse rate. Come back down quickly and keep going for at least 20 minutes. Buttocks and legs get the most workout here.

In the gym or at home, a stair-climbing machine will bring the same benefits with better predictability and sustainability. A machine also takes out the downhill part, which is good if you're after continuous aerobic conditioning but not so good if you're interested in interval training effects. Avoid stair-climbing machine injuries such as wrist damage. Follow instructions closely and do not support your body with your arms. Take a break or slow down if you feel that your legs need a rest. Keep your actions smooth, without bouncing or letting your knees hit your chest.

Jumping Rope

Fun and convenient to do anywhere, jumping rope can bring more aerobic benefit per minute than jogging. Build up to a moderate pace, jumping low to avoid stressing feet, ankles, and knees. This is my personal favorite exercise to do when I'm traveling. Since jumping rope is a high-impact activity, be sure to wear shoes with good cushioning. Avoid jumping on hard surfaces such as pavement or concrete. Instead, opt for grass, dirt, carpet, or a sprung hardwood floor.

Hiking

Hiking avoids the distractions and dangers of urban exercise, but it brings a few dangers of its own. Be alert to changes in trail surfaces and obstacles, and carry a map and survival gear if you're out in remote back country. Be prepared for the weather and for any sudden changes. If you're in a sunny climate or not used to the sun, it's a good idea to wear sun protection, such as a hat with a brim and sunblock. For long, even trails, trail shoes are a wise investment, but reserve a good pair of hiking boots for rocky, hilly trails. If you're on a smooth trail or dirt road, you can have fun altering your pace from fast walking to jogging and back to walking as trail gradation changes.

Cycling

Sustained cycling is a great workout for the legs and buttocks. Stop-start cycling in traffic won't bring the same degree of fitness. Uninterrupted rides, outside, in high gear but with easy pedaling are recommended. Benefits come from rides of 20 to 45 minutes. Beginners should work up their speed gradually from 6 to 7 miles per hour, remembering that cycling at 11 miles per hour burns about four times as many calories per minute as pedaling at 5.5 miles per hour.

Don't be tempted to downshift and put pressure on your thighs. Aerobic conditioning is not achieved through high-intensity exercise. Keep pedals spinning freely with an easy knee action. Get expert advice on saddle and handlebar adjustments to ensure ideal body position. Wear safety gear, and stay alert to avoid accidents.

Stationary bikes bring less danger and a better chance of a sustained workout. Proper adjustments and position are still essential. Boredom can be a major disadvantage, which is why many stationary bike exercisers listen to music or watch TV.

Swimming

Swimming can be a low-stress introduction to aerobic exercise. It's a useful choice for anyone who is overweight or interested in shaping up arms, chest, and stomach. As with all aerobic conditioning, sustained exercise is needed, so use those length lanes at the pool. Aim for a moderate stroke rate for at least 20 minutes.

Rollerblading and Skating

Safety measures are of prime importance to avoid risk of crash injuries with this type of exercise. Never use in-line or other skates for aerobic workouts until you are fully practiced and at ease with the boots. The same rule for sustained exercise applies as for any other aerobic activity, so a suitable location is important. Skate long and hard enough and you'll see and feel muscle tone improve, especially in the thighs and buttocks.

Racquetball, Tennis, and Squash

Keep yourself in motion for half an hour and the fast pace of racquetball and squash brings good overall toning. It's easy to overdo it at first, and next-day muscle soreness can be severe, especially in legs and buttocks. Avoid this by performing thorough warm-ups and by playing with a partner at your own level or one who's willing to take it slowly if you're new to the sport.

The stops and starts of tennis and the shared play of doubles mean that not all tennis meets the requirements for aerobic conditioning. Half an hour's sustained pace at medium intensity is more

likely to come with a singles match and at least a fair degree of experience.

Rowing

Do you have access to an open stretch of water that will allow you at least an uninterrupted half hour's rowing? Because of the equipment and logistics involved, outdoor rowing is not as common a choice as other aerobic sports. It certainly requires good boating skills and water safety practice.

Indoor rowing machines are more useful for this exercise. As with cycling, if you're not looking for that extra sense of recreation and fresh air, then a machine makes good exercise sense. A rowing machine makes your workout predictable and easy to sustain. No life vest needed, either! The popularity of rowing machines stems from the excellent all-around toning brought by rowing moderately at a steady pace. In most exercises, the locomotive power comes from the legs and hips. In rowing, the arms and back are involved to a much higher degree. For this reason, take it gently at first, for you'll be taxing muscle groups unused to the type of work demanded. Make sure your rowing action is smooth, allowing for a full stretch first on arms as you reach, then on your legs as you pull.

Cross-Country Skiing

This is possibly the number one aerobic exercise, but not for the beginner or anyone fainthearted or in ill health. Inherent in cross-country skiing are extreme conditions. The risks of snow and remote locations should be taken seriously. Catch the bug, though, and you'll find that this exercise is one of the most challenging and fun ways to tone up arms, buttocks, calves, and thighs. Of course, there is always the tamer, indoor machine if the real thing doesn't appeal. A machine will result in the same benefit but without the scenery.

One major advantage of cross-country skiing over activities such as running and walking is the reduced stress on feet and ankles. As the skier moves over the snow, the action is a glide, without any pounding of the legs. However, don't let the ease of movement coax you out of warm-ups and cool-downs; these are still essential.

Midnight Aerobics

By this I mean sex. Why not? Sex can be excellent aerobic exercise. Remember the need for sustained work in an aerobic regimen, and you'll burn over 300 calories in one session. Don't neglect warm-ups and cool-downs, especially as they could be more fun than usual. Select your exercise partner wisely, and apply all safety rules!

INJURIES: HOW TO AVOID THEM AND HOW TO TREAT THEM

When you're committed to staying fit, an injury can really cramp your style. If you are careful and don't push too hard, injuries can be avoided. If you do end up hurting, however, turn to supplements that speed healing and natural alternatives to painkilling drugs.

Preventing Injury

Mere fear of injury will eventually probably lead to it, but a working knowledge of its causes can help you to avoid injury. Harm can be done in a variety of ways, including poor or no warm-ups, too much repetition, misuse of weights, and just plain overdoing it.

A warm-up ensures that your muscles will not be jarred by sudden stress. However, the biggest rule of stretching is that muscles should not be overstretched. When you do a warm-up stretch, go as far as you can without straining, breathe into it for at least 10 seconds, and then see if it will stretch a little further. Some trainers advocate holding a stretch for up to 30 seconds. The rule about not overstretching muscles also applies to resistance training or aerobic workouts, when you should not be tempted to take muscles past their limits. This will avoid overextension, which is a common cause of injury.

Repetition, such as unvaried runs or exercise routines, means continued stress on the same body parts. This can lead to unnecessary wear and tear, especially if done without a warm-up.

Muscle pulls and sprains are almost inevitable if weights are used incorrectly. Joints can be wrenched, too, by the severe sudden stress of a carelessly raised or lowered weight. Make sure that you have proper instruction before embarking on a weight-lifting program.

Athletes frequently try to tough out initial warning signs. Working past pain often leads to much more serious conditions. In addition, old injuries will flare up if they are not allowed a full recovery. Too much stress too soon can also result from insufficient rest. Without full attention, whether through tiredness or distraction, you increase the chance of an accident.

Awareness of the risks leads to these positive guidelines:

- *Always warm up.* This prevents injury indirectly by increasing resistance. Oxygen flow is increased, flexibility is enhanced, and muscle pain and cramping become less likely.
- *Respect the structure of your body.* Keep joint and muscle movements within their natural ranges. Remember that movement is transmitted right through your body. How your foot falls affects kneecaps, hips, and spine, for example. Good shoes are a must.
- *Never use equipment on which you are not fully trained.* Always make the necessary adjustments to equipment, such as seats, handlebars, and weights. Tailor the equipment to you, not the other way around.
- *Avoid fatigue.* Take the occasional day off from training. Get enough sleep. Stop exercising when you feel tiredness set in. Relaxation is part of fitness.
- *Pay attention to pain.* Heed your body's signals. It's better to ease off for a day or two with a minor strain than to be out of action for weeks with a severe sprain.
- *Allow for full recovery.* After major injury, ease back into training very gently and under professional supervision. Nurse minor injuries and do not tax painful areas.
- *Take it slowly!* Do not try to do too much too soon. Patience pays with exercise.

Injury prevention is linked to background health. Good nutrition with plenty of fruits and vegetables keeps body systems strong and resistant to injury. It also helps not to eat for 3 hours before a long event. This contributes to an even, distraction-free run without cramps or muscle aches. And when you do eat, eat well.

Minerals are lost in perspiration, particularly in endurance events like triathlons. This can cause muscle cramps. Keep your levels up by drinking vegetable juices and taking selected supplements after and between events. This will aid specifically in maintaining levels of potassium, sodium, and calcium as well as vitamins and other nutrients.

Treating Pain and Injury

The rule for exercise is short and sweet: No gain in pain. No matter what you've heard or what is fashionable, exercise isn't meant to hurt. Pain means injury.

The first approach to pain should be to find out what is causing the pain and eliminate that. If you have an acute pain, such as a muscle sprain, you may need to warm up before you exercise in the future. If you have chronic pain, such as back pain, you may need to do exercises to strengthen your back muscles. Exercise is the single best cure for chronic back pain. (If you have back pain, don't exercise without consulting a doctor. If a sprain or ruptured disk is the cause, the wrong kind of exercise could do further damage.)

Muscle shakes and trembles are signs that the muscles need at least a few minutes' break before you continue exercising. Going past this indication of weakness risks loss of control and therefore injury.

Minimize your use of painkillers. They can mask the scale of an injury, making recovery seem more complete than it really is. There are natural, safe, and effective ways to manage most chronic pain that will allow you to avoid the NSAIDs (nonsteroidal anti-inflammatory drugs) such as ibuprofen, acetaminophen (Tylenol), and aspirin. Ibuprofen and aspirin are very hard on the digestive system, and acetaminophen is very hard on the liver.

Ice is one of the best and simplest remedies for pain caused by inflammation. The cold very effectively reduces the inflammation. Use a cold pack for 20 minutes every few hours for sprains and strains.

For a muscle sprain or strain that's been around for a few days or for swelling caused by a bruise, first use a 20-minute cold pack, then a 20-minute hot pack. The cold will reduce the inflammation, and the heat will encourage blood flow into the area and help break up damaged tissue so the healing can take place.

One of the simplest, cheapest, and most effective ways to relieve chronic pain (with the exception of headaches) is with moist heat. You can apply moist heat by taking a long, hot shower and aiming the shower head at the area that hurts. You can take a long, hot bath with relaxing herbal oils, or you can use a hot pack or a hot water bottle. If you have access to a Jacuzzi, you can aim the jets of water at the places that are painful. Sometimes we resist the simple remedies, but this one is important to use daily if you're suffering from chronic pain.

There are many supplements that can help an athlete deal with the pain of an injury and also help speed repair of tissues. Here are the supplements you should be taking to speed repair after an injury. You can find them at your health food store. Follow the directions on the bottle.

Vitamins and Minerals

Those that can play a part in reducing inflammation include vitamin C (to help repair collagen tissue and reduce inflammation), vitamin E (to speed wound healing) and the B-complex vitamins (to aid in protein synthesis). Taking a magnesium/calcium supplement can relieve the pain of muscle spasms and often relieves chronic headaches.

Digestive Enzymes

Enzymes tend to speed up the rate at which many bodily processes work, and injury repair is no exception. Enzymes working at the site of an injury go to work to remove damaged tissue, which reduces swelling, and to help the body repair itself. As the enzymes do their work, they also become an effective pain reliever. Enzymes help reduce inflammation caused by arthritis as well as injuries to joints and other connective tissues (such as muscle strains) and can even relieve back pain. The enzymes trypsin, chymotrypsin, papain, and bromelain have been most commonly used in the studies involving enzymes and pain relief.

DL-Phenylalanine (DLPA)

This is a combination of L-phenylalanine, an essential amino acid, and D-phenylalanine, a nonnutrient amino acid that helps promote the production of endorphins, natural painkillers made in the brain. DLPA is very effective in the relief of chronic pain, such as back pain. Don't use DLPA in combination with antidepressant drugs or if you have phenylketonuria (PKU).

Glucosamine Sulfate

This naturally occurring compound in the body helps keep cartilage strong and flexible and can also play a role in repairing damaged cartilage. Like bones, the cartilage found in tendons, ligaments, and other connective tissue is very much alive. When it becomes damaged in a healthy person, it is slowly but surely replaced by new cartilage. Glucosamine sulfate is a key substance in the cartilage-rebuilding process. It provides basic cartilage building blocks and stimulates the growth of cartilage. Animal studies have also shown that glucosamine sulfate reduces inflammation. Take one 500 mg capsule three times a day for eight weeks, and then taper down to one 500 mg capsule daily for maintenance.

White Willow Bark

White willow bark was used as a pain reliever long before a chemist at the Bayer Company in Germany synthesized acetylsalicylic acid, or aspirin, from one of its active ingredients in 1897. Aspirin is a synthetic drug (not found in nature), but various teas, decoctions, tinctures, and poultices of the trees of the genus *Salix*, most commonly known as willow or poplar, have been used to relieve pain for many centuries. White willow bark doesn't cause gastric bleeding or ringing in the ears the way aspirin does but is a very effective pain reliever, especially for headaches and arthritis pain. You can drink it as a tea or take it in capsule or tincture form. A bath, wash, or poultice was once used to treat aches and pains in the joints.

Kava (Piper methysticum)

Kava is best known as a drink used in the South Pacific that is relaxing and that tends to reduce anxiety and depression. However, kava is also an effective pain reliever and can often be used in place of the NSAIDs. The best way to take kava is powdered, in a capsule, or as an extract.

Cayenne Pepper

Powdered and taken in capsule form, this powerful spice can be a surprisingly effective remedy for pain caused by inflammation or bruising. The capsaicin in cayenne has the effect of blocking nerve pain transmissions, producing a pain-relieving effect. Capsaicin also has an anti-inflammatory effect, both internally and externally. Studies have shown that taken internally, capsaicin also reduces triglyceride levels, lowers blood pressure, and increases metabolism, making it easier to burn fat and lose weight.

Dried, ground cayenne is used to reduce pain and swelling internally and externally. There are also a variety of ointments containing capsaicin that can be used on painful joints and swellings. Do not apply these ointments to open sores.

Recovering from Injury

Patience is the key to recovery. The body needs time to heal and rebuild. Rest is needed not just for the injured area but for the entire body in the form of plenty of sleep.

Sound nutrition is a must for complete healing. Minor injuries may take less healing time but require good-quality attention to ensure they stay minor. Self-massage is helpful for light aches, and it's wise to follow up with an ice pack on the area for 10 to 20 minutes.

If you use weights, warm up only with a very light weight and low intensity but with a high number of repetitions. Really feel the affected muscles work as you test stretch any recovering muscles.

If you're a runner, road test your fitness: Make sure you experience no pain when walking. Next, venture out on a *slow* 20-minute run on gentle surfaces. Ease back at any sign of pain.

Don't hesitate to consult a doctor for any persistent pain that is not a usual muscle soreness. Deep tissue massage is often helpful for serious injuries. It is essential to rest the injured body part, taking time off from exercise if necessary. As you ease it back into use, apply heat before exercise and ice afterward. Keep intensity low and repetitions high. It can be useful to change workouts altogether to keep intensity levels down for a while, switching, say, from running to walking. As you get back into your normal exercise routine or activity, see if it should be adjusted to gradually train the area that was injured. In this way, the injured area will be better prepared for stresses that might have been the original cause of injury. Above all, do not push too hard too soon.

ISOMETRICS AND ISOTONICS

Isometric exercises require no equipment or special location. They are a start for the reluctant fitness beginner, good for recuperating patients, and a wise measure for any athlete who finds him- or herself chairbound for any length of time at work or traveling.

In contrast to the high degree of movement seen in most exercise, isometrics strengthen and shape muscles by pitting them against one another or against an object such as a chair or table. In this way, they are a specialized and very simple form of resistance exercise. The word *isometric* comes from the Greek for "equal measure." In isometrics, muscles match resisting forces without movement. The idea is to exactly meet the resisting force, not to overcome it. An example would be to press your hands palm down on a desktop and hold for 5 seconds or to hold your head straight for the same amount of time against the light pressure of two fingers on your forehead.

A full isometric program would be a series of exercises, each repeated five times as part of a series working down from head to toe and the series repeated five times a day. Lighter isometric workloads can be devised to suit or used as a highly constructive form of fidgeting and stretching whenever the need arises and movement exercise is impossible. An excellent guide to isometric exercises can be found in *The Lazy Person's Guide to Fitness* by Charles Swencionis (St. Martin's Press, 1996).

Isotonics ask muscles to produce movement and overcome forces by lifting loads, such as wrist or belt weights. Like isometrics, isotonics are a simple form of resistance training. As with isometrics, cardiovascular benefits are minimal, but muscles will increase in endurance as well as strength.

ENLIGHTENED EXERCISE: FITNESS FROM THE EAST

Stress relief is often a natural result of a fitness program. It makes sense, however, particularly for the competitive athlete, to consciously build in stress-relieving workouts that also tone the body, and none are better suited than those from the ancient East. There are aerobic benefits, too, since there is so much emphasis on breathing techniques.

Yoga

Yoga strengthens the spine, increases flexibility, tones flabby muscles, and helps increase their endurance characteristics. The exercises themselves are designed to rest rather than exhaust the body, with yoga moves increasing in difficulty for more advanced fitness goals.

Yoga addresses posture, mental attitude and focus, and diet and is one of the most popular tension-lifting activities in the world. It can be either very gentle or very vigorous and demanding, depending on the instructor and the student. Yoga classes are very common throughout North America these days. Just check the yellow pages of your phone book or call your local hospital; many of them sponsor yoga classes.

Chi Gong

Agility, balance, and coordination combined with mental and emotional focus are the main elements of this Eastern art. There are dozens of types of chi gong, of which tai chi is the best known. Some are used for specific purposes, such as curing illness or healing specific parts of the body. *Chi* means "life energy," and chi gong moves are designed to balance the flow of chi around the body.

Chi gong uses a series of movements, either predetermined or spontaneous, to achieve balance, coordination, and mental and physical fitness. It looks like a series of graceful movements performed in slow motion, but there is much going on mentally as well (or little, an equal discipline).

In China and other Asian countries, people commonly begin their day with a chi gong routine in a public park or on the factory floor. It stretches muscles, stimulates the lymphatic system, improves circulation, and exercises muscles. The result is relaxation as well as enhanced flexibility, balance, and overall health.

11 BEAUTIFUL SKIN, HAIR, AND NAILS ∾

GETTING UNDER YOUR SKIN

Think of chapped lips, skinned knees, scalds, and burns. The memories can make us wince. Think, too, though, of stroking, the warmth of sunlight, and kissing. It is through our skin that we experience all these things, painful or pleasing. Skin, living and breathing between the worlds inside and outside our body, is messenger to them both. It's minus 5 degrees and hailstones are pelting, or the cat, soft and heavy on our lap, needs a claw trim: Our skin can tell you both. When our nose turns blue with cold or we feel a stinging sensation, our skin is letting us know that our body reacts to these things. Our skin relays the changes, external or internal, and responses are triggered that restore the balance. We wrap a scarf around our face, rub on the lip balm, put the cat out, and find an antiseptic lotion. This kind of basic functioning is easy to take for granted, and it is usually issues of health and appearance that bring skin more fully to our attention.

Have you ever worried about a friend looking pale and ragged, with dark rims and bags beneath the eyes? Or perhaps you've comforted a feverish child, cooling the child's reddened cheeks and forehead? We instinctively recognize that skin condition is a sign of general state of health. Because skin is linked to so many bodily functions, from blood circulation to excretion, it's no wonder that it can be a very clear indicator when things go wrong internally. Observing skin symptoms is sometimes the first step leading to treatment of major underlying conditions.

Of course, as a physical container and protector of flesh and blood, skin can have its own problems, too. Then the body has the skin repaired: Cuts are plugged, scabs are formed, and splinters and living invaders like bacteria are engulfed by extra blood flow, bombarding the site of injury with white blood cells and nutrients.

Technology may advance, and fashions may change, but human fascination for skin and its appearance is constant. Ancient Britons used a blue dye from the woad plant as horrifying war paint; empresses are said to have bathed in asses' milk; European ladies and gentlemen of the eighteenth century powdered and rouged their faces; skin tattoos are popular the world over; plastic surgery is now big business; and modern skin grafts are grown in lab dishes. This is not surprising, considering that looks are tied to emotions and sexual attraction. We go pale with shock and red with rage, and we blush with embarrassment. Such indicators of emotional state combined with clues to health mean that skin becomes a physical factor in our relationships and also in the selection of a mate. In sex itself, skin plays a role, conveying and expressing the physical signals that lead to arousal. In fact, skin is easily the organ with which we are most intimately acquainted.

Our language ties qualities and values of skin to character traits and emotional reactions. We might refer to someone as "thick skinned" or "thin skinned," or someone might get "under your skin." If something is of no consequence, you can say that it's "no skin off my nose" or you might "scrape through" a serious situation and "save your skin." Recognition of the importance of skin is built into our everyday lives. Often, however, our understanding and appreciation of its true work and nature are only "skin deep."

Applying in-depth knowledge of skin functions can lead not only to improving its condition and appearance but also to overall well-being. Surface

267

effects are resolved as deeper causes are addressed. In this way, healthy nutrition is a major factor in promoting healthy skin—a case of treatment from the inside producing real benefit on the outside. The scope and details of how this is achieved may vary, but with skin, looking good usually means feeling good, too.

Skin Facts

- Dermatologists estimate that the skin of an adult weighs about 8 pounds and measures about 20 square feet when stretched out.
- The eyelids are covered by skin at its thinnest—only about ⅕ of an inch.
- Skin can be around ⅛-inch-thick at sites like the soles of the feet.
- We shed around 40 pounds of skin over a lifetime.
- Men really *are* thicker-skinned than women!

Your Skin from the Outside In

Nothing beats skin when it comes to waterproof protection for your entire body. This function alone and the fact that it is a differentiated body part would qualify skin as an organ. Yet its intricate structure performs many tasks. Skin has two main layers, an outer band called the epidermis and an inner layer that is about four times thicker and known as the dermis.

The epidermis itself consists of three sublayers. The topmost consists of scaly, dead cells, rich in protective keratin. Dead cells are shed constantly and are actually the major component of household dust. Newly generated cells move toward the surface, constantly replenished from the deepest layer of the epidermis called the basal layer. The basal layer also contains the pigment, or melanin, that gives skin its color.

New skin lies over the dermis, the skin's inner supportive layer. The dermis anchors blood vessels, sweat glands, sense receptor cells, hair follicles, and oil-producing sebaceous glands. Sebaceous glands open out onto hair follicles, while sweat glands release their fluids through other holes in the skin known as pores. Beneath the dermis is a final layer called the subcutis, which is an insulating layer of fat.

Collagen Is Your Skin Glue

Something has to bind all the structures of skin together, and this is done by a tough protein called collagen. Collagen is a major component of connective tissue, which is found wherever different tissues and body parts need to be bound. This protein is produced by cells in the connective tissue called fibroblasts. Collagen is formed in fibers that configure themselves in various ways, such as bundles ideal for the twisting and flexing of tendons joining muscle and bone. In skin, collagen fibers lie in a flat, crisscross position.

Collagen is the most abundant protein in the body. It is high in silicon, a mineral that forms long, complex molecules, suitable for parts of the body that need to be strong and flexible. Collagen works with fibers of another protein called elastin, which, as its name suggests, gives skin its elasticity. The two types of fiber together bring resilience and skin tone. Unfortunately, many people seem to produce less of these proteins as they get older, and factors such as sun and smoking contribute to their destruction. The result is aged skin, the target of numerous marketing campaigns for antiaging cosmetics.

Some dermatologists recommend collagen injections for minimizing wrinkles and scars, and collagen-boosted lips have been acquired by some rich and famous women. Injected collagen is broken down by enzymes in about two years. Money spent on cosmetics with added collagen is also misguided, since skin cannot absorb the protein. Nutritional support of our body's own collagen is a much more sound approach, and it can be delicious, too. Copper, found in dark leafy vegetables, shellfish, and whole grains, and vitamin C, abundant in fruits and vegetables, are both required for the production of collagen. Iron is needed, too, and is found in organ meats, poultry, fish, and parsley. In addition, research from the 1980s shows that bioflavonoids, particularly PCOs, the powerful antioxidants, are very effective in stabilizing collagen structures.

Skin Is Your Body's First Line of Defense

It's true, microorganisms are crawling all over us, new ones arriving every second! But thanks to our trusty skin, very few penetrate to levels where they can do any harm. Germs from public contact are held off by healthy, intact skin. Bugs for illnesses such as colds and flu can only do their work if transferred to sites like our eyes and nose. Skin also filters the sun's rays and keeps out water and toxic substances. A more sophisticated barrier could not be invented.

Yet, besides its physical blocking qualities, skin forms an essential part of the immune system. In healthy people, the mildly acidic film of oil and sweat that coats the skin is itself slightly harmful to bacteria and fungus. Internally, many special cells called Langerhans' cells are sprinkled throughout the skin. The job of these cells is to catch viruses and bacteria and hand them over to white blood cells called T cells. Recent research shows that Langerhans' cells also interact with lymphatic fluid, or lymph, the clear watery fluid that transports white blood cells and other vital substances to blood and tissues.

New discoveries also show that a fascinating range of immune-related substances, such as growth factors, are produced by the cells lining the tiny blood vessels in the dermis. The interaction of all these agents has been observed to trigger complex signals and responses that provide protection against infections, abnormal tissue growth, and external environmental toxins. As studies continue, it may be revealed that conditions like psoriasis may in fact lie in the skin's immune system turning against itself.

Why Skin Is Your Number Two Detoxifier

The skin has been called a second kidney, as its millions of sweat glands excrete many substances that are toxic to the body. With vigorous exercise and high temperatures, our sweat output increases from an average of about a pint a day to around 8 quarts. It's no wonder saunas have become part of detoxification programs.

There are two types of sweat glands. Eccrine glands eliminate mostly water and excess mineral salts, including sodium chloride, which is why sweat tastes salty. These sweat glands work hardest with exercise, high temperature, or stress. Apocrine sweat glands are found in the genital region and armpits. They excrete nitrogen-containing wastes, as well as water and salts, through the pores of our skin. Apocrine glands are the ones to blame for body odor. The sweat from these glands creates body odor when mixed with bacteria and is produced at times of stress.

Poor diet can be a contributory factor in sweat glands becoming overproductive and clogged up. Sweat itself can become laden with material delicious to bacteria. Good nutrition helps the skin carry out its detoxification role and keeps down the levels of toxins it has to deal with.

Skin, Source of Natural Toner and Conditioner

You may have watched birds preening their feathers, spreading natural oils along the shafts and hairs to keep them waterproof and deter pests. When we brush our hair, we are doing the same thing. Our sebaceous glands produce a waterproof skin oil called sebum that is released along the hair shafts. The highest concentration of sebaceous glands is on the face, followed by the back, chest, and shoulders, which is why these are the major sites for acne.

Sebum helps protect hair and keep it glossy while also preventing damage to skin from such factors as wind and dust. Sebum also lubricates the skin and prevents the loss of too much water. When skin retains the right amount of water, this helps it to stay supple. Most simple moisturizers work by supplementing the effect of sebum, sealing in the water content of skin and preventing its evaporation. Beware of too much washing or harsh cleansers, as these can strip away sebum, leaving the skin open to infection as well as dryness.

COMMON SKIN PROBLEMS

So many mechanisms are active in skin that it's easy to understand how their breakdown can result in numerous health conditions. Given the importance we attach to our skin's appearance, it's also not hard to understand that skin problems often cause considerable distress, even when the associated discomfort is not great. The psychological relief gained from solving a skin problem is real and valid. The key is not to be pushed into harsh and desperate measures by the strong emotional drive to find solutions to conditions like acne. There are many gentle, natural remedies and supplements that help bring the chemistry of the skin back into balance. Try these first and aim at a lifestyle without emotional roller coasters and low in stress—your skin reflects both!

Skin Types

What skin type are you? Although you are born with certain basic tendencies, your answer may change throughout your life. Skin is in constant renewal, responding to internal and external influences. Aging may bring drying and thinning as your skin functions slow down. An extreme climate and indoor heating can also dry out your skin. Dietary changes can bring vitamin and mineral deficiencies and sensitivities. Hormone changes, from puberty and pregnancy to menopause, can also affect skin condition. Normal skin is skin that is in balance—smooth, "plump," soft, and blemish free. Fresh, even tone goes along with small to medium pores.

Sensitive skin is delicate, easily irritated by external agents. This skin type is typical of blondes with blue eyes and also redheads. Prone to rashing and stinging, this sort of skin also burns easily in the sun.

Blemished skin is typical of teenagers and is characterized by an overproduction of oil. In later life, contributory factors can include diet, stress, poor elimination, intestinal flora that is out of balance, environmental conditions, allergies, and cosmetics.

Fair-skinned people are prone to dry skin, which involves an underproduction of oil. If skin is thick but pores are visible, water is called for. If skin is fine with barely visible pores, oil, and possibly water, is lacking. Dry skin can be rough and scaly, too, without any shine.

Oily skin is often thicker than other types and has medium to large pores and a shiny appearance. A disadvantage is a tendency to clogged pores. Olive skin is typically quite oily, enjoying the benefits of youthful appearance and less vulnerability to environmental damage.

Combination skin can see a mixture of oily and dry characteristics on the face. Often the forehead, nose, and chin are greasy, while the cheeks and eyes are dry.

Your skin care regimen may change as you add supplements, change your diet, and increase sun and cold protection. Simple observation will tell you when to put away or take out the astringents or moisturizers. Keep in mind that skin condition is the result of many different processes. If you are not troubled by a specific skin problem, it's a good idea to use the supplements and dietary changes recommended generally for healthy, youthful-looking skin. Bringing the functions of your skin back into balance will often result in a skin type closer to ideal.

Acne

Acne is the most common skin problem. Psychologically, acne can be a real downer, often striking teenagers who are already going through emotional turmoil at puberty. Its main features are blackheads, whiteheads, pustules, inflamed red bumps called nodules or papules, and cysts under the skin surface. Scarring can occur when nodules break down the surrounding tissue; it can also be the result of damage done by tampering fingers. Acne breaks out mostly on the face but also frequently on the back, chest, and shoulders.

Acne sites, the most dense locations of sebaceous glands, give a clue to the nature of the condition, which involves overproduction of sebum. Male sex hormones (androgens) such as testosterone stimulate the production of keratin and sebum. They also enlarge sebaceous glands. Levels of these hormones increase in puberty in both boys and girls and are higher in males, which is why acne afflicts mainly teenagers and is most common in males.

Research shows that higher blood levels of testosterone do not always lead to more severe outbreaks. The underlying factor may instead be increased activity, seen in the skin of acne patients, of an enzyme that changes normal testosterone into a more powerful form. Bacterial balance also seems to be very important, with one study revealing increased blood levels of toxins absorbed from the intestines in people with bad acne. This results in more inflammation and tissue destruction because it disturbs the ratio of copper to zinc. Makeup, drugs, and pollutants also aggravate acne.

Although the condition is complicated, a thorough understanding actually opens more doors to the treatment of acne. Nutrition, as always, is important. Although diet, including items like chocolate and fried food, is not a direct cause of acne, sticking to a diet low in fat, sugar, and refined carbohydrates such as cookies and cakes will greatly ease the body's toxic load. Stick to unrefined whole foods and high levels of vitamin-rich vegetables and fruit. Avoid milk, too, as it is frequently high in hormones. Steer clear of iodine, as it can worsen acne. These measures boost the body's ability to fight the bacterial infection and repair skin tissue. Herbal remedies make effective topical treatments:

- Lavender or calendula. Cleanse with rinses made from extracts of the essential oils of these plants.
- Tea tree oil. Apply this essential oil to inflamed areas, as this herb has proven as effective, without the side effects, as benzoyl peroxide.

For further recommendations on lotions, see the section "Natural Preparations for Beautiful Skin," page 284.

Supplements for Acne

No matter how many creams or lotions you slather on, skin won't be at its best without proper nourishment from the inside out. Try these nutrients to promote clear, glowing, blemish-free skin:

- Beta-carotene, 25,000 IU daily to help boost skin immune functions and increase skin tone
- B-complex stress formula, 100 mg daily after eating. The stress formula is recommended, as it includes extra amounts of B_6 and B_5. Vitamin B_6 is particularly helpful to women with premenstrual worsening of acne, as it plays a role in steroid hormone metabolism. A deficiency is itself associated with red and greasy skin. B_5 boosts the adrenal glands and helps to lessen psychological stress.

- Vitamin C, 1,000–3,000 mg daily, the dose spread throughout the day, to boost the immune system
- Vitamin E (dry form), 400 IU, and selenium, 100 mcg, once a day. These are antioxidants working in partnership with zinc and vitamin A. A brazil nut daily is a good source of selenium.
- Zinc, 15 mg daily between meals and apart from other supplements. Do not exceed 30 mg daily, as larger doses can depress the immune system. Low levels of zinc are typical for thirteen- and fourteen-year-old boys and are associated generally with the change of testosterone to its more active form.
- Black currant oil, 1,000–2,000 mg daily, as a supply of essential fatty acids (EFAs) hard to come by in food but required for healthy skin function
- L-cysteine, 500 mg daily with vitamin C, half an hour before meals. This amino acid is a powerful detoxifier and immune system booster.
- Herbal infusions, such as red clover, dandelion, and burdock root. Red clover boosts the immune system, while dandelion is a good source of vitamin A, a known skin healer. Burdock and dandelion both cleanse tissue, working against acne-promoting microbes and the damage they do.

It can take up to twelve weeks to really bring acne under control, although some sufferers find that relief comes quickly. Patience and consistency with a whole-food diet and supplements bring a safer and more thorough remedy than resorting to long-term doses of antibiotics or treatment with vitamin A–based medicines that deplete the body and can lead to toxic side effects. Echinacea, taken internally two weeks on and two weeks off, also helps fight infection. Persistence and a hands-off policy really pay off with acne.

Body Odor

Body odor is produced when sweat from the apocrine sweat glands is broken down by bacteria. Armpits get particularly odoriferous because they, as well as the genital region, are where apocrine glands are found. Antiperspirants work by inhibiting the action of the glands. Most commercial products do this with harmful ingredients like aluminum salts or dyes and are best avoided. America has seen at least eight common ingredients of deodorants and antiperspirants withdrawn in recent years because of health risks. Deodorants usually mask or partly neutralize the offending smells.

Natural ways to reduce the amount of armpit bacteria include:

- Splashing with rubbing alcohol or the most gentle witch hazel
- Herbal antiperspirants with antibacterial ingredients, such as extract of green tea

Supplements that help keep body odor under control include:

- Vitamin B complex, 100 mg daily
- Zinc, 15 mg daily
- Acidophilus, as per directions on container, to keep intestinal toxins down
- Chlorophyll tablets or capsules, one tablet or capsule three times daily, to help control intestinal bacteria

Cutting down on coffee is an additional measure that can help with body odor. If body odor is serious, chronic, and does not resolve using the suggestions given here combined with a good, whole-food diet, get a medical checkup, as an underlying cause may indicate a more serious illness.

Burns

Immediate immersion in ice water for 5 to 10 minutes, with brief breaks, is the best treatment for burns. Head for the hospital in the case of severe burns. In minor cases, after ice water immersion, apply an ice pack intermittently over 24 hours to maintain a low temperature. The cold reduces blood flow, helps prevent leakage of fluid from injured tissues, and lessens pain. Natural topical treatments for burns include:

- Vitamin E. Apply the oil to help reduce scar formation.

- Aloe vera. Apply directly from a cut split leaf. This herb is very soothing and cooling. It is also packed with skin-healing agents.
- Calendula tincture/ointment. Apply to the burn for pain relief and antibacterial and antiseptic action.
- Arnica tincture. Apply directly or in a compress to *unbroken* skin in cases of burns and stings. Arnica is a natural pain reliever.
- Raw honey. Apply to the site. This burn therapy is being used in China and gaining much attention from Western doctors. Honey is antiseptic, soothing, and healing.
- Ginger. Mash the root, soak up the juice with a cotton ball, and apply to the burn to relieve pain.

To speed the process of recovery from burns, the following supplements are useful:

- Beta-carotene, 25,000 IU daily, for immune stimulation and tissue restoration
- Vitamin B complex, 100 mg daily (PABA, or para-aminobenzoic acid, in particular, can reduce the pain of burns.)
- Vitamin C with bioflavonoids, 1,000 mg three times daily, to help new tissue growth and help prevent infection
- Vitamin E, 1,000 IU daily, to promote healing and lessen scarring
- Zinc, chelated or picolinate, 50 mg daily, apart from other supplements, to stimulate wound healing

Victims of serious burns may have a fortunate encounter with a paramedic team equipped with a new product developed in Australia called Water-Jel. A thick, slimy mixture of plant extracts, including eucalyptus oil, it fights infection and is applied in sterile dressing. It is also water-soluble, which helps in the cleaning of wounds. Its main use is in products like fire protection blankets, since it resists temperatures of up to 2,000 degrees Fahrenheit—a staggering example of the potential of natural substances.

Cellulite

Cellulite is not a disease as such. It is a poor skin condition, unwanted due to its unsightly appearance.

When skin affected by cellulite is pinched, it bulges and pits in what is known as the mattress phenomenon. Cellulite becomes a problem when the bulging and pitting are evident without a pinch test when the person is standing or even lying down.

More than 90 percent of cellulite is seen in women. In men, cellulite can be a sign of a deficiency in certain hormones. Female skin is structurally different: The fat cells underlying the skin are larger, more plentiful, and arranged vertically rather than horizontally. The second layer of skin, the dermis, is thinner in females. These facts matter because cellulite is the result of excessive fat cells and a deterioration in the connective tissue made up of collagen and elastin, which bind the layers of our skin together. How many fat cells we have is largely determined by what our mothers ate when we were in the womb!

One of the best ways to prevent cellulite is to keep only a thin layer of fat under our skin. Gentle weight reduction (gentle to avoid stressing connective tissue even more, which would worsen cellulite) and exercise can help lessen the condition. We can also do something about the state of the tissue. Lack of vitamins and minerals, aging, and too much sun are all factors that cause connective tissue to weaken and the dermis to thin. Without strong boundaries in place, fat cells can move up into the dermis, causing the skin to deform. In fact, cellulite develops mostly on the parts of the body that show weight gain (increased fat) first, like thighs and buttocks.

To tackle cellulite, try the suggestions for improving varicose veins (page 278), watch the weight, and exercise. Massaging affected areas helps by stimulating blood circulation and smoothing disrupted skin structure. Work from the outside in toward the heart. Look for creams containing the plant bladder wrack for its soothing, softening, and toning effects. Steer clear of fats and refined carbohydrates, and try these supplements, which, unlike many, have confirmed beneficial effects on cellulite:

- Cola vera cream. Apply to affected areas for a caffeine-induced breakdown of fats that will help improve the skin structure.

- *Centella asiatica*, 30 mg three times a day. This will stimulate the growth of stable connective tissue and blood flow.
- Horse chestnut *(Aesculus hippocastanum)* in two forms—aescin, 10 mg three times a day, and the bark of the root, 500 mg three times a day. These compounds are anti-inflammatory, build up the strength of blood vessels in the skin, and tone the blood.
- Glucosamine sulfate or glucosamine/ mucopolysaccharide complex, 1,000 mg daily

Cuts, Scrapes, and Other Wounds

Always follow first-aid procedures when skin is damaged, and visit the emergency room if in doubt. Once general health and safety is assured, there are several herbal remedies for use on the spot, *externally only* unless otherwise specified:

- Aloe vera. Apply gel directly from split leaf to cuts and scrapes. Aloe contains astringent and antiseptic agents among others necessary for wound healing. Its polysaccharides are thought to lie behind its ability to stimulate growth and repair of the outer layer of the skin.
- Calendula tincture/ointment. Bathe cuts and stings with tincture, or apply the ointment for pain relief and faster healing through its antiseptic and antibacterial action.
- Echinacea tincture. Apply tincture to insect bites and take one dropperful in water. This herb is an effective immune booster with a traditional use in America as a snakebite treatment. It also helps to prevent destruction of a natural barrier between harmful agents and healthy cells.
- Gotu kola tincture. Apply to cuts to set in action a powerful combination of wound-healing compounds used successfully in many clinical studies, especially with surgical incisions. Gotu kola was even used in India and Indonesia to relieve leprosy.

If a wound is dry, a cream or ointment is usually best, whereas a lotion of liquid is called for if the wound is oozing.

Once first aid has been completed, a healthy diet and supplements are a big help in healing skin. These three nutrients are key:

- Vitamin C with bioflavonoids, 1,000 mg twice daily
- Vitamin E (dry form), 400 IU daily
- Zinc, 15 mg daily

These can be taken together, but apart from other supplements to avoid interfering with absorption of other nutrients. All three aid tissue repair. The vitamins work together and are both excellent antioxidants, helping to keep toxins at bay. Vitamin C is essential for tissue growth and repair as well as for fighting infections, and vitamin E and zinc are both wound healers. Recent studies have shown that another supplement, vitamin K, is useful in reducing bruising. It encourages leaky blood vessels to heal faster and is now available in cream form.

Once again, a good healthy diet is called for, as recognized by doctors of the American Academy of Cosmetic Surgery, who recently reported that even mild malnutrition can delay healing and increase scarring.

Dry Skin

Sun, wind, soaps, cosmetics, medications—all causes of dry skin, right? True, but they all do damage in basically the same way. Our skin's natural lubricator and water conserver is sebum, the oil produced by sebaceous glands. External agents wear away this vital substance. In addition, our skin tends to produce less sebum with age. Sebum production declines in most people as early as their twenties. Less sebum means less moisture retention, which leads to dry skin with its typical features of stiffness, scaliness, and flakiness. Some people have a genetic low-oil tendency leading to dry skin, which often carries the advantage of fine texture and clear complexion. Naturally dry skin, however, tends to develop wrinkles and lines earlier than other skin types.

Skin in general will also sacrifice its need for water, as the major organs have first call on supplies. In this way, simple dehydration rather than lack of oil can also cause dry skin. Poor digestion of fats and oils or a simple lack of essential fatty acids will also contribute to dry skin, which can be tackled with dietary adjustment and supplements. Always seek medical attention for severe, chronic dry skin that does not respond to dietary and topical remedies. Occasionally, a more serious condition, such as thyroid malfunction, is an underlying cause.

Preventing Dry Skin

Usually, you can prevent dry skin, technically known as xerosis, by preserving your skin's natural oil with these simple steps:

- Don't bathe or wash too often, and avoid very hot water, which can lead to the release of inflammatory substances in the skin, promoting dryness and soreness. Sponge-bathe odor-producing areas between less frequent baths or showers. Wash your face with a gentle cleanser at night, but only splash with cool water in the morning. This way, you encourage your skin's repair work, out of the sun and wind, at night.
- Avoid long soaks in hot tubs. Hot water can irritate skin, and we've all seen shriveled, prune-like skin from staying in the bath. This wrinkly effect is caused, ironically, by dehydration—the worst thing for dry skin.
- Do not scrub or rub. Scrubbing removes the skin's protective layers, and rubbing can irritate dry skin. Avoid washcloths, and always pat your skin dry.
- Always rinse well, especially your face. It is important to remove all soapy residues, as these can leave a drying film on your skin.
- Avoid astringents and product ingredients that dehydrate the skin. Examples are talc and alcohol. There are now alcohol-free aftershave lotions for men.
- Use mild, herbal cleansers. Strong soaps and lotions, especially ones containing deodorants, actually strip away sebum. Lavender and chamomile, used for centuries in herbal baths, are soothing and antibacterial. Comfrey in particular helps skin to rejuvenate.

Moisturizers

As well as preserving sebum, you can support its action by applying moisturizers. It's important to find one that is allergen free. If you are prone to allergies, be wary of lanolin, an oil from sheep's wool that is known to cause reactions in some people. Test the moisturizer on a small portion of your skin before using it generally.

The most common moisturizers are emollients—softening, soothing agents that usually contain fat. These work like sebum in that they seal in water already in the skin.

Other moisturizers contain humectants, substances that attract and hold water. Sodium hyaluronate (hyaluronic acid) is a humectant that can bind up to a thousand times its own weight in water. Another good humectant ingredient to look for is known as NAPCA. Our skin has its own moisturizers of this type, but because of slowing cellular processes, these moisturizers are frequently not produced in great enough number to prevent dryness.

Various claims are made for creams loaded with much-hyped ingredients, from liposomes to amino acids. Ingredients like alpha-hydroxy acids (AHAs) are now being touted as valuable additions to moisturizers. Research published in *Cosmetics and Toiletries Magazine* shows that AHAs are not in fact particularly useful for skin hydration.

The most effective ingredients are not necessarily the most expensive. So before you hit your pocketbook hard, try these proven natural remedies, and remember—moisturizers work best when applied to damp skin:

- Vitamin E, borage, black currant, flaxseed, and evening primrose oils can work wonders as natural oils that moisturize and supply the skin with nutrients.
- Egg-rich mayonnaise is a very good dry skin moisturizer.
- For really parched skin, mix up a moisturizing mask, using an egg yolk whisked with 1 teaspoon of canola or sesame oil and 1 tablespoon of honey. Ripe avocado also makes a beneficial mask. It can be mashed with egg yolk or an equal amount of sour cream or ripe banana.

Nutrition and Supplements to Treat Dry Skin

Working from the inside to maintain your skin's natural protective coating is just as important as topical treatments. There is just no substitute for a nutritious whole-food diet, high in grains, fruit, and vegetables. And keep hydrated! Aim at about eight glasses of unpolluted water a day, including herbal teas. In today's fast-paced, high-stress world, supplements like the following are also helpful in treating dry skin:

- B complex, 100 mg daily after any meal. Deficiencies of vitamins B_1 or B_2, pantothenic acid, or biotin can lead to dry skin problems and scaliness around the mouth and nose.
- Beta-carotene, 25,000 IU daily, split between breakfast and after dinner. Your body makes vitamin A from beta-carotene without the risk of toxic overdoses. The benefits include soft, smooth, and disease-free skin (a deficiency can itself produce dry, scaly skin).
- Vitamin C with bioflavonoids, 1,000 mg two to three times daily after meals and at bedtime. This vitamin is always a good idea, as it is required for tissue growth and repair.
- Vitamin E (dry form), 400 IU, one to two times daily after meals. This supplement helps to replace cells on the skin's outer layer and works with vitamin C.
- Black currant oil, 1,000–2,000 mg daily for essential fatty acids that promote good skin condition
- Zinc, 15 mg daily taken between meals and apart from other supplements, to aid skin tissue growth and repair. Zinc deficiency itself can cause dry skin with a rough, scaly appearance. Excessive sweating can result in a loss of as much as 3 mg of zinc a day.
- Glucosamine sulfate or glucosamine/ mucopolysaccharide complex, 1,000 mg daily

Black currant oil, beta-carotene, and zinc are probably the three most effective supplements for dry skin. It is also wise to consume plenty of omega-3 fatty acids by eating fatty fish. With good nutrition and cleansing under way, don't forget that you still need to protect your skin from drying out as a result of the elements—so wear those gloves and scarves in wind and cold, and use sunscreen on bright days. Check out the section on winter sun for some tips on dry skin.

Itches, Rashes, and Allergies

A rash is the appearance of skin irritation in the form of redness and blisters. Many rashes itch as the skin gives its lowest pain signal. The instinctive response of scratching increases blood flow to the region. This can be beneficial, although it also sometimes spreads rashes. Some scientists believe that scratching produces a stronger nerve signal, which serves to drown out the original, more distracting itch. Rashes and itching are common symptoms of allergies. When the body responds to a substance that is normally harmless, skin cells release histamines, which make fluid leak from tiny blood vessels into skin tissue. This is called an allergic reaction and in turn causes swelling, rashes, and itching. Supplementation, topical treatments, and dietary changes are used to bring the body's immune system back into balance or simply to calm symptoms like inflammation and itching.

Dermatitis, Eczema, and Hives

Dermatitis is inflammation of the skin. It has many causes. Hives, inflamed weals, or welts are an allergic reaction, lasting a few hours or days, to things like sun, shellfish, or berries. Hives are much less serious than eczema, which is a chronic inflammation of the skin, named from the Greek word for "to boil out." Itching, redness, small blisters, weeping, and swelling are all features of eczema. Crustiness, scaliness, and thickening follow. Eczema is the end result of many internal reactions to allergens. Children and young adults are most affected by eczema as a chronic condition, also known as atopic dermatitis, which is thought to be due to inherited hypersensitivities.

The results of a study in recent years at the Middlesex Hospital in London led researchers to conclude that excluding certain foods from the diet would alleviate moderate to severe cases of eczema in children. If eliminating cow's milk, eggs, tomatoes, artificial colors, and food preservatives doesn't do the trick, look for another frequently eaten food to cross off.

Another study of atopic dermatitis at the University of California at San Francisco showed that sufferers can be helped by taking extra vitamin C. Patients taking the supplement for three months saw the number and severity of symptoms, as well as infections, reduced. If you have eczema, be sure to eat those fruits and vegetables!

Sensitivities—From Plants to Antiperspirants

Eczemalike rashes are seen in cases of poison ivy, poison oak, and reactions to other plants as well as to things like solvents, nickel, lanolin, antiperspirants, and soaps, which can all be allergens. These kinds of reactions are known as contact dermatitis. They are caused by sensitivities and are not true allergies. Stress, heat, soaps, scratching, and rubbing can worsen rashes. Diet, especially milk, can play a role, particularly with children. Always avoid an allergen once it is identified. Plant oils, in particular, are very long lasting. Contact with plant oils brushed onto clothing, tools, and so on, will cause further reactions, so be sure to thoroughly wash any items possibly contaminated. Nickel jewelry can be varnished with clear nail polish, or the skin under watches or bracelets can be dusted with talc to lessen contact. Always ensure that ear piercing is done with stainless steel needles.

Bringing Relief from Itches, Rashes, and Allergies

When it comes to treatment of severe rashes, steroid creams and oral antihistamines are often administered and do bring relief. However, they do not address underlying causes and do create side effects. They are for short-term use only. Herbal treatments, supplements, and dietary adjustments are much safer and gentler. For topical relief try these:

- Zinc ointment (nonoily). Apply to the skin three times daily.
- Aloe vera. Apply gel from leaf to skin to cool, soothe, and aid healing.

- Herbal ointment containing licorice or German chamomile for their anti-inflammatory, corti- sonelike actions.
- Herbal baths of chamomile, lavender, and even oatmeal are all soothing and healing.
- Mugwort plant for poison oak prevention and relief. After washing off the affected area (if pos- sible), rub leaves on skin as soon as possible after contact. Steep fresh leaves in just-boiled water for 10 to 15 minutes. While the remedy is brew- ing, take a shower, followed by a 10-minute soak in a bath containing the mugwort infusion. Avoid contacting clothes as much as possible while removing them, and place them directly where they can be washed separately from other items.

For internal support, the following supplements can be taken:

- Vitamin B complex, stress combination, with breakfast and dinner
- Pantothenic acid (vitamin B₅), 500 mg one to two times daily to support the body's anti- inflammatory actions launched by the adrenal glands
- Vitamin C, 500 mg four times a day as a natural antihistamine and also because histamines destroy vitamin C

For severe rashes and eczema in particular, the preceding and following supplements are useful:

- Beta-carotene, 25,000 IU daily, for up to a month for skin repair, reducing to 15,000 IU for maintenance
- Bioflavonoids, 500 mg daily as antioxidant support
- Vitamin E (dry form), 400 IU daily, as a skin repairer and anti-inflammatory
- Zinc, 15 mg daily, for tissue repair
- Evening primrose oil, 1,000–3,000 mg daily
- Herbal infusions of yellow dock, burdock, red clover, figwort, fumitory, heartsease, or echi- nacea (purple coneflower) all help to nourish and cool the blood and skin. Borage and licorice aid the adrenal glands.

Oil of evening primrose is recommended for eczema sufferers, as they appear to be low on essential fatty acids, which are needed for the body's anti- inflammatory mechanisms. Omega-3 oils also supply fatty acids, and a diet rich in foods like mackerel, her- ring, and salmon as well as nuts and seeds is a good idea for anyone prone to rashes, allergies, and itching.

Liver Spots

Often confused with age spots, liver spots are yellow, brown, or black flat frecklelike marks on the skin, most prevalent in elderly people, although they also frequently appear around age forty. Age spots look similar but have irregular surfaces and look "pasted on." They are thickened areas of skin involving seba- ceous glands, which means that they arise on the face, neck, chest, or upper back. Age spots often itch and are usually harmless, although they are removed by doctors, since they can be precancerous.

A true liver spot is called an *actinic lentigo*, from the Latin for "ray" and "lentil"—in other words, a spot, small and round like a lentil, caused by too much exposure to the sun's rays. They can actually be up to an inch in diameter and do sometimes resemble liver in color and shape. Liver spots are seen mostly on the face or the back of the hands. They involve irregular- ities of the skin's pigment, melanin. The coloration of a liver spot goes deeper than a freckle.

Although liver spots are not usually a sign of dis- ease, seek medical advice if any begin to change in any way. Research is ongoing into drugs that may lighten or remove liver spots, since many people feel they are unsightly. You might have heard of Retin-A or Tretinoin, brand names for retinoic acid. This drug is a vitamin A derivative much hyped in the 1980s. In fact, although there are positive results in studies with creams containing this drug, improvement tends to be modest and brings the risks of an increased tendency to sunburn, dryness, acne flare-ups, and irritated skin.

If you find liver spots hard to live with, remem- ber that they are a useful warning of too much sun. Eat a carrot a day or take a beta-carotene supplement to help your body produce its own vitamin A, and follow the advice for keeping your skin healthy in the sun. Avoiding excessive sun exposure is the best treat- ment of all, according to the American Academy of Dermatology.

Varicose Veins

When the delicate walls of veins are damaged, the veins widen and the valves inside them become faulty. Veins then become varicose—that is, twisted as well as further widened. As well as being unsightly when they show through the skin, varicose veins can be accompanied by fatigue, aching, and a feeling of heaviness. They are seen mostly on the legs, affecting almost half of middle-aged adults and four times more women than men. Pregnancy is a major cause of varicose veins, due to increased pressure in the veins of the legs. The condition is serious when it affects veins deep in the leg, bringing risks of clotting, heart attacks, and strokes.

Genetic weakness of valves is thought to contribute to varicose veins, but there are also theories concerning various factors that may cause the walls of the veins to become weakened. Keeping the skin conditioned is important, since skin helps to support and anchor many veins. Take note that the condition is rare in areas of the world where whole-food, high-fiber diets are the norm. Use the effective herbal remedies proven to relieve cellulite, as these also work well on varicose veins. The following steps will help you keep your venous system healthy:

- Get plenty of exercise.
- Eat lots of fruit (especially berries), fiber, garlic, ginger, onions, and cayenne—all good food for the circulatory system.
- Keep your weight down.

Recommended supplements include:

- Vitamin E (dry form), 400–800 IU daily
- RNA/DNA, 100 mg daily
- Grapeseed extract, 150–300 mg daily, as a rich source of PCOs, which are powerful antioxidants that help to strengthen blood vessels
- Zinc, 15–30 mg daily, to help keep tissues strong

HEALTHY SKIN BY THE SEASON

Healthy Winter Skin

Winter skin problems are not caused by lack of sunlight. In fact, this time of year can be a good opportunity for your skin to rest and recover from long doses of high ultraviolet summer light. So don't bask under tanning lamps as a solution to winter skin problems! They will definitely do more harm than good. The most common unwanted winter skin condition, especially for older people, is dryness. Read the section on dry skin for some general hints on care and prevention of this condition. Winter brings particular challenges, though, which are worth attention.

Winter, Vitamin C, and Collagen

The immune system benefits of vitamin C make it a useful supplement in winter. It's a wise measure for your skin, too, since vitamin C is essential for the production of collagen. Researchers looking not at skin but at vascular disease have actually found a seasonal connection for vitamin C. Their yearlong study, published in the *Scottish Medical Journal*, found that levels of vitamin C in the white blood cells of subjects dropped in winter. Boost your skin's collagen with a generous supply of vitamin C in your winter diet. Eat plenty of oranges, and take a vitamin C supplement of 500 mg at least three times a day.

Winter, Antibiotics, and Biotin

Fall and winter typically bring bouts of illness all too often treated with antibiotics. Antibiotics destroy B vitamins, including biotin, and hamper the ability of intestinal flora to make this essential nutrient. This makes antibiotics the most likely cause of a biotin deficiency, and one of its signs is dry skin. As always, then, be very certain of the need for antibiotics before you take them. If antibiotics are necessary, a vitamin B complex supplement is, too, for general health as well as dry skin. Take a B complex, because all the B vitamins work together in balanced partnership. Good general insurance against a biotin deficiency is to eat foods like eggs, peas, nuts, molasses, and whole-grain cereals. Also keep intestinal flora in good shape with acidophilus supplements to aid synthesis of biotin in the gut.

Winter and Humidity

A snap of cold winter air can be bracing and refreshing, but it is also drying. At the same time, the indoor comfort of central heating only increases the wrinkling, shriveling effect, as dry air and heat both promote the loss of water from the skin. Chapped skin, as seen, for instance, in cracked and peeling lips, is a telltale sign of winter dryness. Applying lip balm and moisturizers helps prevent symptoms, and measures previously suggested for cuts and scrapes make effective remedies for chapped skin. To counter skin dehydration, take the steps recommended for dry skin, including moisturizers, supplements, healthy diet, and protective clothing.

Avoid extremes. Keeping your house at 85 degrees Fahrenheit and going out in your slippers and housecoat when it's below freezing are both ways to promote dry skin. In some homes, relative humidity is similar to that of deserts! The Consumer Product Safety Commission recommends an air moisture level of 30 to 50 percent. This is usually comfortable, and plants and furniture will benefit, too. Keep temperatures reasonable, mist-water plants, and if you do use a humidifier, keep it scrupulously clean.

Winter, Light, and Vitamin D

Typically, only a small amount of vitamin D comes from dietary sources, including liver, egg yolks, fresh milk, and fatty fish. More is produced when a particular kind of cholesterol is converted by the action of ultraviolet rays in sunlight on the skin. In a study on vitamin D, just 200 IU daily of vitamin D was shown to be enough to promote anticancer activity in the blood. Young children on a vegetarian diet might need a vitamin D supplement, especially in winter. Usually, however, deficiency of vitamin D tends to be a problem only for those who don't get out or who live in far northern countries.

Ten Tips for Healthy Winter Skin

1. Drink plenty of clean water, about six to eight glasses a day. Dehydration is hard on the entire body, but it shows first on your skin. Your body is more than two-thirds water, and your skin is the largest organ of your body. Skin is constantly handling incoming bacteria and releasing toxins through perspiration. Giving it plenty of water helps it do the job of housecleaning. At the cellular level, plenty of water is essential for fluid balance and the exchange of waste material.

2. If you're breathing very dry air, get a humidifier. Indoor heating systems tend to dry the air, which dries your mucous membranes, making them more susceptible to infection. A humidifier is good for your sinuses, for your lungs, and for cold prevention. You should have one in the room you spend the most time in during the day (which may mean taking one to the office) and one in the bedroom.

3. Use moisturizing lotions with vegetable oils. Avoid mineral oils, which clog pores. Try the new lotions containing NAPCA, a humectant that helps the skin retain moisture.

4. For rough, chapped spots, open a vitamin E capsule and rub directly on the area.

5. Get plenty of omega-3 fatty acids by eating fish such as salmon, mackerel, cod, halibut, albacore tuna, sardines, and herring at least twice a week, and omega-6 fatty acids by taking supplements of borage oil, black currant oil, or evening primrose oil. These beneficial oils work at the cell level to keep skin smooth and supple.

6. Try lecithin to keep skin cells flexible. You can sprinkle lecithin granules on cereals or salads or eat them straight.

7. Avoid the hydrogenated oils and *trans*-fatty acids found in refined vegetable oils (not including canola oil or olive oil) and margarine, which contain toxic oxidative molecules that cause aging and compete with the beneficial omega-3 fatty acids for cell receptors.

8. Wear gloves whenever it's cold out. Cold, dry air pulls moisture out of the skin, aging it faster.

9. Drink alcohol in moderation. It's a vitamin robber and skin ager.

10. White snow is a highly reflective surface for bright sunlight. If you're spending more than 30 minutes outside in the snow, be sure to wear a sunblock with an SPF of 15 and sunglasses.

Healthy Summer Skin

Summer: We welcome its warmth and brightness on our skin. Increasingly, though, we set limits on that welcome, recognizing sunlight as wonderful in small doses and harmful in large ones. Now that pollution has thinned the ozone layer, caution is even more our summer skin watchword.

Keeping Your Skin Healthy in the Sun

The most important step you can take to preserve the health of your skin is to protect it from damage by sunlight. The American Academy of Dermatology is convinced by research evidence that exposure to the sun, rather than aging, is what causes most wrinkles. Sunburn afflicts millions of people every year, and skin cancer is on the rise. All this harm is caused by invisible rays known as ultraviolet (UV) light. Some researchers also believe that infrared or heat rays may increase the damage done by UV light.

The shorter, less numerous UV rays are called UVB, while UVA rays are greater in number and less intense. UVB attacks the top layer of skin and is the most important cause of skin aging, skin cancer, and sunburn. UVA is now thought also to be a major factor in skin aging, skin cancer, and immune damage. It does not cause sunburn but penetrates the deepest layer of skin, causing harm to elastin and collagen and damaging surface blood vessels. In this way, it destroys protective antibodies in the skin, causes older-looking, wrinkled skin, and initiates disease. Sunscreens that block only UVB may lead to users staying far too long in the sun without the burn caused by UVB but with the initially invisible harm done by UVA.

UV light is most intense at the hottest times of the day in summer months, UVA in particular increasing in intensity by about one hundred times. Levels of UVA remain potentially dangerous all year round, even in colder months. Beware of water, too. UV rays penetrate water to a depth of at least 3 feet, and water's reflective power amplifies sunlight. Snow also reflects UV rays, and glass is no barrier to them. In addition, fog, smog, and clouds do not provide an adequate block to the sun's harmful UV rays. As much as 80 percent of UV light still penetrates on overcast days. These are the reasons many skin experts now advocate the use of sun protection all year.

Medications and Other Products Can Increase Sun Sensitivity

It's not well known, but harm caused by sunlight can be magnified in some people taking medications such as antibiotics, antihistamines, diuretics, oral contraceptives, and tranquilizers. Beware of aftershave products, colognes, cosmetics, and soaps as well as products containing sulphur, benzoyl peroxide, salicylic acid, or resorcinol. After just a few minutes in the sun, these can sometimes trigger a burnlike rash.

Unfortunately, sunscreens can also act as allergens. PABA, for instance, is a recent sunscreen ingredient to which some people are sensitive. If you develop a rash or burn when using a sunscreen, change it immediately.

Some Facts About Skin Cancer

Skin cancers usually start as tumors in the outer layer of skin, but they can grow and spread beyond their point of origin. The tumors are formed from cells that have been triggered into abnormal, out-of-control growth. UV light is the usual trigger for skin cancer. There is little doubt that more of the sun's damaging ultraviolet rays are reaching us as pollution has thinned the earth's protective ozone layer. Skin cancer incidence has been rising, particularly in countries like Australia, where the ozone layer is thinnest.

Although sun exposure is responsible for some skin cancer, an individual's risk also depends on skin color, sex, and location. For example, skin cancer is more common in men, presumably because more men work outside. Rates of malignancies of the lips and face are lower in women, probably due to protection from lipstick and other makeup. Skin cancer in Minnesota is 5.7 times less common than in Texas. This is because rates of skin cancer double every 4 degrees closer to the equator. Living at a high altitude also increases risk, since it increases exposure to high-density ultraviolet light, which can trigger skin cancer.

However, cure rates for skin cancer are high. Different types of skin cancer are named after the type of skin cells they affect. About 95 percent of skin cancers are basal and squamous forms, which have a matching cure rate of over 95 percent. Squamous cancers are potentially more dangerous, since they are more likely to spread. The most serious form of skin cancer, malignant melanoma, is responsible for 75 percent of all skin cancer deaths. Note, though, that only about 5 percent of skin cancers are this type, and it has a cure rate of 90 percent when caught in its early stages.

While cure rates may be reassuring, they don't mean that skin cancer rates are not alarming. They are a definite indication of the increasing need to protect our skin from sunlight. Prevention of skin cancer is a matter of taking the sun in low doses. Chronic overexposure does the really serious damage. However, avoid even the occasional burn, as just three blistering burns in your teenage years, for example, can increase your risk of skin cancer even five to twenty years after the original exposure.

No Such Thing as a "Safe" Tan

Dark, dusty, cramped surroundings became the norm for millions of workers with the coming of the industrial revolution in Europe. The wealthy were not con-fined to factories and could take vacations. A tan was no longer the mark of a farmworker or peasant. Instead, it became a mark of affluence and fashion. This reversed the glamorous associations previously made with milky-white skin. Working conditions have long since improved, but the psychology of tanning has stuck, despite the ever-increasing evidence that sun is the number one cause of skin damage. A tan does signify the body's own protection against the sun's rays, but it is simply not enough, particularly in the face of environmental degradation.

Melanocytes are skin cells that produce the pigment melanin that colors our hair, eyes, and skin. Uneven melanin distribution is the cause of freckles and liver spots. Sunlight stimulates melanin production, which leads to tanning. The permanently high levels of melanin enjoyed by people with dark skin is the reason they suffer from much lower rates of skin cancer. (Whites contract twenty-seven times more skin cancer than blacks.)

The Sun's Effects on the Immune System

A report in *Cancer Weekly* covers research from the University of Texas and Oregon State University on the effects of sun on the immune system. Studies with mice showed a 100 percent increase in tumor incidence in animals subjected to chronic UV exposure. One of

---

Some Warning Signs of Skin Cancer

Older people should always check their skin all over at least once a year. Those who have had skin cancer should check every six months. Everyone needs to keep an eye on any skin abnormalities, watching for new ones and changes in old ones. There are five basic warning signs for the most common type of skin cancer:

- An open sore that will not heal for three weeks or more
- A persistent painful or itchy reddened area that may crust over from time to time
- A smooth growth with a raised edge
- A pearly or semitransparent molelike nodule that can be red, white, pink, brown, or black
- A white or yellow scarlike area

The earlier skin cancer is caught, the better the chance of a cure, so be sure to visit a doctor if you develop any of these symptoms.

the conclusions of the research was that sunlight can knock out some of the body's immune response to cancer. This, combined with UV damage to cell DNA, could allow cancer to form. Research of this kind leads many dermatologists to argue that a tan is actually a sign of skin damage and a warning to lessen exposure to the sun.

It also supports observations about skin cancer and the state of the atmosphere. As the ozone layer has thinned, the age of patients with skin cancer has dropped, as those seeking treatment are often in their late twenties and early thirties rather than their late forties and fifties. This has been a finding at the Department of Immunology of the M. D. Anderson Cancer Center at the University of Texas. The chairman of this department also warns that thinning ozone will lead to exposure to more intense UV and further weakening of the body's immune system. In turn, this could result in more people becoming susceptible to different diseases and allergies. Sunscreen with both UVB and UVA blockers is highly recommended to help prevent immune impairment. Keep taking your antioxidants, too, for it is thought that sunlight stimulates the production of harmful free radicals, which are neutralized or scavenged by antioxidants.

Sun Protection

Your first priority in sun protection are physical and chemical barriers to UV light. If you have children, remember that protection should begin early in life, not simply to avoid the pain of sunburn but also because childhood burns can set the scene for trouble in later life. Follow these suggestions to increase your sun protection:

- Avoid the sun. I don't mean that you should avoid the sun completely. For optimal health, you need some direct sunlight on your skin on a regular basis. Just make those sessions short and during times of the day when the sun is less intense.
- If you're going to be out in the sun for a long time, wear a long-sleeved shirt and long pants.
- Wear a hat and sunglasses. A large brim cap is a good shield for shoulders and neck. Sunglasses

with UV-protective lenses are the only really effective choice and worth the extra expense. But again, don't go to extremes. Your eyes need some direct exposure to sunlight. Don't wear your shades 100 percent of the time.
- Avoid sun-sensitizing substances, as mentioned earlier.
- Use sunscreen routinely, even in the shade, with a sun protection factor (SPF) of at least 15.

Use a good, natural sunscreen, as some of the ingredients in cheap sunscreens can actually harm the skin with long-term use. It is essential to buy a sunscreen that blocks both UVA and UVB. Good sunscreens not only absorb both types of UV rays but also supply the skin with nutrients and help it to repair. Look for sunblocks containing free-radical fighters and healers like zinc and vitamins C, A, and E. A report in *Medical World News* focused on studies of the sunscreen effects of topical vitamin C. Studies show that this vitamin has sunscreening properties that last three days in animals, even after scrubbing. Vitamin C also seems able to provide protection without blocking the skin's ability to make vitamin D and may also stimulate the production of melanin. While a safe, workable form of vitamin C as a sunscreen has not yet been developed, sunscreens enriched with this nutrient are a worthwhile investment.

Summer Supplements

Taking supplements will not protect you from the sun's damaging rays. Only clothing and sunscreen can do that. What supplements can do is strengthen your skin's immune response and its tissue growth and repair mechanisms. There is no substitute for avoiding sun exposure, but a healthy diet and supplements, together with sunscreens and good sun gear, will help keep your skin healthy outdoors. All the following nutrients are needed for tissue repair, healing, and reduction of scar tissue:

- Beta-carotene, 10,000 IU daily
- Vitamin C with bioflavonoids, 2,000 mg daily
- Vitamin E (dry form), 400 IU daily
- Zinc, 15 mg daily at night

- Selenium, in the form of a Brazil nut daily or as a 200 mcg supplement
- B complex, 100 mg daily, particularly pyridoxine (vitamin B$_6$), which has been shown in mice to increase resistance to melanoma tumors and, in cream form, to reverse the development of human malignant melanoma nodules

HOW TO HAVE BEAUTIFUL SKIN

Look to Mother Nature's medicine cabinet for your skin-care solutions. Nourishing your body inside and out will bring out the best in your skin.

Foods for Beautiful Skin

Fresh fruits, vegetables, and whole grains are definitely indicated to keep skin looking beautiful. They are an excellent source of nutrients, including the antioxidant carotenes and also vitamin C, which is essential for the manufacture of collagen. The following foods in particular will help to ensure a regular supply of skin-enriching substances:

- Cauliflower, lentils, peanut butter, and soybeans for a supply of biotin, a B-complex vitamin. A deficiency can lead to dry skin and scaliness around the mouth and nose.
- Molasses, tofu, broccoli, and sesame seeds, rich sources of calcium. An enzyme in skin is calcium sensitive, making calcium an aid in controlling cell functions.
- Whole-grain breads and cereals, beans, shellfish, and dark leafy vegetables. These foods supply a host of useful substances, including copper, which boosts red blood cells and enhances skin tone and texture because it aids the synthesis of both elastin and collagen in skin.
- Brazil nuts, organ meats, and whole grains, particularly for selenium, which works well with vitamin E. Selenium binds with an antioxidant enzyme, helping to prevent free-radical damage. Brazil nuts are grown in selenium-rich soil, and one nut daily should provide enough of this mineral. Soil conditions make other foods a more variable source.

- Salmon, sardines, mackerel, herring, and tuna. Two to three servings per week of these fish, especially baked or poached, will help you keep up a supply of omega-3 fatty acids, which are essential for healthy cell function.
- Walnuts and canola oil. These are vegetarian sources of healthy fatty acids but are only about one-fifth as potent as marine omega-3s.
- Berries, especially bilberries, blueberries, and elderberries. These fruits are an excellent source of PCOs, antioxidants that help maintain the structure of collagen.

Supplements for Beautiful Skin

Beautiful skin is healthy skin. A smooth, firm, glowing complexion is the result of millions of cells working efficiently and in balance with each other thanks to a continuing supply of water and valuable nutrients. Skin is repaired through constant renewal of its cells and regulation of their functions.

In a polluted world with a thinning atmosphere, a healthy, whole-food diet, exercise, sunscreen, and sensible use of supplements are essential for beautiful skin. Be persistent. Results can take up to twelve weeks to show. Here are the generally recommended supplements involved in the production or healing of skin cells:

- Beta-carotene, 10,000 IU daily. Beta-carotene is converted by the body into vitamin A, an antioxidant that boosts the immune system and is well known for relieving skin problems.
- Vitamin B complex, 100 mg daily. B complex will keep you topped up with several important substances: biotin, to guard against dryness; pyridoxine, to help fight blackheads and whiteheads and protect against cancer; niacin, for maintenance of general skin health indirectly through its role in the healthy metabolism of fats, carbohydrates, and proteins; and riboflavin, which is needed more if you are exercising (a deficiency will lead to dry, cracked lips).
- Vitamin C with bioflavonoids, 2,000 mg daily to promote collagen production
- Vitamin E (dry form), 400 IU daily. This antioxidant antiaging vitamin works with vitamin C.

- Zinc, 15 mg daily as an immune booster involved in the repair of skin tissue
- Black currant oil, 1,000–2,000 mg daily as a supply of essential fatty acids
- Grapeseed extract, 150–300 mg daily. This is a rich source of antioxidant PCOs.
- Glucosamine. This amino sugar occurs naturally in the body. It keeps cartilage strong and flexible and is a foundational building block and strengthener in the tissue between cells in the skin and mucous membranes. Take it in the form of glucosamine sulfate, *N*-acetylglucosamine, or glucosamine/mucopolysaccharide complex.
- Herbal infusions. Red clover, dandelion, and burdock root are particularly helpful. Red clover is often used to treat skin disorders, and it is rich in saponins, which boost the immune system and protect against cancer. Dandelion is a useful source of vitamin A and other vitamins, minerals, and chemicals that cleanse skin tissue. Burdock, another tissue cleanser, is antimicrobial and frequently used to relieve conditions like acne.

Natural Preparations for Beautiful Skin

Moisturizing and nutrients are essential for boosting and maintaining the many important functions of skin, with the bonus that skin working well looks great, too. Homemade skin preparations will often be at least as effective as expensive commercial preparations. If you do prefer the convenience of ready-made products, seek out those with whole and natural rather than synthetic or derived ingredients. This will provide you with nature's own ingenious safeguards. Fruit acids, for example, may well produce the same beneficial effects as vitamin A–derived treatments such as Tretinoin and Retin-A, and without the side effects. Recent research suggests that long-term regular use of natural, effective products brings continuing benefits. But be patient. Allow at least two weeks for benefits to begin to show.

Quick and Easy Lotions

Try the following recipes for skin care lotions, building your favorite into your daily routine (unless your skin proves sensitive to some of the acidic ingredients):

- Aloe. This wonderful natural substance is found in many commercial products but is best scooped fresh from inside the aloe leaf. Full of healing chemicals, aloe is very cooling and soothing. Mix aloe with a little vitamin E if you find it drying.
- Brewer's yeast. This has been found to increase collagen production when mixed with a little water, wheat germ oil, or yogurt and patted gently onto the skin. Rinse off once dry.
- Honey. A daily coating allowed to dry for 5 minutes before rinsing off is a very effective skin cell regenerator.
- Mayonnaise and egg yolk. Mix the yolk with ¼ cup of mayonnaise and apply several times a day as an antiwrinkle lotion.
- White grapes. Cut in half and apply gently to the skin around eyes and mouth. A handful of grapes straight from the blender makes a refreshing and toning mask to leave on for 20 minutes before rinsing off. The French have long used champagne to tighten the skin.

Soaps and Oils

Plant extracts, oils, and essential oils have been used for hundreds of years for cleansing and healing skin. Follow tradition and make your own concoctions, or buy products made with natural, soothing, or stimulating ingredients like these:

- Fruit kernel, jojoba, castor, and olive oils. These are all good for moisture loss. Shake 2 cups of one oil or half a cup each of all four oils together with a drop or two of a natural (not synthetic) oil such as . . .
- Tea tree oil, a powerful antiseptic, healing agent
- Comfrey oil, to encourage new cell growth and healing
- Eucalyptus oil, an antiseptic pain reliever that clears the head and stimulates blood flow
- Lavender oil, used for centuries for its antibacterial, healing, and soothing powers

Add your oil mixture to a warm bath and enjoy not more than a 10-minute soak. Any longer creates dehydration. Alternatively, use one oil at a time to savor its individual properties. Herbal rinses make wonderful facial cleansers. Look for them as ingredients of natural commercial preparations. Use infusions of herbs like those already mentioned, or try the following:

- Lemon balm. Used through the ages as a spirit lifter, this herb has antihistamine and antibacterial actions useful against conditions like acne and eczema.
- Chamomile. Another antiseptic, very soothing to the skin
- Sage. Used by Native Americans as a cleanser and remedy with bear grease for skin sores, sage is antibacterial and antioxidant.

Whether or not you have a skin condition, it's wise to select products with stimulating or healing agents that naturally tone and condition the skin. Take the trouble to learn what nature has to offer, and in just a short time your skin will show the benefits in a firm, smooth, and glowing appearance.

How to Keep Your Skin Looking Young

When it comes to keeping young-looking skin, sorry, but moisturizers alone just won't do it. Moisturizing does plump up dehydrated skin, and this does make wrinkles harder to see. However, simple rehydration doesn't address other major biological processes involved in aging skin. As time passes, it is usual for cell growth and glands to slow down. Typically, this will leave skin drier but also with less immune protection and weakened physical structure. Signs of aging, such as wrinkles, often start to show from around age thirty. This all sounds drastic, but a healthy lifestyle with a whole-food, high-fiber diet, lots of exercise, and appropriate supplements really do promote youthful-looking skin. However, the slowing of cellular and glandular processes over time is not the most important factor in creating aged skin. Studies show that the sun is in fact the number one cause of an aged appearance, some experts reckoning that it lies behind 90 percent of all wrinkles.

Experts say that age-caused wrinkles are fairly subtle, while those caused by UV radiation can be deep and extensive, as abnormal protein growth builds up, often lending a yellowish tinge to the skin. The way the sun's light produces wrinkles and generally damages skin is known as photoaging, and it can accelerate true aging effects by as much as twenty years! Read on for tips about natural aging, but also take the sun seriously and less often, using the suggestions for healthy summer skin to keep those sags and wrinkles at bay.

Signs of Aging Skin

Thinning, fragility, wrinkles, and loss of elasticity are all signs of aging skin. Nerve fibers, circulation, and the connective tissue between skin layers all deteriorate with time. The outer layer of skin can become loosely attached and so more easily scraped and torn. Weakened blood vessels mean a greater tendency to bruise. Thinning of skin layers creates less insulation, bringing increased risk of hypothermia. Overall, less internal quality leads to less resistance to external factors, so older people tend to be prone to skin conditions in general, especially those related to long-term exposure to sun. Malnutrition is frequently seen in the elderly and is often a factor that worsens skin conditions. So begin those good nutrition habits now!

Antioxidants to Combat Aging Skin

Many of the downhill changes associated with aging skin feature the destruction of cell membranes. Behind this biological damage are two substances we cannot do without—light and oxygen. Free radicals, components of oxygen metabolism, damage or inactivate components of cell membranes. And light can loosen the bonds of molecules in skin cells, making them even more prone to free-radical damage.

The body is naturally equipped to reduce harmful levels of oxidizing agents, but the job can only be done well with all the right tools, including good nutrition and nutritional supplements. Some of the best-known antioxidant supplements are the vitamins A, C, and E.

Once again, the spotlight is falling on vitamin C. Trials, such as one at Duke University on a vitamin C cream, will test how well antioxidant substances are absorbed and how effective they are. As an antioxidant, it is thought that vitamin C may help guard against wrinkling, declining collagen synthesis, and skin cancers. The theory is that antioxidants help prevent the breakdown of cell membranes. It's believed that a vitamin C skin application could boost the production of skin-firming collagen by special cells called fibroblasts.

Other members of the cooperative antioxidant group are natural plant pigments known as carotenes. The amount of carotene in tissue is considered the most significant factor in determining life span in mammals, including humans. Keeping up carotene levels works to boost immune functions active in the skin.

Flavonoids, the major coloring agents in plants, are antioxidants supplied by a green and fruit-filled diet. These compounds are unusual in their activity against a wide range of free radicals and oxidants. In skin and elsewhere, flavonoid action works against cancer and is anti-inflammatory, keeping skin's stress load down and appearance up.

Moisturizers enhanced with antioxidants, although not proven, are probably worth trying. An antioxidant-rich diet, however, seems a very worthwhile measure to keep your skin looking young. To boost your dietary intake of antioxidants, try the following supplements:

- Beta-carotene, 15,000 IU daily
- Vitamin C with flavonoids, 1,000–2,000 mg daily
- Vitamin E (dry form), 400 IU daily
- Grapeseed extract, 150–300 mg daily as a rich source of PCOs
- Selenium, 200 mcg daily

Smoking and Wrinkling

A report in the *Annals of Internal Medicine* found that smoking greatly increases the chance of facial wrinkling. Obvious examples are the stark lines produced by puckering the lips to draw on a cigarette. Smoking is thought to cause wrinkling in two ways: first, by damaging collagen and elastin, proteins in skin that keep it supple and firm; and second, by producing changes in the tiny blood vessels of the face. Stopping smoking could well lead to some reversal of these effects—yet another reason to add to the long list of reasons for smokers to quit!

Aging, Immunity, and Skin

In healthy people, the cells' ability to repair themselves declines at a constant rate of about 1 percent per year from age twenty to sixty, an underlying factor in the tendency for skin cancer to develop in middle age. Fresh skin cells in a healthy thirty-year-old typically take about twenty-four days to move to the outermost layer of skin. By the age of sixty, this short journey usually takes twice as long! This means that skin is more vulnerable to environmental damage for double the time, with the worst culprit being the sun. Sun protection from early on in life has potentially huge immunity payoffs in old age, since UV rays have been shown to damage the immune system. It's never too late, however, to take protective measures.

Super Skin Secrets: Fruit, Wine, Milk, and Honey

Cleopatra bathing in asses' milk really wasn't such a silly idea. The same goes for rubbing wrinkly elbows with half a lemon. This is because certain plant and dairy food acids, such as honey and molasses, lactic acid in sour milk, salicylic and citric acids from fruits, tartaric acid in wine, grapes, and other fruits, and malic acid in apples, promote new cell growth. Known as hydroxy acids (HAs), these substances also cause shedding of dead cells.

Research using sophisticated measuring techniques on the effects of hydroxy acids on skin is now widespread. In one study, the researchers had twenty subjects applying a mixture of HAs twice daily over twenty weeks. A control group of fifteen people applied the same mixture but adjusted to neutral rather than acidic. In the unadjusted HA group, a 38 percent increase in cell renewal rates, a 35 percent increase in skin firmness, and a 44 percent improvement in smoothness were seen. Further work shows that HAs seem to achieve most of their moisturizing effect in just two weeks and their cell renewal and firmness effects in ten to twelve weeks. A very promising result was that improvement in wrinkles and thickness was still increasing at twenty-six weeks.

The best-known HAs are AHAs (alpha-hydroxy acids), but research indicates that all types appear to produce benefits. Hydroxy acids seem to work by naturally increasing the acidity of the skin long enough to loosen cells in the outer layer, stimulating shedding and new cell growth. At a deeper layer, the changed skin acidity may affect enzymes associated with the production of new cells and the skin's inflammatory response. In general, the researchers concluded that HAs do seem to be valuable aids in long-term skin rejuvenation.

For all the benefits, use an HA product with a pH between 3 and 4.5. There have been reports that reddening and cysts can result from HA application in some people. This is thought to be caused by the acidity and may be avoided by using natural sources, such as yogurt and honey. The research shows that such natural HAs seem to be combined with soothing agents that can even reverse skin irritation. Try some of the recipes given earlier for soaps, oils, and lotions to experience the benefits of HAs.

HAIR AND NAILS: WHAT THEY ARE AND WHAT THEY DO

Hair and nails are more than mere decoration. The hair on our head protects the skull by cushioning it and protects the scalp from the sun and wind. And the hairs on our eyelids (eyelashes) and in our nose and ears filter out dust and dirt particles. Our fingernails also serve a purpose. At one time, they were probably used as weapons and tools, but they also serve to protect the tips of our fingers and give them extra strength. When we use our hands to grasp something or when we walk and run, our fingernails and toenails provide stability.

The Inner Workings of Hair

Each individual head hair has a life span of between two and six years, with three cycles. The first is a growing cycle; the second is a resting cycle, which lasts for only a few weeks; and the third is the falling cycle, when it dies and falls out, to be replaced by a new hair. Most head hair grows about half an inch per month, faster in the summer, and we normally shed fifty to one hundred hairs a day.

Hair grows from follicles, or sacs beneath the skin that contain the root of the hair, much as a pot contains a plant. The average number of hairs on a head is one hundred thousand. The root of the hair is surrounded by a bulb that feeds it with the tough fibrous protein keratin. Each tiny hair follicle has its own blood supply, making good circulation a key to healthy hair. The size of the opening in the follicle determines the thickness of the hair. Relative to its circumference, hair is very strong—stronger than a copper wire of the same thickness.

Hair color is genetically determined and caused by a pigment called melanin found in the follicle. The basic colors are red, yellow, brown, and black, but most hair is a combination of these colors. It is the decline of melanin production that causes hair to lose its color, turning gray, which is its original color mixed with white, or white, which is a complete absence of melanin.

Attached to each follicle are tiny muscles called erector pili, which contract when you're cold or scared. This is what makes animals' hair stand on end, creating a layer of warm air between the erect hairs. Although we no longer have hair covering our bodies as fur, we still have erector pili, which can be seen in action when we have goose bumps.

Just above the bulb and below the skin are sebaceous glands, which produce an oily substance called sebum, which lubricates and protects the hair.

The shaft of hair is made of three layers: the center core, or medulla; the thicker middle layer, called the cortex; and the tough outer layer, the cuticle. Hair is straight, curly, or wavy, depending on the shape of the hair shaft. Straight hair has a round shaft, curly hair has a kidney-shaped shaft, and wavy hair has a slightly curved shaft.

The Inner Workings of Nails

Fingernails and toenails grow from near the bone about ¼ inch past the base of the nail. This is called the nail root. Forming a protective barrier between the nail and skin is a flap of tissue called the cuticle. Improper trimming of the cuticle can allow bacteria and fungi to enter the sensitive tissue under the nail, causing unsightly nails and painful infections.

Under the nail is the nail bed, which is rich with blood vessels and very sensitive. The pink color of the nail is caused by blood vessels close to the surface.

The nails are made of keratin, a tough protein with a high sulphur content produced by the cells under the nail. Fingernails grow about ⅛ inch per month, and toenails grow about ¹⁄₁₆ inch per month. As with hair, fingernails grow more quickly during the warm, summer months.

At one time it was said that eating gelatin would create strong nails, but this is a myth. Both hair and nails are composed primarily of protein, and gelatin is far from a complete protein. It is also a myth that calcium will build stronger nails. The amount of calcium in nails is minimal. There is very little you can do to create hard nails from the outside. Good nutrition and genetics will determine your nail strength. If you have brittle or soft nails, it is especially important to make sure that you're getting all the B vitamins in abundance, not only by eating enough high-quality protein but also by taking a good supplement.

NUTRITION FOR HEALTHY HAIR AND NAILS

Healthy hair and nails are an outer reflection of inner health. That special shine and vibrancy of healthy hair and well-groomed fingernails and toenails send a message to the world about your well-being. When you're sick, malnourished, or under stress, and also as you age, your hair and nails can become dull and brittle. What's going on? Your hair and nails are made of protein and minerals, and they need special nutrients just as much as the rest of you does. If your body is nutritionally deficient, you can bet that your hair and nails are, too, and may even serve as a warning that something is wrong. When your digestion isn't working or your hormones are out of balance, it will also show up on your head and hands.

Protein

Hair and nails are 98 percent protein, so you can probably guess what your key nutrient is when it comes to healthy hair and nails. Although protein is the basic building block of hair and nails, too much will do more harm than good. And since hair loss is associated with a high-fat diet, you need to get the majority of your protein from low-fat sources such as fish, poultry, and legumes such as soy.

For most of us in Western cultures, getting enough protein is not an issue—in fact, most of us get too much protein. Too much protein can also cause unhealthy hair by making the body too acidic. The kidneys need to buffer acidic substances with calcium before they are excreted in the urine. Too much protein will cause a calcium deficiency, which will deplete it from your hair and nails.

Vitamins A, E, and B

Vitamin A is a key vitamin for healthy skin, hair, and nails. One of the signs of vitamin A deficiency or excess is hair loss and soft or brittle nails. If you're eating your five servings of fruits and vegetables a day, you'll be getting lots of vitamin A in yellow and orange vegetables and fruits, and dark green leafy vegetables such as kale and broccoli. Other sources of vitamin A are liver, egg yolks, milk, and butter. You should be taking 10,000–15,000 IU of beta-carotene in your daily vitamins, which the body will convert to vitamin A as needed.

Vitamin E is the other key vitamin for healthy hair and nails. I recommend that everyone take 400 IU of vitamin E daily. Food sources of vitamin E are unrefined, extra virgin olive oil, whole grains, avocados, and nuts.

All of the B vitamins are important to healthy hair and nails. Biotin is especially important. This member of the B-complex family is actually added to many shampoos. However, it will do you more good on the inside than the outside. Although a biotin deficiency is rare, it can cause hair loss, dry skin, and fragile nails. Biotin can be depleted by low-calorie weight loss diets, oral antibiotics, and a steady diet of raw egg whites. Eating foods high in biotin, such as nuts, whole grains, organ meats (such as liver), and vegetables, can reverse hair loss caused by a biotin deficiency.

Nutrients for a Healthy Thyroid Gland

A healthy thyroid gland is essential for healthy hair and nails. Dull, lifeless hair and fragile nails can be caused by a thyroid deficiency. Iodine is important for proper thyroid metabolism. It's found naturally in fish, and is added to most table salt. The Chinese get their iodine by adding a variety of dried seaweed to their foods. Try adding some wakame, hijiki, or arame seaweed to miso soup, and you'll be getting your iodine and many other minerals, along with your low-fat protein! Excessive estrogen, especially relative to low progesterone, can block thyroid action. If your hair has turned lifeless since menopause, try some natural progesterone cream.

Silicon, Selenium, and Iron

After oxygen, silicon is the most abundant element in the earth's crust. It is also abundant in the human body and plays an important part in maintaining the architecture of hair, skin, and nails. Collagen, the "glue" that holds our tissues together, contains a large proportion of silicon. In our blood, silicon is found in the same concentration as it is found in seawater. Some researchers speculate that a decline in silicon levels in the body contributes significantly to the aging process.

In laboratory studies, deficiencies of silicon in rodents induced cartilage and bone disease and damage. Furthermore, when the diets of rats with broken bones were supplemented with silicon, the bones healed faster than in rats not receiving silicon. Silicon is present in abundance in whole foods, such as whole grains, fresh fruits, and vegetables.

A form of silicon, called silica, is used as a dietary supplement for healthier hair, skin, and nails. The horsetail plant is used as a source of vegetable silica, and silica gel is derived from quartz crystals. If you have brittle nails and hair loss, you may have a silicon deficiency. Try taking silica supplements in the form of horsetail or silica gel for three or four months. You can find it at your health food store.

Selenium, another important mineral, is a potent antioxidant that acts as an enzyme for many important bodily functions. Healthy hair, skin, and nails are all dependent on sufficient selenium in the diet. You should be getting 100–200 mcg of selenium daily.

Iron is yet another important mineral in hair and nail health, but iron deficiencies in adults are actually quite rare, and recent research indicates that too much iron can set up damaging oxidation reactions in the body. I recommend that you get small amounts of iron in your multivitamin. Otherwise, don't be concerned with it unless you are anemic.

Cysteine and Glucosamine

Cysteine is an amino acid (one of the building blocks of protein) found in large amounts in hair and nails. Eggs, meat, and dairy products are good sources of cysteine, but since they are high in fat, you can also take cysteine capsules, up to 1,000 mg daily, on an empty stomach. (If you are diabetic or allergic to monosodium glutamate, do not take cysteine.)

Glucosamine is an amino sugar made in the body from glucose and amino acids. Glucosamine keeps cartilage strong and flexible and is a foundational building block and strengthener in the tissue between cells in the skin and mucous membranes. A deficiency of glucosamine can lead to weakness in these tissues. Take it in the form of glucosamine sulfate, *N*-acetylglucosamine, or glucosamine/mucopolysaccharide complex, 1,000 mg daily in divided doses.

WHAT YOU CAN DO TO PREVENT HAIR LOSS

Both men and women hate to lose the hair on their head, but men suffer from baldness more than women do. Ever since Delilah relieved Sampson of his hair, and thus his manliness, Western cultures have equated men's hair with youth and virility. Studies exploring cultural attitudes about balding show that men with hair loss are seen as more passive, less likely to be successful, and less likable. According to one study, the only characteristic not perceived as diminished by baldness is intelligence.

A single scalp hair has a two- to six-year growth cycle. What happens on your head during that cycle depends on your diet, your health, your genes, and your hormone balance. Most people lose 50 to 150 hairs a day. Lose more than this, and you may find yourself with thinner hair. If you notice when you shower that you're losing more hair than usual, take note of your health.

Some twenty to thirty million men in America alone are bald or balding. The most common type of hair loss in men is known as *androgenetic alopecia*, or male pattern baldness (MPB). Some 95 percent of baldness is MPB, and it is caused by male hormones. It is thought that changes in testosterone cause the hair follicles on the head to begin producing the thin "peach fuzz," or *vellus* hair, that covers much of the body, instead of the heavier, darker *terminal* hairs normally produced on the head. Balding men may lose 150 to 300 hairs daily.

Women may lose hair during pregnancy and after menopause, when androgens, or hormones that confer male attributes, become more dominant than estrogen and progesterone. While men go bald, women's hair tends to thin out over the entire scalp.

The only substance approved by the FDA for treating baldness is minoxidil (Rogaine). This drug was originally sold as an antihypertensive (it lowers blood pressure), but people who took it—men and women alike—began reporting excessive hair growth all over the body. Its maker, Upjohn, quickly put it into clinical trials as a medication to restore hair growth. Although minoxidil has since been approved by the FDA for this use, in truth, minoxidil doesn't work very well and never completely restores hair. Men whose hair is thinning can get a small benefit from the drug as long as they take it, but when they stop, the hair will just fall out again. And meanwhile, minoxidil is a powerful antihypertensive with many side effects of its own and is very expensive.

Hair loss can be caused by many types of illness, including allergies and particularly celiac disease (intolerance for wheat gluten), diabetes, and auto-immune diseases such as lupus. Hair loss can also be associated with a high-fat, high-sugar diet. In Chinese medicine, too much "sweet" consumption is

Possible Causes of Hair Loss

- Aging
- Genetic predisposition
- Prescription drugs (birth control pills, anticoagulants, chemotherapy)
- Fungal infections
- Radiation
- Immune disorders
- Diabetes
- Iron deficiency
- Vitamin C deficiency
- Vitamin B deficiency
- Zinc deficiency
- Excess vitamin A
- Progesterone deficiency in women
- Hypothyroidism (low thyroid)
- Poor diet (especially lack of protein)
- Pregnancy (usually grows back within three months after delivery)
- Silicon deficiency

associated with hair loss. Hair loss can also be caused by skin disorders such as eczema and psoriasis.

If you're a woman of menopausal age and your hair is starting to fall out, you may be deficient in the hormone progesterone. Many women are familiar with the hair loss immediately following pregnancy, which is caused by a dramatic drop in progesterone production. Using some natural progesterone cream will quickly restore hair growth for most women.

Hypothyroidism, or low thyroid, especially in women, can cause hair loss. If you have other symptoms of hypothyroidism, such as cold hands and feet, fatigue, and unexplained weight gain, see your doctor for a thyroid test.

Supplements for Preventing Hair Loss

Because hair follicles are fed by blood vessels, good circulation is a key to good hair. There are many vitamins, herbs, and other supplements that help circulation. Ginkgo biloba, an herb that improves circulation to the extremities, may just improve your outer beauty as well as your inner brainpower! And coenzyme Q10 is an important substance for senior citizens whose circulation isn't as good as it once was. Many people who take coenzyme Q10 every day report that their hair is thicker and shinier. Niacin improves circulation to the scalp, and there is some anecdotal evidence that it slows the process of hair loss in men.

Vitamin E and vitamin C both improve circulation, and the bioflavonoids strengthen the capillaries that feed the scalp. Vitamin E supplementation can also reduce testosterone levels in women, which may halt the process of hair loss. A zinc deficiency can compromise the immune system and contribute to hair loss. Be sure you're taking at least 15 mg of zinc daily. Deficiencies of vitamin A and vitamin C can also contribute to hair loss. Be sure you're taking 15,000 IU daily of beta-carotene to get your vitamin A, and be sure to take at least 1,000 mg daily of vitamin C.

KEEPING YOUR HAIR AND NAILS HEALTHY

Hair and nails are often subjected to what I call "hair abuse" and "nail abuse." This abuse is often dictated by the tyranny of fashion, which drives us to dye our hair, style it with spray and gels, perm it, blow-dry it, and expose it to sun and wind. It also drives women to put strange colors on their nails and subject them to drying polishes and polish removers. The same things that dry out the skin will dry out the hair and nails: low humidity, constant exposure to water and soap from doing dishes and other housecleaning chores, sun, wind, and chlorine.

We've all noticed that our hair is less shiny and lustrous after we've been swimming in a chlorinated pool. Sun, wind, and salt water also take their toll on hair. How can you have fun in the sun and have healthy hair, too? Like all good answers, it's simple: Wear a bathing cap in the ocean or pool and a hat in the sun. And if you're going to be in the wind, either wear a hat or pull your hair back in a ponytail or braid. If you don't want to wear a bathing cap while swimming, be sure to shower as quickly as possible after coming out of the pool or ocean. Just by taking a shower, your hair picks up chlorine. I always recom-

mend that if you have chlorinated tap should use a shower filter that filters out poison absorbed in large amounts throug especially when the pores are enlarged by w

Graying Hair

Graying hair is a natural part of the aging process for most of us, but one we tend to resist mightily, as the booming business in hair colorings will attest. There's essentially nothing you can do to prevent graying hair, but you can avoid premature graying with good nutrition and regular scalp massage and by avoiding "hair abuse" and minimizing stress.

A vitamin B_{12} deficiency can cause graying hair, as can a deficiency of vitamin B_5, pantothenic acid. In rodents, graying caused by a B_5 deficiency is reversible when B_5 is replaced, but this has never been demonstrated in humans. Nevertheless, if you are experiencing premature graying, I recommend that you take an extra B-50 complex supplement.

Premature graying can also be caused by celiac disease, thyroid disease, diabetes, pernicious anemia, and other autoimmune diseases.

Dry Hair

Hair abuse is the primary cause of dry hair, although a lack of essential fatty acids (EFAs) can also contribute. If you're eating plenty of whole grains, nuts, seeds, legumes, and fresh fruits and vegetables, you should be getting plenty of EFAs. However, hydrogenated oils can suppress EFAs and cause deficiencies—yet another good reason to avoid these synthetic oils.

Hair is normally covered with the oily substance called sebum, which makes it lustrous and shiny. Harsh shampoos, shampooing too frequently, sun, wind, low humidity, and chlorine will all pull moisture out of the hair shaft and strip away the sebum. This causes the outer layer, or cuticle, of the hair, to crack, exposing the center and causing it to fray or split, leaving hair dry, frizzy, and brittle. Conditioners do not repair split ends. The only cure for split ends is to cut them off.

If you have dry hair, use a high-quality conditioner every time you shampoo. Giving your hair an oil conditioning treatment once or twice a week will help. Use olive oil, jojoba, castor oil, or sweet almond oil. Gently work it into your hair, and then comb it through to make sure the hair is well coated. Wrap your hair in a towel and leave the oil on for at least 30 minutes.

Dandruff

Dandruff is a common disorder of the scalp that causes the skin to scale and flake off, leaving its embarrassing residue on the shoulders. It causes itching, and the resultant scratching results in further irritation of the skin. Dandruff is caused when the natural process of skin shedding is accelerated, probably from a fungal infection. Dandruff can also be caused by dietary deficiencies, stress, and "hair abuse" in the form of too much hair dye, too many perms, excessive blow-drying, and so forth.

A deficiency of vitamin A can cause hair to become dull and brittle and the scalp to become dry and flaky. A vitamin B_6 deficiency can also cause

dandruff, as can a vitamin C deficiency in its extreme form.

If you have dandruff that doesn't itch, you're probably abusing your hair. Try avoiding hair sprays and gels, blow-drying, dyes, harsh shampoos, perms, and straighteners for six weeks and see what happens. In the meantime, you can try a hair rinse of a few drops of essential oil of rosemary, a few drops of tea tree oil, and half a cup of apple cider vinegar in about 2 cups of water. Massage into your hair after shampooing, and leave there for 2 to 3 minutes. Rinse in cool water and gently pat your dry hair.

You can take 100 mcg of selenium daily to relieve flaking and itching. You can also look for natural dandruff shampoos containing selenium or tea tree oil, which are antifungals.

About Scalp Massage

One of the reasons stress is so damaging to the hair is that when we're tense, we tend to contract our scalp muscles along with all our other muscles. This,

---

Healthy Hair Tips

- Wash your hair in warm water and rinse it in cool water.
- Use shampoos with natural ingredients. (Check with your health food store.)
- Don't apply shampoos or conditioners directly from the bottle. Pour a small amount into the palm of your hand, dilute it with a little water, and then apply it.
- You don't need to wash twice with most shampoos. Washing once will protect the healthy oils in your scalp and on your hair.
- Use a large, thick-toothed comb to comb conditioner through your hair.
- Rinse out conditioner thoroughly, or your hair will be heavy and oily.
- Dry your hair by wrapping it in a towel and blotting it, rather than rubbing it, pulling it, or wringing it.
- When your hair is wet, comb it gently, working from the bottom up.
- Protect your hair from the sun and wind, which will dry it.
- Wear a bathing cap when swimming in chlorinated pools.
- Rinse your hair right away after swimming in the ocean.
- If possible, avoid or go easy on hair dyes (most of them contain coal tar, which is carcinogenic), bleaches, and perms. They will all eventually make your hair dull.
- If possible, dry your hair naturally. The constant use of hot combs, heated rollers, and blow-dryers will make your hair dull.

in turn, contracts the tiny muscles around the hair follicles, causing a reduction in oxygen and other nutrients to the follicle.

Massaging your scalp is a key to healthy hair. It increases the flow of blood and oxygen to the hair follicle, improving hair growth and hair quality. I recommend that you spend 2 to 3 minutes gently massaging your scalp with the tips of your fingers each day in the shower. Be sure to massage the scalp rather than the hair to avoid damaging your hair. It's also wonderful to have someone else massage your scalp for you!

Maintaining Healthy Nails

The condition of your nails can tell you a lot about your health. Yellow nails can indicate respiratory disorders, and white nails can indicate liver problems. White spots may be caused by damage to the nail or may be a sign of folic acid deficiency or zinc deficiency.

Transverse grooves across the nails can be a sign of thyroid deficiency. They may also appear in people who are recovering from a serious illness, such as pneumonia. Lengthwise ridges in the nails can be caused by anemia, by applying too much pressure when manicuring your nails, and by biting your fingernails.

Wearing rubber gloves when you wash dishes or do housecleaning will protect your hands and your nails from the drying effects of water, chlorine, and soaps.

If your cuticles are dry and cracked, try applying vitamin E oil directly to them. You can either break open a gel capsule, or buy a small bottle of vitamin E oil.

If your nails are growing very slowly or are splitting, brittle, or soft, review the nutrients for healthy hair and nails in my Basic Personal Supplement Plan in chapter 1, and the Mindell Healthy Hair, Skin, and Nails Program.

Nail fungus, most often found in the toenails, can be very difficult to treat. It requires daily attention with an antifungal agent. I recommend you use a natural antifungal agent such as tea tree oil, rubbing it into the nails every night before bed.

The Mindell Healthy Hair, Skin, and Nails Program

Here are my recommendations for healthy hair, skin, and nails:

- Follow the Basic Personal Supplement Plan from chapter 1.
- Drink six to eight glasses of clean water daily.
- Get at least 20 minutes of exercise at least five times a week.
- Eat plenty of whole grains (brown rice, whole-grain wheat, millet, and rye), nuts, and seeds, all of which contain "healthy" oils that nourish hair, skin, and nails, as well as providing vitamins and fiber.
- Eat plenty of fresh organic fruits, vegetables, and legumes such as soy, which contain fiber for good digestion and the vitamins, minerals, and hundreds of phytonutrients so basic to good nutrition.
- Keep meat and fat consumption low. Eat red meat once a week at most, or eliminate it from the diet. Eat chicken or turkey two or three times a week, and be sure it's free-range fowl, free of hormones and antibiotics.
- Eat fish at least two times a week, preferably salmon, mackerel, cod, and other cold-water fish.
- Eat eggs two to three times a week.
- Get plenty of sleep.
- If you're living a stressful lifestyle, learn a relaxation response, such as meditation, biofeedback, yoga, chi gong, tai chi, or positive visualization.
- Avoid hydrogenated oils and processed oils. Emphasize extra virgin olive oil.
- Avoid sugar and refined carbohydrates, such as pastries and cookies.
- Avoid fried foods.
- Avoid junk foods, fast foods, canned foods, frozen dinners, and other processed foods, which are generally nutrition free and loaded with additives, preservatives, dyes, salt, sugar, and fat.
- Avoid excess caffeine consumption (more than two cups a day).
- Avoid excess alcohol consumption (more than two drinks a day).

12 THE POWER OF HOMEOPATHIC REMEDIES ~

HOMEOPATHY: TREATING THE WHOLE PERSON

This chapter is intended as a homeopathic guide to nonserious conditions. If you have a condition such as diabetes, heart disease, or severe arthritis, I strongly recommend that you work with an experienced homeopathic practitioner, who can offer you the full benefit of these powerful remedies.

Some homeopathic remedies work very quickly and noticeably. For example, with some types of flu, the flu remedy Oscillococcinum can cure symptoms in a matter of hours. And arnica used promptly on a bruise can keep bruising symptoms to a minimum. But if it has taken you a long time to get an illness, a homeopathic remedy is most likely going to take some time, from a few weeks to a few months, to have its effect.

Like all truly effective forms of alternative medicine, homeopathy takes the whole person into account, including the physical, emotional, mental, and spiritual levels. It is a form of medicine best used, most of the time, with attention to its principles and with awareness of all the details that it is capable of addressing. As you delve into homeopathy and learn to apply its remedies, you will learn more about an entirely new dimension of yourself in fascinating detail. When you or your homeopath come upon the correct remedy, you will be amazed at how accurately the list of symptoms for that remedy fits your specific problem.

This chapter was written with the assistance of homeopathic practitioner, teacher, and author David Dancu, and I recommend that if you want to learn more about homeopathy, you take advantage of his book, *Homeopathic Vibrations: A Guide for Natural Healing* (Sunshine Press, 1996), as well as other relevant works (see bibliography). And as I've already said, when working with serious conditions, it is important that you work with a homeopathic practitioner.

THE HISTORY OF HOMEOPATHY

Homeopathy originated in the nineteenth century as a result of the work of a German doctor, Samuel Hahnemann. It is founded on some very specific principles and an extensive list of tested remedies. The remedies are based on natural substances found to have various effects when taken in medicinal doses. The success of homeopathy as a safe and effective form of healing led to growth in its popularity and use throughout the century. As a practice, it was only overtaken when the developing science of modern medicine came to be favored by the medical establishments of North America and Europe.

Almost a century later, the drawbacks and dangers associated with conventional medicine have become obvious. Tranquilizer addiction, birth defects from pregnancy medications, and side effects of common medicines like aspirin demonstrate the darker side of standard medical treatment. Many patients and doctors alike have been prompted to try approaches of a more consistently safe and compassionate nature, such as homeopathy.

The tide has turned again in favor of the ancient tradition of medicine, which sees the physician in service to the natural power of the body to heal itself. The trend in twentieth-century medicine has been toward control and dominance of physical systems in isolation, treating symptoms and pain over and above underlying conditions and causes. Valuable knowledge and techniques have resulted, but often at great cost to the long-term health of patients. The aim now is to combine modern developments with the understanding and usefulness of older, proven practice, including homeopathy.

The Law of Similars

Has anyone ever recommended that you "swallow a hair of the dog that bit you"? As a hangover cure, it leaves a lot to be desired, but the idea of treating symptoms with a little of a substance that causes them is actually very sound. Known as the *law of similars*, the theory is ancient. It was part of the writings of philosophers and physicians from Hippocrates to St. Augustine. Herbalists long ago applied a primitive version of the law of similars in the form of the the *doctrine of signatures*. Some plants were selected for medicinal use because they resembled in some way the part of the body to be treated. The speckled surface of a lungwort leaf, for instance, looks like a lung. Sure enough, modern science shows that the silica in lungwort restores elasticity to lungs, and extracts of the plant are useful for reducing bronchial mucus.

A more refined concept of similarity was proposed in the 1790s by Samuel Hahnemann. Unhappy with the barbaric medical practices of his times, such as bloodletting, cupping, and mercury poisoning, Hahnemann had quit his medical practice. When he turned to the translation of foreign medical and herbal publications, he began to question their theories and observations and apply them to his own knowledge of healing.

Folk medicine from South America had produced a treatment for malaria, the world's number one killer disease of the seventeenth century. Powdered bark from the pretty cinchona tree proved a potent remedy. Known as quinine, cinchona extract is finding favor again today, as malarial parasites have become resistant to synthetic drugs. In Hahnemann's time, herbalists believed that cinchona's effectiveness was due to its bitterness. Hahnemann was not satisfied with this explanation, since many other bitter herbs were of no help.

Deciding to test the law of similars, he dosed himself with extract of cinchona bark. Remarkably, the healthy doctor was inflicted for a short time with symptoms very like those of malaria. This was the first of what Hahnemann called *provings*. He continued with the help of colleagues, family, and friends to conduct further tests on different substances, keeping detailed records of the results. The provings added further evidence that a cure of symptoms could result from taking herbs, minerals, elements, or certain known toxins that actually induced similar responses in healthy people. To summarize his theory, Dr. Hahnemann coined the word *homeopathy* from the Greek words *homoios*, meaning "similar," and *pathos*, meaning "suffering."

Hahnemann's Philosophy of Homeopathy

Hahnemann's published writings demonstrated a refinement and philosophy that contrasted sharply with the crude thinking behind the common medical practices of the day. Unlike most physicians, he stressed the importance of exercise, diet, and hygiene. He was aware of the pioneering work of contemporaries such as Edward Jenner on the smallpox vaccine and was eager to advance the techniques of the ordinary physician.

Hahnemann's 1796 summary of three main approaches to medical treatment remain valid today. The first type of treatment could remove a known cause of a disease. A second form worked to oppose the effects of a disease, such as antacids to relieve heartburn. The third and superior type, in his view, was treatment with similars designed to support the self-healing capabilities of the body. This was the essence of homeopathy. Hahnemann regarded homeopathic treatment and prevention as the only truly valid approaches to medicine. Each remedy leads to the maintenance or active restoration of health rather than to the removal or suppression of disease factors.

Hahnemann understood the role of disease agents but emphasized the idea that each person has a predisposition, or tendency, to get certain types of illness. He observed that agents act as triggers for disease, but not in all cases, and with worse consequences for some people than for others. For example, the flu may afflict half the people in the office, and the other half may be unaffected. This led him to argue that the condition of the person is of greater importance than the disease agent. Included in this concept was the idea of the *vital force* of the individual, a term used by Hahnemann to explain the constant automatic drive of an organism to stay in a healthy state.

Hahnemann's *Organon* and Materia Medica

Hahnemann's first book on homeopathy, *The Organon of Rational Medical Science*, was published in 1810. The *Organon* set out the ideas and philosophy of homeopathy, and Hahnemann explained his systematic approach and theories. These were developed scientifically, from the perspective of someone with a medical degree and who was also an authority on metal poisoning and toxicology.

The powerful effects observed by Hahnemann in provings were achieved using highly diluted amounts of the substances involved, which, in a few cases, were known poisons. The diluted agents became homeopathic remedies. Over four hundred of them were fully described, complete with provings, in his own materia medica, or medical textbook.

Hahnemann's teachings spread slowly throughout Germany, meeting opposition from the entrenched medical establishment. His work was regarded as a threat to much of the German medical world, since he advocated small and limited doses, which would not generate large pharmaceutical or practice profits. Personality played a role, too, as Hahnemann's blunt, undiplomatic style won him few friends in established circles.

In spite of the opposition, Hahnemann expanded his writings, refining and adding remedies, which led to four further editions of the *Organon* during his lifetime. Through his work with patients, he amassed an additional four volumes of information and cures compiled from cases and patient notes. A sixth *Organon* manuscript lay unpublished until it was found in 1920. This was more than seventy-five years after Hahnemann's death at age eighty-eight in 1843—some time before homeopathy reached its nineteenth-century height. The changes and additions to homeopathic theory contained in the sixth *Organon* are major, yet not widely used by many modern homeopaths. The successful results achieved using the first five editions have created a reluctance to change.

Homeopathy in the Nineteenth Century

An increasing number of followers led to the rapid spread of homeopathy to almost all European countries as well as the United States, Mexico, Cuba, and Russia. Eventually, it would also reach South America and India. One of the main reasons for the growth in homeopathy was its superior effect in the treatment of epidemics such as typhoid fever and cholera, which swept over Europe and America in the nineteenth century. When yellow fever hit the southern states of America in 1878, death rates were one-third fewer in patients treated with homeopathy than in those receiving orthodox treatment. In London, in 1854, over half the cholera patients in conventional hospitals died, in contrast to just over 16 percent in homeopathic hospitals.

Homeopathy was introduced to the United States in 1825. Demand for homeopathy in America stemmed initially from German communities. Philadelphia saw the establishment of the first homeopathic medical school in 1833. The school was founded by Dr. Constantine Hering, who had originally taken up the cause against Hahnemann in Germany. Aimed at disproving the discoveries of homeopathy, Hering's research did the opposite! Convinced by a natural form of healing free of side effects, the former enemy became a dedicated ally. Hering went on to write many books on homeopathy, and he himself worked as a homeopathic practitioner.

Another famous American homeopath was James Kent, MD, who was based in Philadelphia from the early 1890s. Many years of work, involving treatment of over thirty thousand patients as well as lectures and notes from other materia medica, led to the publication in 1897 of *Kent's Repertory*. As a comprehensive listing of symptoms and remedies, this source is still used by homeopaths everywhere.

Leading proponents such as Hering and Kent worked to meet the rising call for homeopathy in

America, which, by the 1880s, had created one hundred hospitals and twenty medical colleges. Homeopathy was taught at Boston, Iowa, Michigan, and Minnesota universities. At that time, 20 percent of physicians were homeopaths. The gentle approach of homeopathy, free of side effects and caring for the patient as a whole, was in contrast to the rising use of synthetic drugs and treatment only of symptoms in standard American medical practice.

Pressures Against Homeopathy

Patients in the eighteenth century were accustomed to brutal techniques like mercury dosing, which frequently caused teeth to fall out, and bloodletting often until four fifths of the blood contained in the body was drawn away. Homeopathy provided an attractive alternative. Ordinary folk and the elite of society, including politicians and the wealthy, patronized homeopaths, competing with standard physicians. The resulting jealousy and fear made homeopathy the target of official repression. The founding of the American Institute of Homeopathy in 1844 was followed, as a direct result, two years later by the formation of the American Medical Association (AMA). Doctors with any connections to homeopathic practices were barred from the AMA. Members of the AMA were not even permitted to consult homeopaths.

The pharmaceutical industry also perceived itself threatened by homeopathy. Scientists in the eighteenth century had discovered that the active chemicals of medicinal plants could be isolated. During the nineteenth century, chemists focused on the extraction and synthesis of these potent substances. In the minds of industry and public alike was the idea of quick-fix, one-stop medicine. Long-term effects and treatment of underlying conditions came to be largely ignored. New, synthesized drugs were often speedily effective against urgent symptoms. Side effects went unidentified, as drugs could treat those, too, masking true medicinal changes in the body.

Additional pressure came when the U.S. government commissioned the Flexner Report in 1910. The intention was to assess medical education and to set standard practices. However, this was in the context of a growing chemical approach fixated on physical symptoms. The report led to the closure of many medical schools, including those teaching homeopathy. Homeopathy fell outside the narrow biochemical framework accepted and promoted by the medical establishment. It has to be added that homeopaths created their own vulnerability to attack. As a developing system, homeopathy accommodated proponents of different views on high and low dilutions and did not offer a consistent front to those attempting to undermine the subject. Millions of dollars' worth of grants were denied to homeopathic medical schools, and homeopathic hospitals became standard medical institutions.

Adding to the decline of homeopathy in the United States was a major lifestyle shift from slow-paced and rural to urban and mobile. Society no longer provided an easy fit for the typical family doctor who often treated the same patients for their entire lives. Finally, the advent of so-called "wonder drugs" in the 1940s saw homeopathy retreat outside the margins of medical practice.

Homeopathy Today

It wasn't until the early 1970s that dissatisfaction within the medical field led to a revival of homeopathy. Recognizing the ineffectiveness and often downright harm of modern drugs, some physicians arranged to study in Greece, where homeopathy was more widely practiced. Greek instructors came to America to lecture on Hahnemann's work, and so began the increase in popularity of homeopathy seen in the United States today.

More than one-third of the U.S. population now use alternative remedies, including homeopathy. Complications from prescription drugs result in 40 percent of hospitalizations and cause twenty thousand to thirty thousand deaths every year in the United States. The comparative effectiveness and safety of homeopathic remedies is being demonstrated by more and more top-notch scientific studies done by respected institutes. Studies done in the United States, England, Germany, Holland, and France include research into homeopathic remedies for cold and flu, skin ailments, allergies, insect bites and stings, menopause, and sports injuries.

In the United States, homeopathic remedies are now recognized as medicines. They are freely available in health stores and drugstores and come under the jurisdiction of the Food and Drug Administration (FDA). Some homeopathic remedies, such as nitroglycerine for certain heart ailments, have been taken up by allopathic medicine and used in medicinal doses.

The Queen of England and Mother Theresa have homeopathy in common! The Queen is attended by a homeopathic physician, and homeopathic remedies are used in Mother Theresa's Calcutta hospital. Homeopathic medicines are used in the practices of a fifth of German physicians and just under a third of French physicians. In 1980, there were nearly 800 homeopathic doctors in France and around 200 in Britain. India boasts at least 120 homeopathic medical schools, and there is a sprinkling of schools and colleges in South America. About 450 homeopathic physicians practice in Argentina alone.

Aside from entrenched medical practice steered to a large degree by drug company interests, there has remained a mainstream reluctance to accept homeopathy. One reason for this is that no complete understanding of what makes homeopathy effective exists. Another factor is the lack of interest on the part of homeopaths to finding classifiable, physical causes for the symptoms homeopathy cures. Allopathic medicine has yet to move on the position that the agents of disease are less important than the paths that lead to recovery and cure.

Those practicing homeopathy have begun to realize the need to move on as well and accept the need for testing that meets the criteria of Western medicine as well as established techniques of proving. Perhaps the time has come for the gentle, proven techniques of homeopathy to gain acceptance alongside the best and safest of current established medical practices.

Putting Homeopathy to the Test

Homeopathy is an ongoing subject of research and an interesting one, because the way it works is not completely understood, although there are some very convincing theories. Impartial and well-executed studies include work on a range of subjects. In an article in the *British Medical Journal*, 107 controlled trials in homeopathy were reviewed by authors who were not themselves homeopaths. Most of the trials did not meet Western medical protocols, but nevertheless, the authors were amazed at the amount of positive evidence that could still be gleaned. Many more trials are needed to satisfy scientific criteria, but headway is already being made.

Examples of recent homeopathic trials include a Harvard clinical study on Similasan Eye Drops #2, an ophthalmic (eye) allergy medication containing extracts of honey bee, eyebright, and cevadilla. Using a well-established test known as the antigen challenge, the drops were found to significantly reduce hay fever symptoms such as itching and bloodshot eyes.

According to a study published in *The Lancet*, a homeopathic remedy was more effective than a placebo in relieving allergy symptoms (mainly due to dust mites) in twenty-eight patients who also continued their conventional care. Patients taking the homeopathic remedy reported 33 percent fewer asthma symptoms, sustained for up to four weeks after the trial. Improvements were seen within one week from the start of the treatment. These results correlated with a 53 percent increase in histamine resistance for the treated group, while the placebo group saw a 7 percent decrease.

In a study of eighty-one children in Nicaragua, reported in the journal *Pediatrics*, children treated with a homeopathic medicine for diarrhea recovered more quickly than those given a placebo.

In a 1995 clinical study of sixty-eight volunteers, published in the *European Journal of Clinical Pharmacology*, a homeopathic gel was found to be significantly superior to a placebo in the treatment of mosquito bites.

Results such as these give a hint of the wide-ranging use and effectiveness of homeopathic medicines. It should be noted, too, that this is without the application of full homeopathic techniques, which require exact tailoring of remedies to the individual affected, not just the physical symptoms in isolation.

HOMEOPATHIC PRINCIPLES AND PRACTICE

A basic, guiding principle of homeopathy was stated by Hahnemann in his *Organon*: "The highest ideal of therapy is to restore health rapidly, gently, permanently; to remove and destroy the whole disease in the shortest, surest, least harmful way, according to clearly comprehensible principles." Used according to its principles, homeopathy is a powerful tool for healing, especially when used in consultation with an experienced homeopath.

The Principles of Homeopathy

The homeopathic principles that Hahnemann developed almost two centuries ago are still followed, shaping the practice of all homeopaths today.

The Principle of the Like Remedy

A homeopathic remedy always follows the law of similars, as it is chosen for its ability to produce symptoms that are most like those of the person to be treated. For instance, the syrup of ipecacuanha will cause vomiting when ingested in its natural form. When diluted and potentized in the homeopathic form (this concept will be explained shortly), it prevents or eliminates vomiting and nausea. This is considered the foundation for homeopathic principles; whatever causes a specific reaction in an individual also cures that disharmony when taken in homeopathic dilution.

In homeopathy, symptoms are investigated in depth, covering physical signs, nature of the illness, underlying level of health and energy, personality, trauma, and inherited tendencies. The aim is always to look at the person as a whole. Remedies are chosen from a range that has been scientifically tested on healthy human beings to determine what symptoms they produce. The resulting list of symptoms is known as a remedy's "drug picture." One of the fundamental discoveries of homeopathy showed that the most effective remedy is the one whose drug picture most closely matches the individual's symptoms, or "clinical picture."

The Single Drug Principle

Many combination homeopathic remedies are effective for acute illnesses or conditions. In our fast-paced lives, when there isn't time to stop and review symptoms in depth, a combination remedy often does the

trick. However, it will leave you without knowledge as to which homeopathic substance in particular was most effective. Combinations are not original homeopathic remedies but derive more from the herbalist approach, where long tradition shows that different agents can enhance the effect of others.

Classic homeopathy calls for one remedy to be tried at a time so that its effects can be clearly seen. If unrelated symptoms or symptoms not experienced before should occur after taking a homeopathic dose, the remedy should be discontinued. Any ill effects, however, will be short lived.

The Principle of the Small Dose and Potentization

One fascinating discovery made by Hahnemann was that the effectiveness of a homeopathic remedy increased the more the dose was diluted. Hahnemann observed that when a match was achieved between symptoms and remedy, the patient would be very sensitive to the remedy. A much lower dose was needed for a positive reaction than in a case without a good symptom match or in a healthy person. This spurred Hahnemann to continue lowering dilutions to find curative doses as well as to eradicate toxicity.

Part of the process of dilution involved vigorous shaking, called succussion, to achieve usable, homogeneous chemical solutions. Hahnemann later named this process *potentization* or *dynamization*. Achieving increased potency with lower doses is in contrast to allopathy, where normally the dose is *increased* to produce more effect.

In his fifth edition of the *Organon*, Hahnemann sets out a range of potencies. The most commonly used dilutions are given in centesimal and decimal amounts. In centesimal potencies, one drop of the active substance is dissolved in ninety-nine drops of distilled water, alcohol, or glycerine. Substances that cannot be dissolved in this way are ground up with lactose (milk sugar). A resulting solution is called the mother tincture, which is then used as the basis for further dilution, producing potency ranges from 1c right up to 100,000c (or cm, not to be confused with centimeters). Decimal, or x, potencies involve water or alcohol. The x potencies range from 1x to 200x.

Much weaker solutions, known as 1M potencies, were recommended by Hahnemann in his sixth *Organon*, but these have not been widely used.

The Principle of the Infrequent Dose

Homeopathic remedies are only administered as necessary. With acute, self-limiting conditions such as bruises or colds, the right remedy can produce changes 4 to 8 hours (or even sooner) after the first dose. Patience, however, is part of the key to homeopathic treatment of more serious conditions. Days and sometimes weeks are allowed for effects to be seen, and doses are not repeated when improvement is maintained. There is no expectation of the long, continuous courses of medicine often seen with allopathic medicine.

The Principle of Noninterference with the Body's Natural Response

This principle recognizes the body's innate ability to heal itself. There is much greater knowledge today than during Hahnemann's time of the numerous repair functions of the body. When struck by illness or injury, the body automatically triggers healing processes on many levels. For example, fever burns off infections, endorphins flow as natural painkillers, and white blood cells destroy foreign agents. Although the exact nature of the healing systems was not known to Hahnemann, he recognized and summarized these kinds of responses and their regulatory mechanism as vital reactions.

We now know how conventional nineteenth-century medical practices, such as bloodletting, would have literally drained the body's ability to respond to infection. Hahnemann observed as much, even though he was unaware of the precise processes being crudely ignored. For this reason, he formulated the principle of noninterference. Homeopathy is designed to support the healing functions of the body, shortening the time needed to restore health.

The Principle of Treatment of the Whole Person

Hahnemann observed that the body's ability to fight disease and repair itself was directed by what he referred to as the *vital force*. This was his description of the capacity of organisms to self-regulate always in the direction of survival and therefore health. Even today, this function is not well understood, but, like Hahnemann, we see it affected by moods and emotions. Today, we can measure how our immune cells decrease with depression or how our body's natural anticancer agents increase with happiness. By acknowledging a vital force, Hahnemann was addressing the large role played by the emotional, mental, and spiritual levels of a person's health.

A good homeopathic assessment reviews a person's vitality and emotional state. If someone has a cold but still feels energetic, a more potent remedy will be tolerated. Similarly, acute symptoms, such as a cold, are not treated homeopathically without regard also to chronic conditions, such as arthritis or indigestion.

Thorough training in all aspects of homeopathy leads to the most comprehensive and effective treatments. This is why it makes good sense to select a trained, experienced homeopath.

How Does Homeopathy Work?

The answer to this question is not fully known. The powerful effect of the very diluted remedies used in homeopathy is a puzzling subject for researchers. Many dilutions are so high that no molecular trace of the original substance can be found. Homeopaths believe that the vigorous shaking at each level of dilution leaves the energy of the original dissolved substance imprinted on the medium of solution, something like an energetic blueprint or fingerprint.

Various theories about the mechanism of homeopathy are being tested. For example, electromagnetism may play a role, as it has been found that allergic manifestations occur in highly sensitive subjects contacting water treated with electromagnetic frequencies. Some investigations suggest that when pure water is treated with electromagnetic waves, it gains new physical and chemical properties that are conserved for some time. It's true that the properties of water are in many ways still a mystery. Results of future work investigating homeopathic dilutions may yield interesting discoveries.

Homeopathy can be seen as influencing the energy fields of the body. Each human being is a unique pattern of energy flows, and each cell has an electromagnetic or "bioelectric" field. A cell is an energy generator, functioning in harmony with every other cell to create an overall level of health. At times of illness, there are disharmonies in energy production and flows in the body.

It is thought that the properties of a correct homeopathic remedy for an ailment in some way resonate with and strengthen the body's efforts to realign its unbalanced energy flows.

Working With, Not Against, Symptoms

When you take a dose of, say, antibiotics, the aim is to kill the organisms that have caused the infection. You might also take other drugs to bring down a fever or kill pain. This, of course, is very different from the approach taken by homeopathy. Allopathic treatment has a vital role in emergency treatment, and it gets results because it often removes the sources of an infection or condition. However, it usually does so with a blast of powerful substances that override the body's own defense mechanisms. In many cases, allopathic medicine simply suppresses symptoms and does not tackle root causes. This is true, for instance, of drugs for heartburn, sinus troubles, and high blood pressure. In addition, the medicinal substances themselves frequently cause unwanted side effects, which not uncommonly lead to the administration of yet more drugs.

In homeopathy, symptoms are regarded as outward signs of the body's efforts to repair itself. By taking tiny amounts of a substance that produces similar symptoms, a cure results because the defense work of the body has been stimulated and reinforced. In allopathic medicine, the disease often becomes harder to treat, as with bacteria that become resistant to antibiotics. The aim of homeopathy is not to bypass the body's own systems but to support them. In this way, the body gains in its ability to fend off disease.

Release of Suppressed Symptoms

Hahnemann's provings showed that a remedy can provoke an "occasional initial aggravation," the release of symptoms that have become suppressed. When a release is seen, it is sometimes referred to as a healing crisis. A release involves the recurrence of old symptoms, usually for just a few hours a day, but sometimes longer if they were originally severe. A trained homeopathic doctor will decide whether to prescribe a different remedy, reduce the potency, or wait out the crisis.

In allopathic medicine, it is unlikely that a patient would be asked to consider past symptoms. A reappearance of old symptoms may be seen as incidental or subject to new treatment or mistaken as a sign that a successful treatment should be changed. Allopathic medicine is unlikely to consider a recurrence of old symptoms as a sign of recovery.

The Holistic Approach: Disease as a Dynamic Condition

The tendency in allopathic medicine is to fit the patient to a known disease. A doctor attempts to pin down symptoms to a generally classified pattern, in which the overall match is more important than any variations shown by an individual. This is what medical doctors are taught in medical school: First they learn how to diagnose a disease, and then they learn which drug to prescribe to treat the disease. We've all seen doctors prescribe a first choice of antibiotics and then a second, even a third, when the first was ineffective. People have become used to being treated in such a general fashion, since modern medicine has established certain "molds" for illness to fit into. At the same time, we accept that people experience disease differently, recovering at different rates, responding to viruses with different symptoms, requiring more or less rest. Yet despite these observed differences, we've learned to accept non-individualized treatment.

Holistic treatment does not single out one physical aspect or body part for treatment. It is an approach that takes the whole person into account, rather than just physical symptoms. As a holistic practice, homeopathy does not place the disease in a compartment separate from the individual. Symptoms are seen to reflect ongoing, dynamic efforts by the body to return to a healthy state, not as unwanted manifestations to be classified and stamped out in isolation from other bodily functions.

In this way, homeopathy recognizes the interdependency of all parts of the body. It also incorporates the role played by personality types, so that homeopathic treatments are tuned to each individual patient.

The Homeopathic Physician

Most physicians are well intentioned and sincere in their vocation. The training of an allopathic doctor, however, is steered toward acceptance of a prescription drug culture, in which the medical world is greatly influenced by the pharmaceutical industry. The homeopath takes a more independent view, although his or her training in medical matters will be just as thorough. A homeopath perceives his or her prescriptions as supplementary rather than superior to the body's own powers. In practicing homeopathy, a physician will usually pay greater attention to the patient's general condition than an allopathic doctor. A desire to know a great deal about individual patients and their symptoms in great detail leads to much more time spent with them than is the norm in conventional medicine. Whereas a standard physician may see about thirty patients a day, spending about 10 minutes with each, a homeopathic doctor typically sees eight to ten patients a day and spends about an hour with each one.

Like any other doctor, a homeopathic physician receives an MD degree and his or her state license to practice medicine. To qualify to practice homeopathy, he or she then goes on to a postgraduate course in the subject, followed by a period of work with a practicing homeopathic physician. Only a few states license homeopathic practitioners. Recommendations from others and experience count equally for conventional and homeopathic doctors.

What to Expect from a Homeopathic Physician

You may understand how a homeopathic doctor is different from an allopathic physician, but how does this affect treatment? Homeopathy sets out certain procedures as standard. As a result, patients can expect a basic similarity in the work of different homeopaths. As with doctors of all kinds, of course, each physician has his or her own style and character, which will influence the way he or she practices.

One of the major preferences expressed by those who choose a homeopathic doctor is over the amount of time the physician is willing to spend with patients. An initial hour-long interview is typical, and feedback from patients is welcome in regard to the changes seen after taking a remedy. Important and specific use is made of patient-doctor time.

A standard element of homeopathy is the collection of information about the patient. This is known as "taking the case." From the first encounter with the patient, a homeopathic doctor is taking note of his or her condition. Factual information is recorded, including age, occupation, marital status, and the patient's reason for visiting. A homeopath goes on from there to consider factors such as posture, complexion, stress level, and emotions as valuable clues to an individual's state of health. Considerable skill is needed for a homeopath to be sure of noting underlying traits, and not simply accepting a doctor's-visit façade.

An interview covers not just physical symptoms, their onset, type, and timing, but also personal history, which provides information about a patient's emotional and mental tendencies—if the patient is ambitious, inhibited, or extroverted, for example. A history of family illness is also covered to indicate any possible inherited conditions and the individual's probable underlying physical strengths and weaknesses.

Symptoms are discussed in detail, determining how they have changed and if they vary over the day. In addition, the patient is asked to describe how the condition affects him or her and if it has changed the way the patient reacts to his or her environment. Food preferences are important here, noting, for instance, if something is disliked that was previously favored.

The result of the initial interview is a comprehensive picture of the patient's state of health, specific symptoms, and personal response to the condition. The homeopathic physician uses the interview notes as the basis for prescribing a remedy without needing to first classify the illness.

Visiting a physician for a full homeopathic review results in the prescription of a single remedy. This is to avoid stimulating multiple responses in the body that cannot be definitely associated with a specific remedy. In other words, a homeopath's initial intention is to find only the remedy that is key to the illness. This approach is very different from an individual's educated purchase of a combination remedy for self-treatment. Someone finding quick relief, say, from hay fever isn't going to mind exactly which substance in a combination remedy produces the result. More severe conditions, however, merit a comprehensive investigation, which leads in traditional homeopathy to one remedy alone.

Diagnosis Comes Second to Symptoms

The pattern of symptoms observed by a homeopathic physician is used to point to a specific remedy rather than to a particular disease. This is called "constitutional prescribing," or matching the treatment to the person as a whole, not just the condition. Homeopaths do provide a diagnosis if one is needed, say, for insurance purposes, but the diagnosis is not used to provide the framework for action.

Out of perhaps a dozen main symptoms, the physician will usually judge five or so to be the strongest. One symptom may point to several remedies. Exactly which remedy is used is determined in cross-reference with the remedies suggested by the other leading symptoms. Usually, one remedy will match most of the symptoms. The physician checks the description of patient and symptoms listed under the remedy to ensure that it is indeed a clear match with the individual being treated. A good match between the "drug picture" and the "clinical picture" is confirmation that the right remedy has been selected. The remedy is prescribed, and any dietary factors, such as coffee, which could interfere with its actions, are considered as possible causes of the problem, too. Most homeopaths provide general advice about diet and lifestyle, since prevention of disease is a high priority in the homeopathic world. The first visit, however, is usually reserved for "taking the case" and dealing with immediate discomfort.

Aggravation as a Common Response

The old adage "You'll feel worse before you feel better" often holds true in homeopathy. A patient is usually very sensitive to the right remedy, which produces symptoms most similar to his or her own. The right remedy will often provoke the defensive measures of the body and often actually increases the intensity of symptoms for as long as a day or two. This syndrome of aggravation can also be the release of earlier, repressed symptoms.

An expert homeopath will be sure to confirm that any increase in symptoms is either a temporary, bearable worsening of symptoms or a renewal of old ones, rather than a new set of responses that are not connected to the original condition being treated.

Keeping Costs Down

One bonus of homeopathic treatment is that it is less costly than allopathic medicine. Visits are made less frequently, and fewer diagnostic tests are ordered. A century and a half of research, provings, and contributions to materia medica means that homeopathic pharmaceutical companies do not have to bear the huge costs of research and development of new drugs. A homeopathic physician prescribes from an established range of about five hundred classically proven homeopathic substances and a total of about twenty-eight hundred substances, which are produced without expensive hype and promotion. The result is medications for prescription and self-treatment that are cheaper than conventional medicines. An allopathic doctor, in contrast, has a prescription list of about ten thousand available drugs, whose high cost reflects the high price of their manufacture and promotion.

Homeopathic drugs are safe. The long history of their production and use has ensured that they are nontoxic. Modern medical drugs, on the other hand, lead to an estimated five to ten million serious reactions every year. The costs of treating adverse drug reactions do not arise with homeopathy.

The Patient's Role

Anyone seeking homeopathic treatment benefits from a willingness to be honest and thorough in communicating with the physician. A homeopathic patient-doctor relationship is a close and active one.

The patient is not a passive recipient of advice and treatment. Finding an effective homeopathic remedy relies on good communication from a patient willing to convey a lot of information about his or her condition. With a remedy in use, the patient's job is to provide feedback about any and all changes. Strong communication creates a close and effective relationship between homeopathic patient and doctor. This helps the doctor ensure that the appropriate medicine is being used and that no condition needing allopathic intervention has been missed. Unlike allopathic patients, who are expected to quietly and passively do as they are told without question, homeopathic patients are expected to speak up loud and clear!

SELF-TREATING USING COMBINATION REMEDIES AND FORMULAS

Combination remedies have been used in homeopathy since its beginnings. One of Samuel Hahnemann's first combinations, Causticum, was a mixture of slaked lime with a solution of potassium sulphate. Its effectiveness was clear and powerful. This unique combination remedy covers many conditions, including joint problems, emotional disharmonies, allergies, fibromyalgia, sinus problems, back pains, and multiple sclerosis.

There are several things to consider when choosing either a combination remedy or a combination of remedies. Most classical homeopaths use only single remedies, simply because they can determine the effect of that remedy without interaction of other forces. With each single remedy, there is a clear proving of what that remedy can cause.

Simplicity is the underlying key for using homeopathy, and single remedies provide the basis for maintaining that simplicity. Combinations, on the other hand, are easy to use for self-treatment but may not be as effective for chronic conditions, such as asthma, arthritis, depression, anxiety, or most other long-term illnesses.

Let's say I have been getting headaches frequently. They usually occur after stress or possibly from a reaction to car exhaust. There are three approaches to consider. The obvious and easy one is the traditional Western philosophy of taki aspirin to eliminate the headache. The sec approach is to try a homeopathic combination cor taining five or six remedies, all generally specific for headaches, such as Nux vomica, Spigelia, Sanguinaria, or Lycopodium. One of these will probably work just fine, much like an aspirin.

The third approach, which is a more classical homeopathic approach, considers the cause of the headache, not just the symptom. One remedy is given based on the whole picture, rarely just the headache alone. This way, a determination is made on both the effect and the result, while also considering reactions in other parts of the body.

The first two approaches look to the symptom without considering the person or the cause. And there are obvious times when this approach is not only effective but necessary. Whenever possible, though, a review of all symptoms will help to establish a deeper, more permanent healing.

In addition to having specific labels for various ailments, ranging from colds to asthma, combination remedies list a series of ingredients. Reputable companies make these combinations based on sound homeopathic principles. They combine remedies that work for the ailment described on the label, specifically derived from established materia medica and provings.

Each homeopathic remedy chosen is based on clear symptoms of mental, emotional, and physical aspects. A good example is a remedy called Pulsatilla. Emotionally, the symptom picture of this remedy is generally a codependent, weepy, timid, depressed, capricious, and soft woman. Physically, she often has PMS, stomach or digestive disorders, hay fever, headaches, and joint problems and is rarely thirsty, despite a dry mouth.

Typically she is also warm-blooded, with most of her symptoms being much worse either in the sun or in a stuffy, warm room. Her skin is frequently fair, she has light-colored hair, and is overweight. Visualize a vine clinging to the side of a building, and you have a good picture of Pulsatilla tendencies. A healthy person taking this remedy may exhibit some of the preceding symptoms. But this also demonstrates what it can cure when taken by someone who has similar symptoms.

...meopathic remedy has its own
... in more depth than others.
...cific to certain ailments, such
...nd bladder problems. There
... hundred proven remedies,
...ed on a regular basis.

...here are also quite a few substances being called homeopathic that have never been proven and that have no relationship to cure other than the fact that they have been diluted. It takes time and effort to weed out the proven from the unproven, but the time taken may prevent ill effects or an unwanted proving on yourself.

All proven remedies are listed in a book called a materia medica. The materia medica gives necessary information about each specific remedy, including its effects. Ask your health food store to carry an inexpensive version for review purposes. You can also use this book and the others recommended in the bibliography for proven recommendations.

Remedies that are proven combinations often naturally occur that way. This list includes calcium and phosphorus, iron and phosphorus, sodium and sulphur, and hundreds of others. The idea is to understand what the combination may create and what effect it will have on the body once created.

For an acute problem or an emergency, combination can be very helpful and effective. In chronic or long-term disharmonies, the combination remedies act much in the same way as an aspirin does, rarely getting to the cause, just giving temporary relief. And continued repetition is necessary to maintain that relief.

The following is a review of specific remedies in relation to general areas of the body. When considering a combination for a certain ailment, one or more of these remedies would generally be included. Keep in mind that each remedy may be valuable for more than one type of illness or ailment. For instance, Arsenicum album is a single remedy used for allergies, sneezing, diarrhea, colitis, skin problems, respiratory ailments, shingles, headaches, food poisoning, fears, anxiety, compulsive disorders, and depression. But it is best used when there is restlessness in conjunction with one of these ailments; otherwise, it may not be as effective or long lasting.

The following conditions and their related remedies should be used as guidelines rather than absolutes. Remember that some substances being sold as homeopathic remedies have never been proven, so unless one of the listed remedies is included, use caution in your selections.

- *The head (including headache, injury, pains, and congestions):* Arnica; Aconite; Belladonna; China; Gelsemium; Glonine; Iris; Kali bichromicum; Lachesis; Natrum muriaticum; Nux vomica; Phosphorus; Pulsatilla; Sepia; Silica; Sulphur
- *The nose (including sinus, pains, congestion, and discharges):* Aconite; Allium cepa; Arsenicum iodatum; Belladonna; Calcarea carbonica; Euphrasia; Hepar; Kali bichromicum; Lycopodium; Mercurius; Natrum muriaticum; Pulsatilla; Silica; Sticta; Thuja
- *The mouth (including abscesses, odor, pains, and infections):* Arsenicum album; Calcarea carbonica and phosphorica; Camphora; China; Carbo vegetabilis; Hepar; Mercurius; Nitricum acidum; Lachesis; Nux vomica; Silica; Sulphur
- *The eyes (including injuries, vision problems, eruptions, discharges, inflammations, pains, and styes):* Apis; Aconite; Euphrasia; Ruta; Staphysagria; Causticum; Phosphorus; Pulsatilla; Natrum muriaticum; Nitricum acidum; Mercurius; Kreosotum; Rhus tox.; Silica
- *The ears (including infections, hearing, pains, and tinnitus):* Aconite; Belladonna; Chamomilla; Pulsatilla; Silica; Hepar sulphuris; Mercurius; Kali bichromicum; Sulphur; Causticum; Petroleum; Lycopodium; Sarsaparilla; China
- *The throat (including infection, inflammation, and pains):* Aconite; Apis; Arsenicum album; Belladonna; Cantharis; Phytolacca; Sulphur; Phosphorus; Pulsatilla; Lycopodium; Mercurius; Lachesis; Natrum muriaticum; Rhus tox.; Silica; Capsicum
- *The lungs (including inflammations, infections, breathing difficulties, coughs, and discharges):* Arsenicum album; Antimonium tart.; Argentum nitricum; Bryonia; Carcinosin; Drosera; Hepar; Kali bichromicum; Lachesis; Phosphorus; Rumex tuberculinum; Spongia; Sambucus; Sulphur

- *The stomach (including digestion, gas, bloating, pains, cramps, poor appetite, hiccups, and nausea):* Antimonium crudum; Argentum nitricum; Arsenicum album; Carbo vegetabilis; Calcarea carbonica; China; Chelidonium; Ipecacuanha; Cocculus indicus; Lachesis; Lycopodium; Nux vomica; Aloe; Natrum muriaticum; Pulsatilla

- *Extremities (including joints, pains, bones, bruises, breaks, arthritis, inflammations, ligaments, and strains):* Arnica; Calcarea carbonica; Calcarea fluorica; Calcarea phosphorica; Causticum; Colchicum; Cuprum; Silica; Symphytum; Phosphorus; Plumbum; Bryonia; Rhus tox.; Ruta; Ledum

- *Female (including PMS, hormonal problems, cysts, herpes, pains, menopause, discharges, and headaches):* Belladonna; Calcarea carbonica; Caulophyllum; Cimicifuga; Cyclamen; Ignacia: Lilium tig.; Natrum muriaticum; Natrum carbonicum; Natrum phosphoricum; Phosphorus; Sepia; Pulsatilla; Platinum; Sabina; Lycopodium; Thuja; Silica; Kreosotum; Medorrhinum; Nitricum acidum

- *Male (including herpes, impotence, erectile difficulty, prostate, pains, desires, infections, and inflammations):* Arsenicum album; Argentum nitricum; Calcarea carbonica; Calcarea sulphurica; Causticum; Conium; Lycopodium; Nux vomica; Medorrhinum; Lachesis; Thuja; Sabal; Sulphur; Mercurius

- *Sleep (including insomnia, thoughts, disturbed, restless, anxious; too short or too long, and unrefreshing):* Arsenicum album; Argentum nitricum; Calcarea carbonica; Calcarea sulphurica; Causticum; Conium; Lycopodium; Nux vomica; Medorrhinum; Lachesis; Thuja; Sabal; Sulphur; Mercurius

- *Fevers (including infections, inflammation, viral, bacterial, malarial, and nervous):* Aconite; Arsenicum album; Baptisia; Belladonna; China; Bryonia; Gelsemium; Hepar sulphuris; Lycopodium; Natrum muriaticum; Nux vomica; Phosphorus; Pyrogenium; Rhus tox.; Silica; Stramonium; Sulphur

- *Organs (including liver, spleen, heart, kidney, bladder, brain, and gallbladder):* Arsenicum album; Apis; Cantharis; Calcarea carbonica; China; Ceanothus; Cardus marianus; Alumina; Crategus; Aurum; Berberis; Equisetum; Chelidonium; Lycopodium; Lachesis; Natrum mur.; Phosphorus; Nux vomica; Belladonna

- *The mind (including anxiety, fears, lack of confidence, anger, despair, confusion, blame, mental exhaustion, grief, guilt, mental restlessness, apathy, impatience, sensitivity, stubborness, shyness, suicidal feelings, and worry):* Aconite; Aurum; Arsenicum album; Argentum nitricum; Causticum; Calcarea carbonica; Calcarea phosphorica; Carcinosin; Kari carbonicum; Ignacia; Lycopodium; Nux vomica; Natrum muriaticum; Natrum phosphoricum; Mercurius; Nitricum acidum; Phosphoricum acidum; Phosphorus; Stramonium; Silica; Sulphur; Thuja

As mentioned earlier, there are over twenty-eight hundred proven remedies, and it would be impossible to include all of the appropriate ones in the preceding list. But generally speaking, you will find that one or more of the remedies mentioned here are frequently included in a combination.

The main reason to take a formula or combination remedy is to get well or recover from an illness or accident. This recovery should be quick, painless, and without side effects. Just as important for some is the low cost of the remedies in comparison to typical medical expenditures.

Using formula remedies essentially covers each of these components, especially in acute or short-acting ailments. The remedy best suited to the illness is often found within the combination, as there may be up to ten remedies combined in a formula. In effect, it is just the one that fits the disharmony that helps to alleviate it, while the others are rendered inert by the very effectiveness of the productive one.

For example, consider the case of a twenty-four-year-old woman who has allergies to ragweed with the following symptoms: sneezing; burning, tearing eyes; itching throat; runny nose with a clear, watery discharge; head feels stuffy or congested; occasional wheezing with cough.

Combination remedies for allergies would generally include Allium cepa, Arsenicum album, Euphrasia,

Arundo, Wyethia, Sabadilla, Ambrosia, and possibly Nux vomica, Arsenicum iodatum, or Natrum muriaticum. But there is only one remedy that stands out above all the others and fits each of the allergic symptoms described in our example: Ambrosia.

As Ambrosia so closely matches these symptoms, it eliminates them, brings about balance in the body, and more or less negates the other listed remedies. Allergies disappear, the immune system becomes stronger, and after a few more doses, the symptoms may not even return—all because the best-suited remedy fit the symptom picture.

However, homeopathic remedies work because they relate to the symptoms and the person, not because they are "magic pills." The body often takes a long time to recover balance, depending, of course, on the duration of illness. Remedies assist in accelerating the healing and balancing process, but not overnight. They work for the simple reason that they elevate the body to exert its fullest potential in recovery. But potential is rarely reached in a single day. Time and perseverance are part of the underlying principles of homeopathy, especially considering the time it takes to reach imbalance.

Combination remedies have a clear advantage over antacids, aspirin, or other pain relievers, as they do not have side effects and can be just as potent. If the intent is to just get better for the moment, without considering the long term, then formula remedies are useful and relatively inexpensive. On the other hand, should your interest be in a more permanent type of healing, then you need to consider deeper, single remedies.

Most of us take pills, whether they are medications, herbs, or homeopathic remedies, to recover our health and eliminate the return of symptoms. Ragweed is more a trigger for allergic reactions than it is the actual cause. The specific cause can relate more to an oversensitive adrenal system, overuse of chemicals, inherited tendencies, processed foods, vaccinations, or even pollution from the environment.

When we just treat allergic reactions, we do not alter the cause or replenish the adrenal system. We have a temporary resolution, and for some that is all that is needed. For others, elimination on a permanent basis is the ultimate goal. We are a nation desirous of the "quick fix," without consideration for the ill effects that such a "fix" has on the body.

Remember: Use combinations for the short term and a single remedy for the long term (for chronic illness). For help choosing single remedies, consult with a homeopath. Fortunately, homeopathic education has increased over the past decade, and there are some excellent practitioners available in North America. Many are nondoctors who specialize in this growing field, allowing the costs to remain reasonable.

In 1990, there were over thirty-seven million people who used alternative medical practices, and combination remedies were considered some of the safest and most reliable ones available. Traditional medicine does not effectively treat certain illnesses, or if it does, side effects are frequently greater than the disease.

A good example is the overuse of antibiotics for children with ear infections. After the antibiotic, the body's natural ability to combat bacteria is diminished, and so infections keep coming back. Combination remedies eliminate this type of recurrence and assist the body in preventing susceptibility to future disharmonies.

HOW TO USE HOMEOPATHIC REMEDIES

Homeopathic remedies in pill form look and taste like little sugar pills. They also come suspended in alcohol or other types of liquid dilution. When you take the pills, it is best not to touch them with your hands. Most homeopathic remedy containers provide a bottle cap or other type of top to make it easy for you to avoid touching the pills. Just pour the pills out into the top and then directly into your mouth. The pills should be dissolved in the mouth rather than chewed or swallowed.

The liquid remedies can be dropped right on the tongue (don't touch the dropper to your mouth) or added to clean water.

The container will suggest the dose. Dosage is not as important in homeopathy as getting the right remedy. When you are self-treating, it is probably best to use potencies of 6–30x or 6–30c.

Most homeopaths recommend that you not eat or drink anything within 20 or 30 minutes of taking a homeopathic remedy. While you are taking a homeopathic remedy, you should not drink coffee or consume anything containing a strong essential oil, such as eucalyptus, tea tree oil, peppermint, menthol, and camphor. Other things that can "antidote," or cancel out, the effectiveness of homeopathic remedies are drugs, nail polish, and any type of strong negative emotional stress. People respond very differently to homeopathic medicines. Some people are very sensitive to them and may have them canceled out by relatively minor tastes, smells, or events, while in others the remedies keep on working almost regardless of what they do. I recommend that you keep a diary of what you experience and how you're feeling.

Homeopathic combinations, when used as directed, and with proven remedies, are safe and effective and rarely have any side effects. You can feel confident that this approach, which has been used for over two hundred years, effectively stimulates the immune system rather than diminishes it. Homeopathy, whether used in combination or as a single remedy, assists the body in rediscovering its natural ability to heal itself. Few other approaches to healing can make that same claim.

SIXTY-TWO OF THE MOST COMMONLY PRESCRIBED HOMEOPATHIC REMEDIES

This section is a listing of sixty-two homeopathic remedies and their "symptoms," as described by homeopath David Dancu. They are only a small portion of the twenty-eight hundred remedies available, but they will give you a very good sense of what is available and what types of symptoms to look for in a homeopathic treatment. According to Dancu, some 70 to 80 percent of all disharmonies treated with homeopathy will be well served by using one of these remedies. Use this as a general guide and as a way to familiarize yourself with the essence and identity of each remedy.

Studying and understanding homeopathic remedies is a long-term process. Many remedies have similar traits and symptoms, but each has some unique component to set it apart from the others. These are the aspects that give a deeper comprehension of its essence and help establish a better grasp of the whole remedy.

Aconite. Anxiety and fears; shock; panic attacks; early or sudden onset of illness; restlessness; worse after cold, wet weather.

Alumina. Anxiety from being hurried; dullness; mental slowness; dryness of all membranes; constipation; disorientation; dizziness; itchiness of the skin without eruptions.

Anacardium. Low self-esteem; abusive; cursing; depression; fears and delusions; controlling; violent and angry; brain fatigue; most symptoms are better from eating; strong sexual desires.

Apis. Redness, itching, swelling; busy; thirstless; right-sided ailments; worse from heat applications.

Argentum nitricum. Anxiety and panic attacks; impulsive; feelings of abandonment; open and excitable; warm-blooded; worse after eating sweets, but craves them; gastrointestinal problems; left-sided ailments; many phobias.

Arnica. Trauma; injuries; concussions; bruises; irritability; prefers to be alone; pain relief; refuses doctor's help.

Arsenicum album. Anxiety; restlessness; avarice; compulsive; fearful; depressed; skin disharmonies; chilly; controlling without spontaneity; right-sided ailments; worse around midnight; asthma; thirst for small sips; burning sensations.

Aurum. Severe suicidal depression; serious; self-condemnation; guilt and abandonment issues; worse with cloudy weather; intense; worse with pain; anger with remorse; moans during sleep.

Baryta carbonica. Slowness in mental development; immature behavior; low self-esteem; shy and yielding; anxious and nervous; chronic tonsillitis; blank facial expression.

Belladonna. Early onset with redness, heat, flushing of the face, and fever; delirium; anger intense with hitting, biting; migraines; thirstless; strep and sore throats.

Bryonia. Irritability; prefers solitude; fear of business or financial failure; dry mucous membranes and dry colon; intense thirst; warm-blooded; joint problems; worse with any movement/motion.

Calcarea carbonica. Overly responsible; bone problems; fear of heights; fear of going insane; overwhelmed; slow development as a child; stubborn; overweight; slow metabolism; head sweats; milk allergy.

Calcarea phosphorica. Complains about everything; loves change and travel; dissatisfied; sensitive; craves smoked foods; state of weakness; grief with sighing; slow development.

Cantharis. Urinary tract infections; burning sensations; strong sexual desires; incontinence; violent emotions.

Carbo vegetabilis. Intense irritability; gastrointestinal problems; negative; prostration and weakness; coma; indifference; coldness; air hunger.

Carcinosin. Intense, sympathetic, passionate; family history of cancer; fastidious; craves chocolate and spicy foods; moles on back; strong libido; loves animals; low energy from 3 to 6 p.m.; loves travel.

Causticum. Idealistic and rebellious; sympathetic; serious; very sensitive to suffering of others; grief; joint and TMJ problems; warts; compulsive; desires smoked foods; chilly; incontinence.

Chamomilla. Peevish when ill; intense irritability; excessive sensitivity to pains; infant desires to be carried; one cheek red, other pale; colic; ear infections; teething problems; worse with travel.

China officinalis. Internal sensitivity; introverted; taciturn; gastrointestinal disharmonies; worse with loss of fluids; anemia; colitis; worse with touch; periodicity of complaints; fear of animals.

Conium. Emotional flatness or indifference; paralysis; cancer; hardness of glands; tumors; fixed ideas; fogginess of the brain.

Cuprum. Spasms and convulsions; appears emotionally closed; sensation of suffocating; flat facial expression; seizures; rigid; intense emotions suppressed.

Ferrum metallicum. Anemia; desires raw meat; overweight; face flushes easily; very sensitive to noise; strong willed; better walking slowly; general weakness and fatigue; demanding.

Gelsemium. Fatigue; heaviness of the eyelids; brain fatigue; stage fright; weakness of will; cowardly; indifference; forgetful; tremble with anticipation; depressed; thirstless; chilly; headaches; diarrhea.

Graphites. Slowness with poor concentration; skin abnormalities; irritable; anxious; herpes; indecisive; many self-doubts; fastidious; overweight tendencies; offensive sweats; restlessness; photophobia.

Hepar sulphuris. Anger when security is threatened; irritable; worse with any draft of air; sensitive; chilly; infections and abscesses; intense and hurried; rarely cheerful; abusive; overreacts to pain.

Hyoscyamus. Paranoia; jealous with violent outbursts; intense sexual desires; worse with touch; hyperactive child; shameless; defiant; delusions; talkative; fear of dogs; wild gestures.

Ignacia. Acute grief or worse since grief; romantic/idealistic; aggravation from consolation; prefers to be alone; stress is better after eating; better with exercise; sighing; disappointed love.

Iodum. Very warm; thyroid dysfunctions; very restless and busy; compulsive; talkative and anxious; impulsive; intense appetite; anger; avoids company; discontent and destruction; general fears.

Kali bichromicum. Sinus disharmonies/headaches; strong sense of right and wrong; thick, yellow, ropy discharges; rigid and proper; self-occupied; suppresses emotional aspect of personality.

Kali carbonicum. Righteous and strong sense of duty; mind rules emotions; fear of losing control; rigid; asthma; possessive; conservative; quarrelsome; self-reproach; worse 2 to 5 a.m.

Lachesis. Left-sided complaints; loquacity; suspicious; jealous; sarcastic; opinionated and can be fanatical; warm-blooded; all types of menstrual disharmonies; intense personality; vindictive; active mind; drug and alcohol addictions; low self-esteem.

Ledum. Prefers solitude; hatred for self and others; joint problems; worse with heat, although chilly; worse with movement or motion; irritable; insect bites, lockjaw, or injuries with bruising; puncture wounds.

Lycopodium. Poor self-confidence; anger and irritability; liver and kidney disharmonies; fears and anxieties; hyperactive children; right-sided ailments; low energy 4 to 8 p.m.; anticipatory anxiety; tendency to dominate or control; opinionated; avoids responsibility; digestive problems; generally chilly but prefers open air and worse with warmth.

Magnesia muriatica. Yielding; aversion to confrontations; feels anxious at night; very responsible; noises annoy; composed, with suppressed inner anger; depression; unrefreshing sleep.

Medorrhinum. Nasal discharges; cruel and aggressive behavior; an extremist; "sex, drugs, and rock 'n' roll"; self-centered and loves danger; obsessive/compulsive; history of STDs; hurried; intense passions; bites fingernails; overwhelmed by impulses; night person; loves sea.

Mercurius. Strong reaction to temperature changes; emotionally closed; stammering speech; conservative; anxious with destructive ideas; paranoia; façade; worse at night; excess saliva; night sweats; serious appearance; metallic taste in mouth; gum infections.

Natrum carbonicum. Very sensitive; craves potatoes; inner turmoil and depression with appearance of cheerfulness; prefers solitude; emotionally closed; sweet and selfless; delicate; poor digestion; worse heat and sun; sadness; milk allergies; sympathetic.

Natrum muriaticum. Fear of being hurt; closed emotionally from past grief; very sensitive; critical; perfectionist; romantic; strong desire for solitude; serious and controlled; introverted; depression; generally worse from being in the sun or heat; hay fever; herpes.

Natrum sulphuricum. Head injuries and concussions; suicidal depressions; very responsible and serious; warm-blooded; feels better after a bowel movement; emotionally closed; asthma; possible past history of STDs; sensitive; practical, with business focus.

Nitricum acidum. Generally negative person; self-discontent and anger; curses; restless; hypersensitive; selfish; anxieties about health and death; vindictive; chilly pains come and go suddenly.

Nux vomica. Type A personality; ambitious; meticulous; hypersensitive, with tendency to overreact; liver and bowel remedy; driven to excess; addictive personality; sensitive nervous system; intense irritation from wind; chilly; increased hunger.

Petroleum. Skin disharmonies of all types, with dryness; quick temper; motion sickness; herpes; offensive perspiration; unable to make decision; chilly; worse in winter; increased hunger.

Phosphoricum acidum. Dullness and slowness; apathy; feels overwhelmed with grief and emotions; intense fatigue and loss of energy; yielding; desires refreshing fruits; dehydration; chilly.

Phosphorus. Expressive and extroverted; prefers consolation and company; impressionable and very sensitive; many fears and anxieties; affectionate; chilly, yet likes cold drinks; craves spicy, salty, and sweets; sympathetic; intuitive; nosebleeds.

Platinum. Primarily a female remedy; haughty to the extreme; is worse with touch; idealistic; dwells on the past; feels abandoned; dislikes children; insolent and rude; pretentious; strong libido.

Plumbum. Taciturn; sad; shy; selfish; difficulty in expressing themselves; indifference; illness slow in development; very chilly; pains tend to radiate; neurological disorders.

Psorinum. Skin dysfunction of all types; periodicity; pessimist; tends to despair with hopelessness; anxiety and fear, especially of poverty; very chilly; low energy; feels forsaken/lost; dirty skin.

Pulsatilla. Warm-blooded; capricious mood swings; PMS; mild and dependent nature; female remedy; abandonment issues; desires consolation; weepy; digestive and sinus (thick yellow/green mucus) problems; worse with heat and craves fresh air; thirstless with dryness.

Rhus toxicodendron. Great internal restlessness; obsessive tendencies; skin and joint remedy; feels better stretching and with motion; withholds affections/feelings; apprehensive at night; timid; herpes with burning and itching; worse with cold/damp.

Ruta. Affects tendons and fibrous tissues; distrustful; startles easily; argumentative; stiffness/pain; strains; sprains; eyestrain; related headaches; worse with motion or lying on painful side.

Sepia. Indifference and desire to be alone; impatience; irritability; low sexual desire; chilly; grief and depression; PMS/menopause; bearing-down sensations; leucorrhea; taciturn and negative; herpes.

Silica. Yielding, timid, and bashful; emotionally dependent; low self-esteem; stubborn; chilly; conscientious about details; constipation; slow development; weakness; perspires easily; recurring infections.

Spigelia. Left-sided ailments; serious; responsible; violent pains; migraines; grief; worse with tobacco smoke; anxiety of pointed objects; pinworms; combination heart and eye symptoms; chilly; worse with touch.

Spongia. Fear of suffocation; heart ailments; increased anxiety; dry mucous membranes; dry, barking, croupy cough; easily frightened; thyroid disharmonies; respiratory conditions; weakness.

Staphysagria. Sweet, yielding person; suppressed emotions; very sensitive; emotionally dependent; fear of losing control; possible history of sexual abuse or humiliation; strong sexual history; grief; suppressed anger; low self-confidence; worse after nap; mild.

Stramonium. Violent tendencies; etiology from a fright; impulsive rage; wild behavior; night terror; desires company and light; intense thirst; flushed face; excitable; stammers; convulsions; promiscuous; hyperactive children; could be mild, gentle, and very sensitive.

Sulphur. Idealistic and philosophical; self-contained; indolent; warm-blooded; burning sensations; desires spicy foods; appearance is not important; collects things; opinionated; desires open air; itch; offensive discharges; offended by others' body odor; aversion to bathing.

Syphilinum. Compulsive tendencies; worse at night; very chilly; alcoholic; excess saliva; fear of disease/germs or going insane; nails are distorted; anxious; indifferent; worse with hot or cold extremes.

Thuja. Low self-confidence; emotionally closed and hard to get to know; secretive; fastidious; hurried; herpes and suppressed venereal disease; ailments after vaccinations; urine stream is forked; runny nose; chilly; left-sided ailments; irritable; warts; oily skin.

Tuberculinum. Desires change and travel; feels unfulfilled; can be mean; compulsive; chilly; respiratory disharmonies; milk and cat allergies; hyperactive children; romantic longings; desires smoked foods; excess perspiration at night; itch, better with heat.

Veratrum album. Self-righteous and haughty; thinking more than feeling; precocious child; hyperactive child; ambitious; deceitful; very chilly; abusive spouse; critical; jealous; restlessness; religious mania; excessive cold sweats; inappropriate kissing or hugging.

Zincum. Hypersensitive and overstimulated; impulsive movements; restlessness; always complaining; mentally overwhelmed and fatigued; worse when drinking wine or alcohol; superstitious; chilly; affected by noises; feels better after eating.

REMEDIES FOR SHORT-TERM, ACUTE ILLNESSES

Homeopathic self-treatment and combination remedies are best suited to acute illnesses. An acute illness is self-limiting, meaning that it has a life span of approximately seven to ten days. Without any treatment, it usually goes away on its own. This section is a compilation of the most common acute remedies, as compiled by homeopath, teacher, and author David Dancu.

Homeopathy is not used for every symptom that arises, as these symptoms are the body's messages of disharmony. A fever is a message that there is an infection, and body heat is a means of disarming or eliminating the infection. By allowing the body to function as much as possible without outside influences, it finds a way to recover and regain its energy, balance, and strength.

The following list of remedies covers a variety of acute illnesses along with some proven remedies. These brief symptoms will help you in using homeopathy for short-term, acute illnesses and can be helpful in some emergencies. Obviously, if there is a crisis or critical situation, common sense dictates that proper medical treatment be obtained. On the other hand, homeopathic remedies are excellent for shock and emergencies while a person is being transported to the hospital or health care provider.

Accidents

Abrasions/Cuts

- Arnica for trauma of all types and bleeding, even coma.
- Calendula for antiseptic use, either internal or external.

- Hypericum for injury to nerve endings or incisions.
- Ledum helps heal puncture and penetration wounds.

Bites

- Belladonna for dog and snake bites.
- Hypericum when pain seems excessive for wound.
- Lachesis for snake bites or with flushes of heat.
- Ledum for all types of bites with coldness around area.

Bleeding

- Ferrum phosphoricum helps coagulate the blood.
- Ipecacuanha for gushing, bright red blood with nausea.
- Lachesis when blood is dark and area is blue.
- Phosphorus for all types of hemorrhaging.

Bruises

- Arnica for bruises or muscle injuries.
- Bellis for trauma, contusions, and soreness.
- Hamamelis helps with internal bleeding and bruising.
- Ruta for stiffness in muscles and tendons from bruising.

Burns

- Belladona for fever, flushing of the face, and delirium.
- Cantharis reduces pain and promotes healing process.
- Hypericum reduces pain when nerve endings are involved, such as spine, fingers, and teeth.
- Urtica urens for first- and second-degree burns.

Head Injuries

- Arnica for all types, conscious or unconscious.
- Cicuta for dilated pupils, muscle spasms, and stiffness.

- Gelsemium for occipital pain and heaviness of the eyes.
- Hypericum for numbness, tingling, and seizures.

Shock

- Aconite after sudden fright or fearful situation.
- Arnica after an injury or trauma, causing shock.
- Carbo vegetabilis for fainting, coldness, and difficulty breathing.
- Veratrum album when skin and perspiration are very cold.

Whiplash

- Bryonia when any movement is painful.
- Causticum when neck muscles and tendons contract.
- Hypericum if nerves and a tingling sensation are involved.
- Rhus tox. for injuries that are better with motion and heat.

Allergies

Anaphylactic Shock

- Apis for constriction, inflammation, swelling, hives, redness of the skin, and soreness; worse with heat.
- Urtica urens for eruptions, itching, blotches, and burning; heat with a stinging sensation.
- *Consider:* Arsenicum album; Natrum mur.; Rhus tox.

To Animals

- Arsenicum album for respiratory-related reactions.
- Allium cepa for clear, burning nasal discharge with runny eyes.
- Euphrasia for profuse, burning discharge from eyes.
- Natrum mur. for egg white–like discharge; cannot smell.

- *Consider:* Sabadilla; Nux vomica; Tuberculinum; Sulphur.

To Chemicals

- Arsenicum when there is a burning sensation after exposure.
- Coffea for excitability of the mind and nervousness.
- Mercurius when you feel worse at night with excess sweat.
- Nitricum acidum for the oversensitive, depressed, and negative types.
- *Consider:* Nux vomica; Phosphorus; Sulphur; Psorinum.

To Dust

- Arsenicum album when respiration/wheezing is involved.
- Bromium when there is a feeling of suffocation and coldness.
- Hepar for heart palpitations and anxious wheezing.
- *Consider:* Silica; Ipecacuanha; Pothos.

To Foods

- Beans: Bryonia; Lycopodium; Petroleum; Calcarea carb.
- Bread: Bryonia; Lycopodium; Natrum mur.; Pulsatilla; Sepia.
- Cheese: Arsenicum; Nux vomica; Phosphorus; Sepia.
- Coffee: Cantharis; Causticum; Chamomilla; Nux vomica.
- Fruit: Arsenicum; Bryonia; China; Colocynthis; Pulsatilla.
- Meat: Arsenicum; Calcarea; China; Ferrum; Kali carb.
- Milk: Calcarea; China; Magnesium mur.; Natrum carb.; Sepia.
- Onions: Lycopodium; Thuja; Sulphur; Ignacia; Pulsatilla.
- Potatoes: Aluminum; Bryonia; Silica; Sepia; Pulsatilla.

- Salt: Carbo vegetabilis; Natrum mur.; Drosera; Phosphorus; Silica.
- Starches: Berberis; Lycopodium; Natrum mur.; Lachesis.
- Sugar: Argentum nit.; Lycopodium; Sulphur; Phosphorus.
- Vegetables: Aluminum; Bryonia; Kali carb.; Natrum sulph.
- Wheat: Allium cepa; Lycopodium; Natrum mur.; Pulsatilla.

Hay Fever

- Arsenicum iod. for profuse watery discharges and tickling.
- Arum for sneezing and tickling sensations; congestion.
- Arundo for burning and itch in nostrils with sneezing.
- Wyethia for itching of the palate and dry mucous membranes.
- *Consider:* Arsenicum; Allium cepa; Sabadilla; Euphrasia.

Insect Bites

- Apis for hot, swollen skin that is worse with heat.
- Hypericum for tingling sensations or numbness.
- Ledum for any puncture wound with coldness around the wound.
- Urtica urens for hives, itching, redness, and worse with heat.
- *Consider:* Arsenicum; Belladonna; Thuja; Lachesis.

Poison Ivy

- Anacardium for intense itch with swelling and redness.
- Bryonia for swelling, heat, dryness, thirst, and irritability.
- Croton tig. for painful scratching and pustules; intense.
- Graphites for a watery discharge from the reaction.

- *Consider:* Clematis; Rhus tox.; Sepia; Sanguinaria.

To Smoke

- Euphrasia for burning in the eyes and nasal discharge.
- Ignacia when breathing is affected; person feels annoyed.
- Sepia for nausea and exhaustion with any left-sidedness.
- Spigelia for dryness, tickling, and constriction in throat.
- *Consider:* Nux vomica; Natrum mur.; Causticum; Sulphur.

Childhood Ailments

Chicken Pox

- Aconite for the first stages of the outbreak.
- Antimonium crudum when overheated and angry.
- Rhus tox. for restless, intense itch with swollen glands.
- Sulphur for a burning itch that is worse in heat and sweat.

Colds

- Aconite for sudden onset from cold, dry winds.
- Belladonna for early stage with fever, redness, and thirst.
- Kali bic. when discharge is thick, yellow-green, and ropy.
- Pulsatilla for thick yellow mucus and clinging to parent.
- *Consider:* Allium cepa; Euphrasia; Hepar; Nux vomica.

Colic

- Chamomilla when desires to be carried, is irritable and angry.
- Colocynthis for a bloated stomach with intense pains.

- Dioscorea for arching back with cramping pains and gas.
- Magnesia phos. when a child feels better bending double with cramps.

Coughs

- Barking: Aconite; Belladonna; Drosera; Spongia.
- Croupy: Aconite; Hepar sulphuris; Spongia; Lachesis; Phosphorus.
- Dry: Belladonna; Bryonia; Drosera; Natrum mur.; Rumex.
- Hacking: Allium cepa; Arsenicum; Drosera; Phosphorus.
- Rattling: Antimonium tart.; Causticum; Dulcamura; Ipecacuanha.
- Violent: Belladonna; Causticum; Cuprum; Lachesis; Phosphorus.
- Whooping: Antimonium tart.; Carbo vegetabilis; Cuprum; Drosera.

Diarrhea

- Arsenicum for a watery, burning stool with nausea.
- China for a painless stool containing undigested food.
- Podophyllum for a frequent, gushing stool that is smelly.
- Rheum for sour-smelling stool resulting from teething.
- *Consider:* Nux vomica; Sulphur; Silica; Rhus tox.

Earache

- Aconite for the early stages with cold symptoms.
- Chamomilla when pain and irritability arise together.
- Hepar for smelly discharges; is worse when cold.
- Pulsatilla for congestion with redness and discharge.
- *Consider:* Lycopodium; Silica; Mercurius; Belladonna.

Fevers

- Aconite for sudden onset with anxiety, heat, and dryness.
- Belladonna for flushed face, burning heat, and delirium.
- Gelsemium for shivering, heat, drowsiness, and no sweat.
- Mercurius for excess saliva; heat alternates with chills.
- *Consider:* Natrum mur.; Nux vomica; Pulsatilla; Sulphur.

Indigestion

- China when gas arises after eating fruit; bloated.
- Ignacia when problem is caused by any type of emotional upset.
- Lycopodium for gas and bloating made worse by eating.
- Nux vomica from overindulgence of food or drink.
- *Consider:* Argentum nitricum; Pulsatilla; Carbo vegetabilis; Sulphur.

Influenza

- Oscillococcinum for the earliest stages, within 24 hours.
- Baptisia for prostration, muscle soreness, and stomachache.
- Eupatorium when there is deep bone ache and debility.
- Gelsemium for drowsiness, aches, chills, and exhaustion.
- *Consider:* Arsenicum; Bryonia; Rhus tox.; Nux vomica.

Measles

- Aconite is excellent for early stages.
- Belladonna for fever; is used in early stages.
- Bryonia for cough, fever, dryness, and intense thirst.
- Pulsatilla if restless and desires attention; no thirst.

- *Consider:* Gelsemium; Apis; Euphrasia; Phosphorus.

Mumps

- Belladonna for swelling, fever, heat, and redness.
- Jaborandi for redness, swollen glands, and excess saliva.
- Mercurius for painful swelling, fever, and profuse sweat.
- Rhus tox. for swelling with fever; better with heat.
- *Consider:* Aconite; Apis; Lachesis; Phytolacca; Pulsatilla.

Rash (Diaper)

- Apis for red, sore, shiny, hot skin; worse with heat.
- Petroleum for dry, red, itching, cracked skin.
- Rhus tox. when it is better with hot baths; skin itches, flakes, and burns.
- Sulphuricum acidum for blotchy, red skin; worse with heat.
- *Consider:* Sulphur; Graphites; Mezereum; Urtica urens.

Sore Throat

- Aconite for heat and fever from dry, cold winds.
- Belladonna is the first choice with heat and redness.
- Causticum for burning, soreness, rawness, and tightness.
- Phytolacca for congestion, redness, and extreme pain.
- *Consider:* Apis; Hepar; Lachesis; Mercurius; Gelsemium.

Teething

- Belladonna for pain, fever, shrieking; restless and flushed.
- Calcarea phos. for slow, difficult dentition.
- Chamomilla for intense pain, irritability, and hot cheeks.

- Pulsatilla for clinginess; painful dentition; better in fresh air.
- *Consider:* Coffea; Silica; Kreosotum; Rheum; Phytolacca.

Headaches

Hormonal

- Cyclamen for a flickering sensation; worse in open air and when chilled.
- Kreosotum for menstrual headaches with irritability.
- Lachesis for burning pain, coming in waves; left-sided with burning.
- Sepia when feels as if there is a band around the head; left side; sad.
- Pulsatilla for when you feel weepy, sad, thirstless, and are sweating; better in open air.
- *Consider:* Lycopodium; Natrum mur.; Belladonna; Lac caninum.

Migraine

- Bryonia for a pressing sensation with thirst; worse with motion.
- Gelsemium for dull, droopy mind fog; blurred vision.
- Glonoinum for throbbing pain, heaviness, and irritability.
- Melilotus for bursting pain with red face and nausea.
- Sanguinaria for right-sided pain that radiates to eye; worse in the morning.
- *Consider:* Belladonna; Iris; Coffea; Apis; Nux vomica; Spigelia.

Periodic

- Arsenicum for one specific time of day with burning; better with heat.
- China when worse from loss of fluids or malaria; liver ailments.
- Nitricum acidum for burning nasal discharge; worse with pressure.
- Silica for radiating pains, head sweats, worse with drafts, chills.

- *Consider:* Natrum mur.; Sanguinaria; Sepia; Lachesis; Ignacia.

Sick

- Chelidonium for liver-related and right-sided sickness with drowsiness.
- Cocculus for motion sickness, loss of sleep, or noise.
- Nux vomica for overindulgence of any kind.
- Picric acidum for mental strain, fatigue, or travel.
- *Consider:* Iris; Ipecacuanha; Sulphur; Arsenicum album; Sanguinaria.

Sinus

- Dulcamara for changes in barometric pressure; worse in damp air.
- Euphrasia for burning sensation in the eyes with tearing.
- Kali bic. for burning sensation at root of nose; pain in one area; sinusitis.
- Mercurius for excess saliva, bad breath, and metallic taste.
- *Consider:* Calcarea sulph.; Hepar; Nux vomica; Thuja; Natrum mur.

Tension

- Argentum nitricum for an enlarged-head feeling with impulsiveness.
- Ignacia when you feel worse from any emotional stress or anxiety.
- Natrum mur. when feels like pounding hammers; worse 10:00 a.m.; throbs.
- Phosphoricum acidum when apathetic; worse from loss of fluids or emotions.
- Zincum when exhausted, nervous, and restless; noise sensitive.
- *Consider:* Coffea; Gelsemium; China; Nux vomica; Thuja; Phosphorus.

Sports Injuries

Broken Bones/Fractures

- Arnica for the earliest stages of trauma or injury.

- Bryonia when pain is intense from any type of motion.
- Calcarea phos. helps in formation of callus in fractures.
- Symphytum helps bones to properly knit after being set.
- *Consider:* Hypericum; Rhus tox.; Ruta; Silica; Calcarea.

Dislocations

- Calcarea when the problem is chronic and fails to heal.
- Carbo animalis for diminished strength and tendon contraction.
- Kali nitricum for numbness, heaviness, and weakness of limbs.
- Ruta when tendons are involved, especially wrist and ankle.
- *Consider:* Arnica; Natrum carb.; Rhus tox.; Lycopodium; Bryonia.

Hip Pointers

- Aesculus for radiating pain that is worse on standing.
- Calcarea phos. for stiffness; worse with motion or air drafts.
- Rhus tox. if stretching reduces pain; better with heat.
- Ruta for lameness and stiffness; better when lying down.
- *Consider:* Arnica; Bellis; Hamamelis; Symphytum; Bryonia.

Pulled Hamstring

- Ambra-G for drawing pain; limb seems shortened; tingling.
- Bellis for soreness, stiffness, coldness, and bruising.
- Causticum for hardness of tendons and contractions; cramps.
- Ledum for swelling and stiffness; better with ice.
- *Consider:* Arnica; Ruta; Rhus tox.; Bryonia; Sulphuricum acidum.

Sprains/Strains

- Asafoetida for hysteria with bone pains and inflammation.
- Bellis for stiffness with a bruised sensation.
- Bryonia when worse from any movement; wants to be alone.
- Millefolium for tearing pains from overexertion; irritable.
- *Consider:* Arnica (first); Rhus tox.; Ruta; Ledum.

Travelers' Ailments

Constipation

- Alumina when patient has no desire for stool or may strain; straining; worse with travel.
- Bryonia for dark, dry, hard stool; very thirsty for cold water.
- Nux vomica when bloated and irritable; never feels fully vacated.
- Silica for ineffectual urging; hard stool that pulls back in.
- *Consider:* Plumbum; Sulphur; Opium; Aloe; Sepia; Nitricum acidum.

Diarrhea

- Aconite after cold, dry wind or fright.
- Arsenicum for prostration, vomiting, restlessness, and anxiety.
- China after eating fruit or a summer chill; painless; fever.
- Colocynthis for intense colicky pains; better with pressure.
- *Consider:* Nux vomica; Veratrum album; Podophyllum; Aloe; Sulphur.

Indigestion

- Anacardium for heartburn 2 hours after eating; pain, fullness.
- Carbo vegetabilis for offensive gas, bloating, pain, and internal heat.
- Lycopodium when bloated with pain; better after passing gas.
- Nux vomica when worse after overeating; gas, bloating, and cramping.

- *Consider:* Arsenicum; Bryonia; China; Pulsatilla; Sulphur; Hepar.

Influenza/Cold

- Baptisia for prostration, cramps, nausea, and confusion.
- Eupatorium perf. for deep bone aches with chills and headache.
- Ferrum phos. for the earliest stages without clear symptoms.
- Gelsemium when achy, chilled, weak, and anxious; heavy eyelids.
- *Consider:* Arsenicum; Bryonia; Nux vomica; Rhus tox.; Hepar.

Jet Lag

- Argentum nitricum for fear and panic when flying; anxious.
- Arnica for being cramped in a seat for a long period.
- Cocculus when lack of sleep causes irritability and fatigue.
- Gelsemium for heavy eyes, headache, weakness, and tired limbs.
- *Consider:* Rescue remedy; Phosphoricum acidum; Zincum; Sulphuricum acidum.

Motion Sickness

- Borax for nausea or vomiting; worse with downward motion.
- Cocculus for queasiness; worse with the thought of food.
- Nux vomica for nausea, headache, and chills; no desire for food.
- Tabacum when chilled, giddy, and sweating; worse with tobacco smoke.
- *Consider:* Rhus tox.; Petroleum; Ipecacuanha.

Sleeplessness

- Arsenicum for restlessness, anxiety, fatigue, and irritability.
- Coffea when nervous, anxious, hypersensitive, and mentally active.

- Ignacia when worse from emotional stress or grief.
- Nux vomica when worse from overeating, alcohol, or mental strain.
- *Consider:* Aconite; Lycopodium; Pulsatilla; Arnica.

Stress

- Natrum mur. for long-term emotional ill effects and solitude.
- Nux vomica when there is mental stress and overstimulation.
- Passiflora when overworked, worried, restless, and exhausted.
- Valeriana when oversensitive, irritable, nervous, and changeable.
- *Consider:* Zincum; Arsenicum; Argentum nitricum; Ignacia; Sepia.

Women's Ailments

Cystitis

- Apis for burning, stinging, and soreness when urinating.
- Cantharis for intense urging, burning.
- Equisetum for bladder fullness, severe pain, and frequent urge.
- Lycopodium for low back pains, straining, and retention.
- *Consider:* Aconite; Belladonna; Lachesis; Sepia; Pulsatilla.

Discharges

- Black: China; Kreosotum; Rhus tox.; Secale.
- Bloody: Calcarea sulph.; China; Cocculus; Nitricum acidum; Sepia.
- Burning: Calcarea; Borax; Kreosotum; Pulsatilla; Sulphur.
- Green: Carbo vegetabilis; Kali bic.; Mercurius; Natrum mur; Sepia.
- Itching: Calcarea; China; Mercurius; Sepia; Kreosotum; Zincum.
- Milky: Calcarea; Kali mur.; Sepia; Silica; Pulsatilla; Lachesis.

- Offensive: Kali; Arsenicum; Kreosotum; Mercurius; Nux vomica.
- Profuse: Calcarea; Graphites; Sepia; Silica; Stannum; Thuja.
- Thick: Arsenicum; Calcarea; Kali bic.; Natrum carb; Thuja; Zinc.
- Thin: Graphites; Nitricum acidum; Pulsatilla; Sulphur; Silica; Sepia.
- White: Borax; Graphites; Natrum mur.; Sepia; Nux vomica; Pulsatilla.
- Yellow: Arsenicum; Calcarea; Chamomilla; Hydrastis; Pulsatilla.

Genital Herpes

- Natrum mur. for tingling sensations; worse in sun or under stress.
- Petroleum for sensations of moisture with crusting and itch.
- Sepia for itching, worse at folds of skin and in spring; odor.
- Thuja for eruptions on covered parts only; sensitive to touch.
- *Consider:* Rhus tox.; Alnus; Medorrhinum; Lachesis; Dulcamara.

Menopause

- Lachesis for hot flashes and fainting; worse with tight clothing.
- Lilium tig. for intensity, depression, irritability, and prolapsed vagina.
- Pulsatilla when clingy, complaining, weepy, and sad; worse with heat.
- Sepia when overwhelmed and irritable; prefers solitude; hot flashes.
- *Consider:* Sulphur; Natrum mur.; Phosphorus; Sabina; Kreosotum.

Menses

- Absent: Aurum; Ferrum; Graphites; Kali carb.; Lycopodium; Pulsatilla.
- Clotted: Belladonna; Calcarea; China; Lachesis; Sabina; Pulsatilla.
- Cramps: Chamomilla; Cocculus; Colocynthis; Magnesia phos.; Sepia.

First-Aid Remedies

Remedy	Used for	Benefits
Arnica (internal and as oil or ointment; use before other remedies to treat the shock of any injury)	Bee, hornet, and wasp stings Bleeding under skin Bruises, ordinary Burns (treatment for shock only) Fractures Injuries from blows or falls Jagged cuts (internal remedies only) Muscular soreness Shin splints Shock Soreness, general Strains, general Strained back muscles Twisted knee (take on first day)	Speeds healing; relieves pain; reduces swelling
Bryonia	Fractured ribs Injured joint (swollen, distended, worse with movement) Twisted knee (take on second day if worse with movement)	Relieves pain; speeds healing
Calendula (nonalcoholic lotion for cuts or ointment for scrapes, etc.; saturate dressing with lotion)	Abrasions Bee, hornet, and wasp stings Bleeding from mouth Burns, first degree (add drops to cold-water treatment)	Cleanses and speeds healing of slight wounds; helps stop bleeding; inhibits infection.
Cantharis	Burns, third degree (internally only)	Speeds healing
Glonoinum	Sunstroke and heat exhaustion	Speeds recovery
Hypericum (lotion for external use)	Burns, second degree (immerse in lotion) Crushed nerves Nerve injuries to extremities and elbows Puncture wounds	Promotes tissue growth; speeds healing; relieves pain
Ledum (lotion for external use)	Bee, hornet, and wasp stings Black eye Bruises (cold, numb, long lasting) Puncture wounds Splinter under nail Swelling	Reduces pain and inflammation, especially when wound relieved by cold
Rhus toxicodendron (use after Arnica)	Blistery itches Injury after lifting/overexertion Joints, creaky Joints, hot, swollen Poison ivy/oak Strained/torn muscles, tendons, ligaments Tendonitis	Relieves aches and itching; speeds healing

(Continued)

Remedy	Used for	Benefits
Ruta (use after Arnica and when Rhus tox. has not helped)	Bruised bone covering Injuries to bones Lame feeling Prolapsed, protruding rectum Soft tissue injuries Sprains to ankle/wrist Strained/torn muscles (when initial swelling has decreased)	Speeds healing

- Frequent: Arsenicum; Belladonna; Cyclamen; Ferrum phos.
- Irregular: Argentum nit.; Nux moschata; Pulsatilla; Sepia; Senecio.
- Late: Causticum; Cuprum; Lachesis; Natrum mur.; Sarsaparilla.
- Painful: Cimicifuga; Magnesia phos.; Millefolium; Cactus; Pulsatilla; Sabina; Sulphur; Caulophyllum; Cyclamen; Chamomilla.
- Profuse: Arsenicum; Ferrum phos.; Phosphorus; Calcarea phos.; Sabina; Senecio; Millefolium; Natrum mur.; Ferrum; Cyclamen.
- Suppressed: Belladonna; Cyclamen; Lachesis; Senecio; Sepia.

Pelvic Inflammatory Disease

- Arsenicum for burning, offensive discharge with anxiety.
- Lac caninum for ovarian pains and vaginal gas; fear of snakes.
- Lachesis for left-sided pains and cysts; worse with tight clothing.
- Sabina for severe PMS, intense pains, gushing flow; leukorrhea.
- *Consider:* Apis; Belladonna; Cantharis; Pulsatilla; Chamomilla; Sepia.

Vaginitis

- Kreosotum for strong itch with burning discharge and odor.
- Medorrhinum for high sex drive and chronic infection; herpes.
- Pulsatilla when needy and capricious; does not tolerate pain.

- Thuja for green discharges, herpes, polyps, and cysts.
- *Consider:* Arsenicum; Graphites; Mercurius; Sepia; Sulphur.

THE HOMEOPATHIC FIRST-AID KIT

Many homeopathic remedies are useful as immediate treatment in the case of injury or accident. Homeopathic treatment for emergencies does not require the detailed taking of a case, as is needed for chronic illnesses. Only a small number of remedies apply. It is important to remember that homeopathic medicines should not be used in place of standard first-aid measures. Always perform these procedures first and summon help when needed.

For on-the-spot treatment, besides pellets and tablets, homeopathic tinctures can be applied directly to injured sites. Tinctures are prepared with alcohol, which can sting cuts and broken skin.

It is always worth using topical applications made from the original substances of certain homeopathic remedies, such as calendula. The creams and lotions make very effective support for remedies taken internally.

First-Aid Doses

Common dosage of homeopathic remedies in first aid is two tablets, three to four times a day. This can increase to two tablets every 30 minutes to 1 hour when pain is severe. Reduce the frequency as improvement begins, but continue dosing until improvement is well established.

GLOSSARY ~

A

absorption The process by which nutrients are passed into the bloodstream.

acetate A derivative of acetic acid.

acetic acid Used as a synthetic flavoring agent, one of the first food additives (vinegar is approximately 4 to 6 percent acetic acid); it is found naturally in cheese, coffee, grapes, peaches, raspberries, and strawberries; generally recognized as safe (GRAS) when used only in packaging.

acetylcholine One of the chemicals involved in the transmission of nerve impulses.

adrenal glands The glands located above each kidney that manufacture adrenaline, noradrenaline, and steroids.

adrenaline A hormone secreted by the adrenal glands into the bloodstream in response to physical or mental stress, such as fear or injury; works with noradrenaline to regulate blood pressure and heart rate.

aldosterone A hormone secreted by the adrenal glands that regulates the salt and water balance in the body; one of the steroids.

alkaline Containing an acid-neutralizing substance; being alkaline, sodium bicarbonate is used for excess acidity in foods.

allergen A substance that causes an allergy.

amenorrhea Absence or suppression of menstruation.

amino acid chelates Chelated minerals that have been produced by many of the same processes that nature uses to chelate minerals in the body; in the digestive tract, nature surrounds the elemental minerals with amino acids, permitting them to be absorbed into the bloodstream.

amino acids The organic compounds from which proteins are constructed; twenty-two amino acids have been identified as necessary to the human body; nine are known as essential—histidine, isoleucine, leucine, lysine, total S-containing amino acids, total aromatic amino acids, threonine, tryptophan, and valine—and must be obtained from food.

androgen Any of the group of hormones that stimulate male characteristics.

angina pectoris A cramping pain in the chest, stemming from the heart and often spreading to the left arm and shoulder.

anorexia Loss of appetite, especially resulting from disease.

anorexia nervosa A psychological disorder featuring an abnormal fear of becoming obese, a persistent aversion to food, a distorted self-image, and severe loss of weight.

antibody A protein substance produced in the blood or tissues in response to a specific antigen, such as a toxin or bacteria; by neutralizing organic poisons and weakening or destroying bacteria, antibodies form the basis of immunity.

antigen Any substance not normally present in the body that stimulates the body to produce antibodies.

antihistimine A drug used to reduce the effects associated with histamine production in allergies and colds.

antineoplastics Drugs that prevent the growth and development of malignant cells.

antioxidant A substance that can protect another substance from oxidation; often added to foods to keep oxygen from changing the food's color.

antitoxin An antibody formed in response to, and capable of neutralizing, a poison of biological origin.

arteriosclerosis A disease of the arteries characterized by hardening, thickening, and loss of elasticity of the arterial walls; results in impaired blood circulation.

arthritis Inflammation of the joints.

assimilation The process whereby nutrients are used by the body and changed into living tissue.

asthma A condition of the lungs characterized by a decrease in diameter of some air passages; a spasm of the bronchial tubes or swelling of their mucous membranes.

ataxia Loss of coordinated movement caused by disease of the nervous system.

atherosclerosis A process whereby fatty deposits in the walls of arteries make the walls thick and hard, narrowing the arteries; a form of arteriosclerosis.

ATP The molecule adenosine triphosphate, the fuel of life; a nucleotide—building block of nucleic acid—that produces biological energy with vitamins B_1, B_2, and B_3, and pantothenic acid, another B-complex vitamin.

autoimmunity An abnormal condition where the body produces antibodies against its own tissue.

avidin A protein in egg white capable of inactivating biotin.

B

bacteriophage A virus that infects bacteria.

basal metabolic rate The body's rate of metabolism when at rest.

basophil A type of white blood cell representing less than 1 percent of the total.

B cells White blood cells, made in bone marrow, that produce antibodies upon instructions from T cells, manufactured in the thymus.

beta-carotene A plant pigment that can be converted into two forms of vitamin A.

BHA Butylated hydroxyanisole; a preservative and antioxidant used in many products; insoluble in water; can be toxic to the kidneys.

BHT Butylated hydroxytoluene; a solid, white crystalline antioxidant used to retard spoilage of many foods; can be more toxic to the kidneys than its nearly identical chemical cousin, BHA.

bioflavonoids A group of compounds needed to maintain healthy blood vessel walls; found chiefly as coloring matter in flowers and fruits, particularly yellow ones; known as vitamin P complex.

biotin A colorless, crystalline B-complex vitamin; essential for the activity of many enzyme systems; helps produce fatty acids; found in large quantities in liver, egg yolk, milk, and yeast.

bursa A pouch, or sac, containing fluid for the lubrication of joints.

bursitis Swelling or inflammation of a bursa.

C

calciferol A colorless, odorless crystalline material, insoluble in water; soluble in fats; a synthetic form of vitamin D made by irradiating ergosterol with ultraviolet light.

calcium gluconate An organic calcium-based compound.

capillary A minute blood vessel, one of many that connect the arteries and veins and deliver oxygen to the tissues.

carcinogen A cancer-causing substance.

cardiotonic A compound that aids the heart.

cardiovascular Relating to the heart and blood vessels.

carotene An orange-yellow pigment occurring in many plants and capable of being converted into vitamin A in the body.

casein The protein in milk that has become the standard by which protein quality is measured.

catabolism The metabolic change of nutrients or complex substances into simpler compounds, accompanied by a release of energy.

catalyst A substance that modifies, especially increases, the rate of chemical reaction without being consumed or changed in the process.

cellulose Carbohydrate found in the outer layers of fruits and vegetables that is undigestible.

cerebrovascular accident A blood clot or bleeding in the brain; a stroke.

chelation A process by which mineral substances are changed into an easily digestible form.

cholesterol A white, crystalline substance, made up of various fats; naturally produced in vertebrate animals and humans; important as a precursor to steroid hormones and as a constituent of cell membranes.

chronic Of long duration; continuing, constant.

CNS Central nervous system.

coenzyme A substance that combines with other substances to form a complete enzyme; nonprotein and usually a B vitamin.

collagen The primary organic constituent of bone, cartilage, and connective tissue.

complex carbohydrate Fibrous molecule of starch or sugar that slowly releases sugar into the bloodstream.

congenital Existing at birth; not hereditary.

coronary occlusion Blockage of a heart artery.

coronary thrombosis Blood clot in a heart artery.

corticosteroids See *steroids*.

D

demineralization The loss of minerals or salts from bone and tissue.

dermatitis An inflammation of the skin; a rash.

diastolic Second number in a blood pressure reading; measures the pressure in arteries between contractions of the heart.

dicalcium phosphate A filler used in pills, that is derived from purified mineral rocks and is a source of calcium and phosphorus.

diluents Fillers; inert material added to tablets to increase their bulk in order to make them a practical size for compression.

disaccharide A sugar that breaks down into two monosaccharides.

diuretic Tending to increase the flow of urine from the body.

DNA Deoxyribonucleic acid; the nucleic acid in chromosomes that is part of the chemical basis for heredity.

E

emulsion A substance with chemical characteristics of both water and oil; aids in mixing and dispersing between the two.

endocrine Producing secretions passed directly to the lymph or blood instead of into a duct; relating to the endocrine glands or the hormones they produce.

endogenous Being produced from within the body.

endorphins Natural opiates produced in the brain; pain suppressants.

enteric coated Describing a tablet that has been coated so that it dissolves in the intestine, not in the acid environment of the stomach.

enzyme A protein substance found in living cells that brings about chemical changes; necessary for digestion of food; compounds with names ending in *-ase*.

epinephrine See *adrenaline*.

ergosterol A vitamin D group steroid; originally found in ergot, a fungal disease of rye; also found in other fungi, yeast, and mushrooms; changed by ultraviolet light into vitamin D_2.

excipient Any inert substance used as a diluent or vehicle for a drug.

exogenous Being derived or developed from external causes.

F

fatty acids Acids produced by the breakdown of fats; essential fatty acids cannot be produced by the body and must be included in the diet.

FDA Food and Drug Administration.

fibrin An insoluble protein that forms the necessary fibrous network in the coagulation of blood; an excess of fibrinogen in the blood increases the risk of heart disease.

free radicals Highly reactive chemical fragments that can beneficially act as chemical messengers but in excess produce an irritation of artery walls and start the arteriosclerotic process if antioxidants are not present.

fructose A natural sugar occurring in fruits and honey, called fruit sugar; often used as a preservative for foodstuffs and an intravenous nutrient.

G

galactosemia A hereditary disorder in which ingested milk becomes toxic.

gland An organ in the body where certain substances in the blood are separated and converted into secretions for use in the body (such as hormones) or to be discharged from the body (such as sweat); nonsecreting structures similar to glands, like lymph nodes, are also known as glands.

glucose Blood sugar; a product of the body's assimilation of carbohydrates and a major source of energy.

glutamic acid An amino acid present in all complete proteins; also manufactured commercially from vegetable protein; used as a salt substitute and flavor-intensifying agent.

glutamine An amino acid that constitutes, with glucose, the major nourishment used by the nervous system.

gluten A mixture of two proteins, gliadin and glutenin, present in wheat, rye, oats, and barley.

glycogen The body's chief form of stored carbohydrate, primarily in the liver; converted to glucose when needed.

GRAS Generally recognized as safe; a list established by Congress to cover substances added to food.

H

HDL High-density lipoprotein; HDL is sometimes called "good" cholesterol because it is the body's major carrier of cholesterol to the liver for excretion in the bile.

hemoglobin Molecule necessary for the transport of oxygen by red blood cells; iron is an essential component.

hesperidin Part of the vitamin C complex.

histamine An organic compound of ammonia released by the body in allergic reactions.

holistic treatment Treatment of the whole person, rather than just parts or symptoms.

homeostasis The body's physiological equilibrium.

hormone A substance formed in endocrine organs and transported by body fluids to activate other specifically receptive organs, cells, or tissues.

humectant A substance that is used to preserve the moisture content of materials.

hydrochloric acid An acid secreted in the stomach; a main part of gastric juice.

hydrolyzed Put into water-soluble form.

hydrolyzed protein chelate Protein that is water-soluble and chelated for easy assimilation.

hyperglycemia Abnormally high blood sugar.

hypoglycemia Abnormally low blood sugar.

I

ichthyosis A condition characterized by a scaliness on the outer layer of skin.

idiopathic A condition whose causes are not yet known.

immune Protected against disease.

infarction Localized tissue death due to lack of oxygen supply.

insulin A hormone, secreted by the pancreas, that helps regulate the metabolism of sugar in the body.

interferon Any of a group of proteins produced by cells in response to infection by a virus; prevents viral replication and can induce resistance to viral antigens.

IU International units.

L

lactating Producing milk.

lactose One of the sugars found in milk.

LDL Low-density lipoprotein; sometimes referred to as "bad" cholesterol, LDLs easily become oxidized and carry cholesterol through the bloodstream; studies show that high levels can increase risk of coronary artery disease (CAD).

lecithin Any of a group of fats rich in phosphorus; essential for transforming fats in the body; rich sources include egg yolk, soybeans, and corn.

linoleic acid One of the polyunsaturated fats; an essential fatty acid; a constituent of lecithin; known as vitamin F; indispensable for life and must be obtained from foods.

lipid A fat or fatty substance.

lipofuscin A group of fats, plentiful in adult cells and associated with aging.

lipotropic Preventing abnormal or excessive accumulation of fat; lipotropin is a hormone that stimulates the conversion of stored fat to usable, liquid form.

lymph The almost clear fluid flowing through the lymphatic vessels; lymph nourishes tissue cells and returns waste matter to the bloodstream.

lymphocyte Any of the almost colorless cells produced in lymphoid tissue, as in the lymph nodes, spleen, thymus, and tonsils; lymphocytes make up between 22 and 28 percent of adult human white blood cells; primarily responsible for antibody production, lymphocytes include B cells and T cells.

M

megavitamin therapy Treatment of illness with massive amounts of vitamins.

metabolism The processes of physical and chemical change whereby food is broken down into simpler substances or waste matter; energy is produced by these processes.

monosaccharide A simple sugar with one molecular unit, such as glucose.

mucopolysaccharide Thick gelatinous material found in many places in the body; it glues cells together and lubricates joints.

N

naturopathy The use of herbs and other methods to stimulate the body's innate defenses without using drugs.

neuropathy Symptoms caused by abnormalities in sensory or motor nerves.

neurotransmitter A chemical substance that transmits or changes nerve impulses.

nitrites Substances used as fixatives in cured meats; can combine with natural stomach and food chemicals to cause dangerous cancer-causing agents called nitrosamines.

noradrenaline A hormone produced in the adrenal glands that increases blood pressure by narrowing blood vessels without affecting the heart's output; works with epinephrine.

norepinephrine See *noradrenaline*.

nucleic acid Any of a group of complex compounds that form a major part of DNA and RNA; found in all living cells and viruses.

O

oncologist Specialist in tumors; cancer specialist.

organic Describing any chemical containing carbon; also describing any food or supplement made with animal or vegetable fertilizers and produced without synthetic fertilizers or pesticides and free from chemical injections or additives.

orthomolecular Referring to the right molecule used for the right treatment; doctors who practice preventive medicine and use vitamin therapies are known as orthomolecular physicians.

OSHA Occupational Safety and Health Administration.

oxalates Organic chemicals found in certain foods, especially spinach, that can combine with calcium to form calcium oxalate, an insoluble chemical that the body cannot use.

oxidation The way certain types of altered oxygen molecules cause biochemical reactions; examples are browning of apples and rancidity in oil.

P

PABA Para-aminobenzoic acid; a member of the vitamin B complex.

palmitate Water-solubilized vitamin A.

peroxides Free radicals formed as by-products when oxygen reacts with molecules of fat.

phytoestrogen Any of a number of compounds found in plants that occupy estrogen receptors and may help protect the body from the negative effects of excess estrogen.

PKU (phenylketonuria) A hereditary disease caused by the lack of an enzyme needed to convert an essential amino acid (phenylalanine) into a form usable by the body; can cause mental retardation unless detected early.

placebo A substance that produces no pharmacological activity; one used instead of and alongside an active substance for comparison.

polysaccharide A molecule made up of many sugar molecules joined together.

polyunsaturated fats Highly nonsaturated fats from vegetable sources; can dissolve or absorb other substances.

precancerous lesion Tissue that is abnormal but not yet malignant.

predigested protein Protein that has been processed for fast assimilation and can go directly into the bloodstream.

prostaglandins Hormonelike substances that aid in regulation of the immune system.

protein A complex substance containing nitrogen that is essential to plant and animal cells; ingested proteins are changed to amino acids in the body.

provitamin A vitamin precursor; a chemical substance necessary to produce a vitamin.

PUFA Polyunsaturated fatty acid.

R

RDA Recommended dietary allowance, as established by the Food and Nutrition Board, National Academy of Sciences, National Research Council.

retrovirus A virus containing RNA.

riboflavin Vitamin B$_2$; part of the B vitamin complex; yellow, crystal-like coenzyme involved in the breakdown of proteins, fats, and carbohydrates; must be obtained from food.

ribonucleic acid (RNA) A constituent of all living cells and many viruses; its structure determines protein synthesis and genetic transmission.

rose hip A rich source of vitamin C; the nodule underneath the bud of a rose called a hip, in which the plant produces vitamin C.

rutin A substance often extracted from buckwheat; part of the vitamin C complex.

S

saturated fatty acids Fatty acids that are usually solid at room temperature; higher proportions found in foods from animal sources.

sclerosis The hardening or thickening of a part of the body, such as an artery.

sequestrant A substance that absorbs some of the products of chemical reactions; it prevents changes that would affect flavor, texture, and color of food; used for water softening.

serotonin A neurotransmitter considered essential for mood and concentration.

serum Any thin, watery fluid; especially the clear, sticky part of blood that remains after clotting.

simple carbohydrate Simple sugar molecule, such as glucose, that is rapidly absorbed by the bloodstream.

steroids Hormones produced by the adrenal glands that influence or control key functions of the body; formed from cholesterol; three major types influencing (1) skin, muscle, fat, and metabolism of glucose, (2) sexual functions and characteristics, and (3) processing of minerals; used as drugs such as cortisone to suppress the immune system, reduce inflammation, and treat allergies.

syncope Brief loss of consciousness; fainting.

synergistic The way two or more substances produce an effect that neither alone could accomplish.

synthetic Produced artificially; not found in nature.

systemic Capable of spreading through the entire body.

systolic First number in a blood pressure reading; measures the pressure in arteries as the heart contracts.

T

T cells White blood cells, manufactured in the thymus, that protect the body from bacteria, viruses, and cancer-causing agents.

teratological Referring to monstrous or abnormal formations in animals or plants.

thymus Major gland of the immune system situated behind the top of the breastbone; site of T cell production.

tocopherols The group of compounds (alpha, beta, delta, epsilon, eta, gamma, and zeta) that make vitamin E; obtained through vacuum distillation of edible vegetable oils.

toxicity The quality or condition of being poisonous, harmful, or destructive.

toxin An organic poison produced in living or dead organisms.

triglycerides Fatty substances in the blood.

U

unsaturated fatty acids Fatty acids most often liquid at room temperature; primarily found in vegetable fats.

US RDA United States recommended dietary allowance.

V

virus Any of a large group of minute organisms that can only reproduce in the cells of plants and animals.

vitamin Any of about fifteen natural compounds essential in small amounts as catalysts for processes in the body; most cannot be made by the body and must come from the diet.

X

xerosis Skin condition characterized by dryness, lacking moisture or oil; often resulting in a pattern of fine lines, scaling, and itching.

Y

yeast Single-celled fungus that can cause infections in the body.

Z

zyme A fermenting substance.

RESOURCES ~

For more information on herbal medicines

The American Botanical Council
P.O. Box 201660
Austin, TX 78720
(512) 331-8868
www.herbalgram.org

The Herb Research Foundation
1007 Pearl Street, Suite 200
Boulder, CO 80302
(303) 449-2265
www.herbs.org

An excellent guide to alternative medicine health care professionals

The Alternative Medicine Yellow Pages, $12.95
    (Available in many bookstores)
Published by:
Future Medicine Publishing
98 Main Street, Suite 209
Tiburon, CA 94920

For referrals to naturopathic physicians

American Association of Naturopathic Physicians
P.O. Box 20386
Seattle, WA 98102
(206) 323-7610

For referrals to Chinese medicine doctors

American Association of Acupuncture and Oriental
    Medicine
4101 Lake Boone Trail, Suite 201
Raleigh, NC 27607
(919) 787-5181

BIBLIOGRAPHY ~

Abbott, Lisa, et al. "Magnesium Deficiency in Alcoholism: Possible Contribution to Osteoporosis and Cardiovascular Disease in Alcoholics." *Alcoholism: Clinical and Experimental Research* 118, no. 5 (Sept./Oct. 1994): 1076–82.

Aebi, S., and B. H. Lauterburg. "Divergent Effects of Intravenous GSH and Cysteine on Renal and Hepatic GSH." *American Journal of Physiology* 263 (Aug. 1992): 348–52.

Alberts, D. S., et al. "Randomized, Double-Blinded, Placebo-Controlled Study of Effect of Wheat Bran Fiber and Calcium on Fecal Bile Acids in Patients with Resected Adenomatous Colon Polyps." *Journal of the National Cancer Institute* 887, no. 2 (Jan. 17, 1996): 81–91.

Austin, Steve, and Cathy Hitchcock. *Breast Cancer: What You Should Know (But May Not Be Told) About Prevention, Diagnosis, and Treatment.* Rocklin, Calif.: Prima Publishing, 1992.

Aw, T. Y., et al. "Absorption and Lymphatic Transport of Peroxidized Lipids by Rat Small Intestine in Vivo: Role of Mucosal GSH." *American Journal of Physiology* 262 (Jan. 1992): 99–106.

Aw, T. Y., et al. "Intestinal Absorption and Lymphatic Transport of Peroxidized Lipids in Rats: Effect of Exogenous GSH." *American Journal of Physiology* 263 (Nov. 1992): G665–72.

Bagga, D., et al. "Effects of a Very Low Fat, High Fiber Diet on Serum Hormones and Menstrual Function." *Cancer* 76, no. 12 (Dec. 15, 1995): 2491–96.

Baghurst, P. A., et al. "Dietary Fiber and Risk of Benign Proliferative Epithelial Disorders of the Breast." *International Journal of Cancer* 63 (1995): 481–85.

Baird, I., et al. "The Effects of Ascorbic Acid and Flavonoids on the Occurrence of Symptoms Normally Associated with the Common Cold." *American Journal of Clinical Nutrition* 32 (1979): 1686–90.

Balasubramaniyan, N., et al. "Status of Antioxidant Systems in Human Carcinoma of Uterine Cervix." *Cancer Letters* 87 (1994): 187–92.

Barnes, R. M. R. "IgG and IgA Antibodies to Dietary Antigens in Food Allergy and Intolerance." *Clinical and Experimental Allergy* 25 (1995) (Suppl. 1): 7–9.

Barrie, N. D. "Effects of Garlic Oil on Platelet Aggregation, Serum Lipids and Blood Pressure in Humans." *Journal of Orthomolecular Medicine* 2, no. 1 (1987): 15–21.

Bauer, J., et al. "Cytokines, Neuropeptides, and Other Factors in Cutaneous Immune Responses." *Western Journal of Medicine* 160, no. 2 (Feb. 1994): 181–83.

Bellavite, P., and A. Signorini. *Homeopathy, A Frontier in Medical Science.* Berkeley, Calif.: North Atlantic Books, 1995.

Bellizzi, M., et al. "Vitamin E and Coronary Heart Disease: The European Paradox." *European Journal of Clinical Nutrition* 48 (1994): 822–31.

Bengmark, S., and B. Jeppsson. "Gastrointestinal Surface Protection and Mucosa Reconditioning." *Journal of Parenteral and Enteral Nutrition* 19 (1995): 410–15.

Bigazzi, Pierluigi E. "Autoimmunity and Heavy Metals." *Lupus* 3 (1994): 449–53.

Bland, J. "The Nutritional Effects of Free Radical Pathology." In *1986—A Year in Nutritional Medicine.* Los Angeles: Keats Publishing, 1986.

Blomqvist, B. I., et al. "Glutamine and Alpha-Ketoglutarate Prevent the Decrease in Muscle Free Glutamine Concentration and Influence Protein Synthesis After Total Hip Replacement." *Metabolism* 44 (1995): 1215–22.

Boericke, W. and Tafel. *The Family Guide to Self-Medication, Homeopathic*. Boericke & Tafel, Inc., 1988.

Bordia, A. "The Effect of Vitamin C on Blood Lipids, Fibrinolytic Activity and Platelet Adhesiveness in Patients with Coronary Artery Disease." *Atherosclerosis* 35 (1980): 181–87.

Bragg, P., et al. *The Complete Triathlon Endurance Training Manual*. Santa Barbara, Calif.: Health Science, 1985.

Braverman, E., et al. *The Healing Nutrients Within: Facts, Findings, and New Research on Amino Acids*. Los Angeles: Keats Publishing, 1987, p. 90.

Buchman, A. L. "Glutamine: Is It a Conditionally Required Nutrient for Human Gastrointestinal System?" *Journal of the American College of Nutrition* 15, no. 3 (1996): 199–205.

Bulpitt, C. "Vitamin and Blood Pressure." *Journal of Hypertension Theory and Practice* A14, nos. 1 and 2 (1992): 119–38.

Burr, M. L., et al. "Effects of Changes in Fat, Fish, and Fiber Intakes on Death and Myocardial Reinfraction." *The Lancet* 2 (1989): 757–61.

Byrnes, P. "Wild Medicine." *Wilderness* 59, no. 210 (1995): 28–33.

Cameron, M. *Lifetime Encyclopedia of Natural Remedies*. Parker Publishing, 1993.

Cara, L., et al. "Effects of Oat Bran, Rice Bran, Wheat Fiber, and Wheat Germ on Postprandial Lipemia in Healthy Adults." *American Journal of Clinical Nutrition* 55 (1992): 81–88.

Carlotti, P., et al. "The Cellular Aging Process and Free Radicals." *Drug & Cosmetic Industry Magazine* 144, no. 2 (Feb. 1989): 22–23.

Carper, J. *Food: Your Miracle Medicine*. New York: Harper Perennial, 1994, pp. 14–16, 240–41.

Carter, C. "Dietary Treatment of Food Allergy and Intolerance." *Clinical and Experimental Allergy* 25 (1995) (Suppl 1.): 34–42.

Ceconi, C., et al. "The Role of Glutathione Status in the Protection Against Ischaemic and Reperfusion Damage: Effects of *N*-Acetyl Cysteine." *Journal of Molecular and Cellular Cardiology* 20, no. 1 (Jan. 1988): 5–13.

Chaitow, L. *Prostate Troubles*. London: Thorsons, Harper Collins, 1988.

Challem, J. "Dietary Changes Can Protect Against Prostate Problems." *Let's Live* (July 1994): 14–15, 18–20.

Chope, H., et al. "Nutritional Status of the Aging." *American Journal of Public Health* 44 (1955): 61–67.

Cichoke, Anthony J. *Enzymes and Enzyme Therapy*. Los Angeles: Keats Publishing, 2000.

Clark, N. *Sports Nutrition Guidebook*. New York: Leisure Press, 1990.

Colgan, Michael. *Optimum Sports Nutrition*. New York: Advanced Research Press, 1993.

Cowan, L. D., L. Gordis, J. A. Tonascia, and G. S. Jones. "Breast Cancer Incidence in Women with a History of Progesterone Deficiency." *American Journal of Cardiology* 114 (1981): 209–17.

Cummings, S., and D. Ullman. *Everybody's Guide to Homeopathic Medicines*. New York: Putnam, 1991.

Dancu, D. A. *Homeopathic Vibrations, A Guide to Natural Healing*. Boulder, Colo.: Sunshine Press, 1996.

Davies, S., et al. *Nutritional Medicine*. New York: Avon Books, 1990.

Deakin, L. "Summer Tan? New Evidence—Finally Change Your Mind." *Total Health* 15, no. 4 (Aug. 1993): 54–62.

DiCyan, E. *A Beginner's Introduction to Trace Minerals*. Los Angeles: Keats Publishing, 1984.

Donahue, P. *Relief from Chronic Skin Problems*. New York: Dell, 1992.

Donsbach, K. "Benign Prostatic Hypertrophy & Prostate Cancer." Rockland Corporation, 1994.

"Don't Be Stupid Under the Sun." *USA Today* 122, no. 2578 (July 1993): 6.

The Dorling Kindersley Visual Encyclopedia. New York: Dorling Kindersley, 1995.

Dragoo, J. *Handbook of Sports Medicine*. Ariz.: Renaissance Publishing, 1993.

Droge, W., et al. "Functions of Glutathione and Glutathione Disulfide in Immunology and Immunopathology." *FASEB Journal* 8 (1994): 1131–38.

Earth Matters, Issue #30. London: Friends of the Earth, summer 1996.

Eaton, K. K., et al. "Gut Permeability Measured by Polyethylene Glycol Absorption in Abnormal Gut Fermentation as Compared with Food Intolerance." *Journal of the Royal Society of Medicine* 88 (Feb. 1995): 63–66.

"Effects of Estrogen or Estrogen/Progestin Regimens on Heart Disease Risk Factors in Postmenopausal Women." The postmenopausal estrogen/progestins interventions (PEPI) trial. *JAMA* 273, no. 3 (Jan. 18, 1995): 240–41.

Elin, R. "Magnesium: The Fifth But Forgotten Electrolyte." *American Journal of Clinical Pathology* 102, no. 25 (1994): 616–22.

Ellison, P. T., C. Panter-Brick, S. F. Lipson, and M. T. O'Rourke. "The Ecological Context of Human Ovarian Function." *Human Reproduction* 8, no. 22 (1993): 48–58.

Enwonwu, C. O., and V. I. Meeks. "Bionutrition and Oral Cancer in Humans." *Critical Reviews in Oral Biology and Medicine* 6, no. 1 (1995): 5–17.

Farnsworth, N., et al. "Medicinal Plants in Therapy." *Bulletin World Health Organization* 63 (1985): 965–81.

Fehily, A. M., et al. "Diet and Incident Ischaemic Heart Disease: The Caerphilly Study." *British Journal of Nutrition* 69 (1993): 303–14.

Felson, D. T., Y. Zhang, M. T. Hannan, D. P. Kiel, P. W. F. Wilson, and J. J. Anderson. "The Effect of Postmenopausal Estrogen Therapy on Bone Density in Elderly Women." *New England Journal of Medicine* 329 (1993): 1141–46.

Fenske, N. "Common Problems of Aging Skin." Special issue: "Caring for the Aging Patient." *Patient Care* 23, no. 7 (April 15, 1989): 225–28.

Flagg, E. W., et al. "Plasma Total Glutathione in Humans and Its Association with Demographic and Health-Related Factors." *British Journal of Nutrition* 70, no. 3 (Nov. 1993): 797–808.

Fletcher, R. H., and S. W. Fletcher. "Glutathione and Ageing: Ideas and Evidence." *The Lancet* 344 (Nov. 19, 1994): 1379–80.

Fogarty, M. "Garlic's Potential Role in Reducing Heart Disease." *British Journal of Clinical Practice* 47, no. 2 (1993): 64–65.

Gaby, Alan R. *Preventing and Reversing Osteoporosis*. Rocklin, Calif.: Prima Publishing, 1993.

Gadkari, J. V. "The Effect of Ingestion of Raw Garlic on Serum Cholesterol Level, Clotting Time and Fibrinolytic Activity in Normal Subjects." *Journal of Postgraduate Medicine* 37, no. 3 (1991): 128–31.

Ganske, M. "Feed Your Face: Why Your Complexion Needs Vitamins." *Redbook* 185, no. 1 (May 1995): 59–63.

Gelbard, M. *Solving Prostate Problems*. New York: Fireside, Simon & Schuster, 1995.

Gilchrest, B. "At Last! A Medical Treatment for Skin Aging." *Journal of the American Medical Association* 259, no. 4 (Jan. 22, 1988): 569–72.

Gillum, Richard F. "Dental Disease and Coronary Artery Disease." *American Heart Journal* (Dec. 1994): 1267.

Giovannucci, E., et al. "Intake of Fat, Meat, and Fiber in Relation to Risk of Colon Cancer in Men." *Cancer Research* 54 (May 1, 1994): 2390–97.

Gittleman, Ann Louise. *Guess What Came to Dinner: Parasites and Your Health*. Garden City Park, N.Y.: Avery Publishing, 1993.

Golan, Ralph. *Optional Wellness*. New York: Ballantine Books, 1995.

Gorman, C. "Does Sunscreen Save Your Skin?" *Time* 141, no. 21 (May 24, 1993): 69–71.

Green, J. *The Male Herbal*. Freedom, Calif.: The Crossing Press, 1991.

Hallfrisch, J., et al. "Diets Containing Soluble Oat Extracts Improve Glucose and Insulin Responses of Moderately Hypercholesterolemic Men and Women." *American Journal of Clinical Nutrition* 61 (1995): 369–84.

Hamilton, S. "What You Should Know About Homeopathy." *American Health* (Dec. 1995).

Hammond, C. B., F. R. Jelvsek, K. L. Lee, W. T. Creasman, and R. T. Parker. "Effects of Long-Term Estrogen Replacement Therapy. I. Metabolic Effects." *American Journal of Obstetrics and Gynecology* 133 (1979): 525–36.

Hauser, Robert A., et al. "Blood Manganese Correlates with Brain Magnetic Resonance Imaging Changes in Patients with Liver Disease." *Canadian Journal of Neurological Science* 23, no. 2 (May 1996): 95–98.

Hawk, J. L.,"Ultraviolet A Radiation: Staying Within the Pale." *British Medical Journal* 302, no. 6784 (May 4, 1991): 1036–37.

He, J., et al. "Dietary Macronutrients and Blood Pressure in Southwestern China." *Journal of Hypertension* 13, no. 11 (1995): 1267–74.

Health Letter Associates. *The New Wellness Encyclopedia.* Boston: Houghton Mifflin, 1995, pp. 296–97, 549.

Hedlund, L. R., and J. C. Gallagher. "Increased Incidence of Hip Fracture in Osteoporotic Women Treated with Sodium Fluoride." *Journal of Bone and Mineral Research* 4 (1989): 223–25.

Hendler, S. *The Doctors' Vitamin and Mineral Encyclopedia.* New York: Fireside, Simon & Schuster, 1991.

Hickey, M. "The Beauty Diet: Foods That Help Improve Appearance." *Ladies' Home Journal* 112, no. 7 (July 1995): 96.

Hileman, B. "Reproductive Estrogens Linked to Reproductive Abnormalities, Cancer." *Chemical and Engineering News* (Jan. 31, 1994): 19–23.

Hill, N., et al. "A Placebo Controlled Clinical Trial Investigating the Efficacy of a Homeopathic After-Bite Gel in Reducing Mosquito Bite Induced Erythema." *European Journal of Clinical Pharmacology* 49 (1995): 103–8.

Hobbs, C. *The Echinacea Handbook.* Portland, Oreg.: Eclectic Medical Publications, 1989.

"Homeopathy Scores Again." *Townsend Letter for Doctors & Patients* (June 1996): 27.

Hu, Howard, et al. "The Relationship of Bone and Blood Lead to Hypertension: The Normative Aging Study." *JAMA* 275, no. 15 (April 17, 1996): 1171–76.

Humble, C. G., et al. "Dietary Fiber and Coronary Heart Disease in Middle-Aged Hypercholesterolemic Men." *American Journal of Preventive Medicine* 9 (1993): 97–202.

Hunninghake, D. B., et al. "Hypocholesterolemic Effects of a Dietary Fiber Supplement." *American Journal of Clinical Nutrition* 59 (1994): 1050–54.

Hunninghake, D. B., et al. "Long-Term Treatment of Hypercholesterolemia with Dietary Fiber." *American Journal of Medicine* 97 (Dec. 1994): 504–8.

Hunter, C. *Vitamins, What They Are and Why We Need Them.* London: Thorsons, 1978, pp. 63–72, 90.

Iantomasi, T., et al. "Glutathione Metabolism in Crohn's Disease." *Biochemical Medicine and Metabolic Biology* 53 (1994): 87–91.

"If You Don't Succeed the First Time." *Medical Update* 14, no. 10 (April 1999): 4.

Jacques, P. "Effects of Vitamin C on HDL and Blood Pressure." *Journal of the American College of Nutrition* 9, no. 5 (1990): 554/Abstract 106.

Jendryczko, A., et al. "Effects of Two Low-Dose Oral Contraceptives on Erythrocyte Superoxide Dismutase, Catalase and Glutathione Peroxidase activities." *Zentralbl Gynakol* 115, no. 11 (1993): 469–72.

Jenkins, D. J., et al. "Effects on Blood Lipids of Very High Intakes of Fiber in Diets Low in Saturated Fat and Cholesterol." *New England Journal of Medicine* 329, no. 1 (July 1, 1993): 21–26.

Jensen, B., et al. *Empty Harvest.* Garden City Park, N.Y.: Avery Publishing, 1990.

Julius, M. "Glutathione and Morbidity in a Community-Based Sample of Elderly." *Journal of Clinical Epidemiology* 47, no. 9 (1994): 1021–26.

Kaaks, R., et al. "Dietary Intake of Fiber and Decreased Risk of Cancers of the Colon and Rectum: Evidence from the Combined Analysis of 13 Case-Control Studies." *Journal of the National Cancer Institute* 84, no. 24 (Dec. 1992): 1887–96.

Kadunce, D., et al. "Cigarette Smoking: Risk Factor for Premature Wrinkling." *Annals of Internal Medicine* 114, no. 10 (May 15, 1991): 840–45.

Kahn, J. "Homeopathic Remedy Relieves Allergic Asthma Symptoms." *Medical Tribune* 11 (Jan. 5, 1995).

Kalimi, M., and W. Regelson, eds. *The Biologic Role of Dehydroepiandrosterone.* Walter de Gruyter, 1990.

Kamen, Betty. *Hormone Replacement Therapy: Yes or No?* Novato, Calif.: Nutrition Encounter, Inc., 1993.

Kanazawa, T., et al. "Anti-Atherogenicity of Soybean Protein." *Annals of New York Academy of Science* 676 (1993): 202–14.

Khaw, K.T., and E. Barrett-Connor. "Dietary Fiber and Reduced Ischemic Heart Disease Mortality Rates in Men and Women: A 12-Year Prospective Study." *American Journal of Epidemiology* 126 (1987): 1093–102.

Kim, Rokho, et al. "A Longitudinal Study of Low-Level Lead Exposure and Impairment of Renal Function: The Normative Aging Study." *JAMA* 275, no. 15 (April 17, 1996): 1177–81.

Kinscherf, R., et al. "Effects of Glutathione Depletion and Oral *N*-Acetyl-Cysteine Treatment on CD4+ and CD8+ Cells." *FASEB Journal* 8, no. 6 (April 1, 1994): 338–51.

Kleerekoper, M. E., et al. "Continuous Sodium Fluoride Therapy Does Not Reduce Vertebral Fracture Rate in Postmenopausal Osteoporosis." Abstract. *Journal of Bone and Mineral Research* (1989) Res. 4 (Suppl. 1): S376.

Kowalchik, C., et al. *Rodale's Illustrated Encyclopedia of Herbs.* Emmaus, Pa.: Rodale Press, 1987.

Kromhout, D., et al. "Dietary Fiber and 10-Year Mortality from Coronary Heart Disease, Cancer and All Causes: The Zutphen Study." *The Lancet* 2 (1982): 518–21.

Laing, C. "City Air Pollution Linked to Male Infertility." *Medical Tribune* (Nov. 9, 1995): 14.

———. "Abdominal Obesity Linked to BPH." *Medical Tribune* (Jan. 1, 1993).

Lanza, E., et al. "Dietary Fiber Intake in the U.S. Population." *American Journal of Clinical Nutrition* (1987): 790–97.

Lassen, K. O., and M. Horder. "Selenium Status and the Effect of Organic and Inorganic Selenium Supplementation in a Group of Elderly People in Denmark." *Scandinavian Journal of Clinical Laboratory Investigation* 54 (1994): 585–90.

Lee, John R., with Virginia Hopkins. *What Your Doctor May Not Tell You About Menopause: The Breakthrough Book on Natural Progesterone.* New York: Warner Books, 1996.

Lemley, B. Interview with Andrew Weil. *New Age Journal* (Dec. 1995): 68.

Lessof, M. H., et al. "Reactions to Food Additives." *Clinical and Experimental Allergy* 25 (1995) (Suppl. 1): 27–28.

Li, J., et al. "Glutamine Prevents Parenteral Nutrition-Induced Increases in Intestinal Permeability." *Journal of Parenteral and Enteral Nutrition* 18 (1994): 303–7.

Liberty, M. "The Best Skin Protection Under the Sun." *Better Nutrition for Today's Living* 56, no. 7 (July 1994): 56.

Lip, G. Y. H. "Fibrinogen and Cardiovascular Disorders." *Quarterly Journal of Medicine* 88 (1995): 155–65.

Lipkin, R. "Vegemania—Scientists Tout the Health Benefits of Saponins." *Science News* 148 (Dec. 9, 1995): 392–93.

Loguercio, C., et al. "Effect of *S*-adenosyl-L-methionine Administration on Red Blood Cell Cysteine and Glutathione Levels in Alcoholic Patients with and Without Liver Disease." *Alcohol and Alcoholism* 29, no. 5 (1994): 597–604.

Lou, F., et al. "A Study on Tea Pigment in the Prevention of Atherosclerosis." *Preventive Medicine* 21, no. 3 (1992): 333.

Loughram, J. "Skin Care Basics." *Let's Live* 55 (Jan. 1996).

Lust, J. *The Herb Book.* New York: Bantam Books, 1974.

Mabey, R. *The New Age Herbalist.* New York: Collier Books, Macmillan Publishing, 1988.

McClanahan, Mark A. "Mercury Contamination in the Home." *The Lancet* 347 (April 13, 1996): 1044–45.

Macolo, N., et al. "Ethnopharmalogic Investigation of Ginger (*Zingiber Officinale*)." *Journal of Ethnopharmacology* 27 (1989): 129–40.

MacLennan, R., et al. "Randomized Trial of Intake of Fat, Fiber, and Beta-Carotene to Prevent Colorectal Adenomas." *Journal of the National Cancer Institute* 87, no. 23 (Dec. 6, 1995): 1760–66.

MacRury, S., et al. "Seasonal and Climatic Variation in Cholesterol and Vitamin C: Effect of Vitamin C Supplementation." *Scottish Medical Journal* 37, no. 2 (1992): 49–52.

Mann, C. et al. "The Chemistry, Pharmacology, and Commercial Formulations of Chamomile." *Herbs, Spices, and Medicinal Plants* 1 (1985): 235–80.

Marlett, J. A. "Content and Composition of Dietary Fiber in 117 Frequently Consumed Foods."

Journal of the American Dietetic Association (1992): 175–86.

Martlew, G. *Electrolytes, the Spark of Life.* Murdock, Fla.: Nature's Publishing, 1994.

Mesch, U., et al. "Lead Poisoning Masquerading as Chronic Fatigue Syndrome." *The Lancet* 347 (April 27, 1996): 1193.

Mindell, Earl. *Earl Mindell's Anti-Aging Bible.* New York: Simon & Schuster, 1996.

———. *Earl Mindell's Food as Medicine.* New York: Simon & Schuster, 1994.

———. *Earl Mindell's Herb Bible.* New York: Simon & Schuster, 1992.

———. *Earl Mindell's Shaping Up with Vitamins.* New York: Warner Books, 1985.

———. *Earl Mindell's Soy Miracle.* New York: Simon & Schuster, 1995.

———. *Earl Mindell's Vitamin Bible.* New York: Warner Books, 1991.

———. *The Mindell Letter,* a monthly newsletter published by Phillips Publishing, Potomac, Md. (1-800-787-3003).

———. *Parent's Nutrition Bible.* Carson, Calif.: Hay House, 1992.

Miura, K., et al. "Cystine Uptake and Glutathione Level in Endothelial Cells Exposed to Oxidative Stress." *American Journal of Physiology* 262 (Jan. 1992): C50–58.

Moore, Michael. *Medicinal Plants of the Mountain West.* Santa Fe, N. Mex.: Museum of New Mexico Press, 1979.

———. *Medicinal Plants of the Pacific West.* Santa Fe, N. Mex.: Red Crane Books, 1993.

Mowrey, Daniel B. *The Scientific Validation of Herbal Medicine.* Los Angeles: Keats Publishing, 1986.

Murray, Michael. *The Healing Power of Herbs.* Rocklin, Calif.: Prima Publishing, 1995.

———. *Male Sexual Vitality.* Rocklin, Calif.: Prima Publishing, 1994.

———. *The Saw Palmetto Story.* Wash.: Vital Communications, 1990.

Murray, Michael, and Joseph Pizzorno. *Encyclopedia of Natural Medicine.* Rocklin, Calif.: Prima Publishing, 1991.

Natural Pest Control, by Andrew Lopez, The Invisible Gardener of Malibu, 29161 Heathercliff Road, Ste. 216-408, Malibu, CA 90265 (1-800-354-9296).

Needleman, Herbert L., et al. "Bone Lead Levels and Delinquent Behavior." *JAMA* 275, no. 5 (Feb. 7, 1996): 363–69.

Newsome, D. "Role of Antioxidants in Macular Degeneration: An Update." *Ophthalmic Practice* 12, no. 4 (1994): 169–71.

Northrup, Christiane. *Women's Bodies, Women's Wisdom.* New York: Bantam Books, 1994.

Norwell, D. Y., et al. "Garlic, Vampires and CHD." *Osteopathy Annual* 12 (1984): 276–80.

O'Keefe, James H., Jr., et al. "Insights into the Pathogenesis and Prevention of Coronary Artery Disease." *Mayo Clinic Proceedings* 70 (Jan. 1995): 69–79.

"Out, Out, Darned Spot! Reducing Liver Spots & Wrinkles with Tretinoin." *Executive Health's Good Health Report* 28, no. 9 (June 1992): 8.

Panos, M. D., and J. Heimlich. *Homeopathic Medicine at Home.* New York: Putnam, 1980.

Paolisso, G., et al. "Plasma GSH/GSSG Affects Glucose Homeostasis in Healthy Subjects and Non-Insulin-Dependent Diabetics." *American Journal of Physiology* 262 (Sept. 1992).

Paris, B. *Natural Fitness.* New York: Warner Books, 1996.

Pejaver, R., et al. "High-Dose Vitamin E Therapy in Glutathione Synthetase Deficiency." *Journal of Inherited Metabolic Disorders* 17 (1994): 1749–50.

Potts, R., et al. "Changes with Age in the Moisture Content of Human Skin." *Journal of Investigative Dermatology* 82 (1984): 97–100.

Prior, J. C. "Postmenopausal Estrogen Therapy and Cardiovascular Disease." Letter. *New England Journal of Medicine* 326 (1991): 705–6.

———. "Progesterone as a Bone-Tropic Hormone." *Endocrine Reviews* 11 (1990): 386–98.

Prior, J. C., Y. M. Vigna, and N. Alojado. "Progesterone and the Prevention of Osteoporosis." *Canadian Journal of Obstetrics/Gynecology and Women's Health Care* 3 (1991): 168–84.

Probert, C. S. H., et al. "Some Determinates of Whole-Cut Transit Time: A Population Based Study." *Quarterly Journal of Medicine* 88 (1995): 311–15.

Rader, J. I. "Anti-Nutritive Effects of Dietary Tin." *Advances in Experimental Medicine and Biology* 289 (1991): 509–24.

Rafal, E., et al. "Topical Tretinoin (Retinoic Acid) Treatment for Liver Spots Associated with Photodamage." *New England Journal of Medicine* 326, no. 6 (Feb. 6, 1992): 368.

Rahman, Mahfuzar, and Olav Axelson. "Diabetes Mellitus and Arsenic Exposure: A Second Look at Case-Control Data from a Swedish Copper Smelter." *Occupational and Environmental Medicine* 52 (1995): 773–74.

Rainsford, K. D. "Leukotrienes in the Pathogenesis of NSAID-Induced Gastric and Intestinal Mucosal Damage." Special Conference Issue. *Agents Actions* 39 (1993): C24–26.

Raloff, J. "Ecocancers." *Science News* 144 (July 3, 1993): 10–13.

———. "The Gender Benders." *Science News* 145 (Jan. 8, 1994): 24–27.

———. "That Feminine Touch." *Science News* 145 (Jan. 22, 1994): 56–59.

Reilly, D., et al. "Is Evidence for Homeopathy Reproducible?" *The Lancet* 344 (Dec. 10, 1994): 1601–6.

"Research Offers Evidence of Vitamin E Cardiac Benefit." *Medical Tribune* 8 (Nov. 21, 1994).

Reuben, C. "No More Dry Skin." *Let's Live* (Jan. 1996).

Riemersma, R. "Risk of Angina Pectoris and Plasma Concentrations of Vitamins A, C, and E and Carotene." *The Lancet* 337 (1991): 1–5.

Rimm F., et al. "Vegetable, Fruit and Cereal Fiber Intake and Risk of Coronary Heart Disease Among Men." *JAMA* 275 (1996): 446–51.

———. "Vitamin E Consumption and the Risk of Coronary Heart Disease in Men." *New England Journal of Medicine* 328 (1993): 1450–56.

Ripsin, C. M., et al. "Oat Products and Lipid Lowering: A Meta-Analysis." *JAMA* 267, no. 24 (1992): 3317–25

Rose, Jeanne. *Jeanne Rose's Herbal Body Book*. New York: Perigree, Putnam Publishing, 1976.

Rosenbaum, A. "To Each His Own—Gentle Herbal Remedies for Men." *Vegetarian Times* no. 186 (Feb. 1993): 75.

Sastre, J., et al. "Exhaustive Physical Exercise Causes Oxidation of Glutathione Status in Blood: Prevention by Antioxidant Administration." *American Journal of Physiology* 263 (Nov. 1992): (5 Pt 2) pR992–5.

"Save Your Skin." *The Edell Health Letter* 10, no. 1 (Dec./Jan. 1990): 7.

Schmidt, Michael. *Tired of Being Tired*. Berkeley, Calif.: Frog, 1995.

Schmitt, Nicholas. "Could Zinc Help Protect Children from Lead Poisoning?" *Canadian Medical Association Journal* 154, no. 1 (Jan. 1, 1996): 13–14.

Schroeder, H. *The Trace Elements and Man*. Greenwich, Conn.: Devin-Adair, 1973.

Sears, Barry, with Bill Lawren. *Enter the Zone*. New York: Regan Books, 1995.

Sehnert, K. W., A. F. Clague, and E. Chearskin. "Improvement in Renal Function Following EDTA Chelation and Multi-Vitamin-Trace Mineral Therapy: A Study in Creatinine Clearance." *Medical Hypotheses* 15, no. 3 (Nov. 1984): 301–4.

Serna, Gaspar De La. "Fibrinogen: A New Major Risk Factor for Cardiovascular Disease: A Review of the Literature." *Journal of Family Practice* 39, no. 5 (Nov. 1994): 468–77.

Shepherd, S. "Smoothing Skin Wrinkles: What's New Under the Sun?" *Executive Health Report* 26, no. 7 (April 1990): 2.

Sherman, B. M., J. H. West, and S. G. Korenmam. "The Menopausal Transition: Analysis of LH, FSH, Estradiol and Progesterone Concentrations During Menstrual Cycles of Older Women." *Journal of Clinical Endocrinology and Metabolism* 42 (1976): 629–36.

Simons, A., et al. *Before You Call the Doctor*. New York: Ballantine Books, 1992.

"Skin Problems Among the Elderly." *Medical Update* 14, no. 7 (Jan. 1991): 4.

Slavin, J. "Nutritional Benefits of Soy Protein and Soy Fiber." *Journal of the American Dietetic Association* 91 (1991): 816–19.

Smith, U. "Carbohydrates, Fat, and Insulin Action." *American Journal of Clinical Nutrition* 59 (1994) (Suppl.): 686S–689S.

Smith, W. "Hydroxy Acids and Skin Aging." *Cosmetics and Toiletries Magazine* 109, no. 9 (Sept. 1994): 41–46.

Somer, E. *The Essential Guide to Vitamins and Minerals.* New York: HarperCollins, 1995.

Stadtler, Von P. "Amalgam." *Occupation and Environment* 43 (1995): 163–71.

Stampfer, M. J., et al. "Vitamin E Consumption and the Risk of Coronary Disease in Women." *New England Journal of Medicine* 328, no. 20 (1993): 1444–49.

Stampfer, M. J., et al. "Postmenopausal Estrogen Therapy and Cardiovascular Disease—Ten-Year Follow-up from the Nurses' Health Study." *New England Journal of Medicine* 325 (1991): 756–62.

Steiner, M., et al. "Vitamin E—An Inhibitor of Platelet Release Action." *Journal of Clinical Investigation* 57 (1996): 732–37.

Steinman, D. "Enlarged Prostate? Try Tree Bark." *Natural Health* (July/Aug. 1994), pp. 44–46.

———. "Treating Prostate Troubles." *Natural Health,* (Nov./Dec. 1993): 56–59.

Stenson, J. "Prostate Cancer—Aggressive Treatment Unneeded for Patients with Low-Grade Tumors." *Medical Tribune* (Sept. 21, 1995): 15.

Stoll, B. A., et al. "Can Supplementary Dietary Fiber Suppress Breast Cancer Growth?" *British Journal of Cancer* 73 (1996): 557–59.

Swain, J. F., et al. "Comparison of the Effects of Oat Bran and Low-Fiber Wheat on Serum Lipoprotein Levels and Blood Pressure." *New England Journal of Medicine* 322 (1990): 193–95.

Swencionis, C. *The Lazy Person's Guide to Fitness.* New York: St. Martin's Press, 1994.

"Tanned Look Grows Old Fast." *The Edell Health Letter* 11, no. 5 (May 1992): 6.

Terho, E. O., and J. Savolainen. "Diagnosis of Food Allergy." *European Journal of Clinical Nutrition* 50 (1996): 1–5.

Thomas, P. "Vitamin C Eyed for Topical Use as Skin Preserver." *Medical World News* 32, no. 3 (March 1991): 12.

Tierra, Lesley. *The Herbs of Life: Health and Healing Using Western and Chinese Techniques.* Freedom, Calif.: The Crossing Press, 1992.

Trowell, H. C., and D. P. Burkitt, eds. *Western Diseases: Their Emergency and Prevention.* London: Edward Arnold Publishers, 1981.

Ullman, D. *The Consumer's Guide to Homeopathy.* New York: Putnam, 1995.

University of Texas/Oregon State University. "Immune Suppression Caused by Sun Exposure." *NCI Cancer Weekly* 4 (Sept. 4, 1989): 2.

Vanderhoek, J., et al. "Inhibition of Fatty Acid Lipoxygenases by Onion and Garlic Oils. Evidence for the Mechanism by Which These Oils Inhibit Platelet Aggregation." *Biochemistry and Psychopharmacology* 29, no. 3 (1980): 169–73.

Van Poppel, Geert, et al. "Antioxidants and Coronary Heart Disease." *Annals of Medicine* 26 (1994): 429–34.

Van Zandwijk, N. C. "N-Acetylcysteine for Lung Cancer Prevention." *Chest* 107, no. 5 (May 1995): 1436–41.

Vaughn, L., et al. *Prevention Magazine's Complete Book of Vitamins and Minerals.* Avenel, N.J.: Wings Books, 1994.

Verschuren, W. M. "Serum Total Cholesterol and Long-Term Coronary Heart Disease Mortality in Different Cultures: Twenty-Five-Year Follow-Up of the Seven Countries Study." *JAMA* 274, no. 2 (July 12, 1995): 131–36.

"Vitamin E Supplementation and Skin Photoprotection." *American Family Physician* 51, no. 4 (March 1995): 956.

Walsh, P., et al. *The Prostate.* Baltimore: Johns Hopkins University Press, 1995.

Warner, J. O. "Food and Behavior." *Clinical and Experimental Allergy* 25 (1995) (Suppl. 1): 23–26.

———. "Food Intolerance and Asthma." *Clinical and Experimental Allergy* 25 (1995) (Suppl. 1): 29–30.

Watson, W. "Food Allergy in Children." *Clinical Reviews in Allergy and Immunology* 13 (1995): 347–59.

Weil, Andrew. *Natural Health, Natural Medicine.* Boston: Houghton Mifflin, 1995.

Weiner, M. *Earth Medicine—Earth Food.* New York: Fawcett Columbine, 1980.

Werbach, Melvyn R., and Michael T. Murray. *Botanical Influences on Illness.* Tarzana, Calif.: Third Line Press, 1994.

West, Stanley. *The Hysterectomy Hoax.* New York: Doubleday, 1994.

Wilcox, G., et al. "Oestrogenic Effects of Plant Foods in Postmenopausal Women." *British Medical Journal* 30 (1990): 905–6.

Willard, Terry. *The Wild Rose Scientific Herbal.* Calgary, Alberta, Canada: Wild Rose College of Natural Healing, 1991.

Willet, W. C., et al. "Dietary Fat and Fiber in Relation to Risk of Breast Cancer: An 8-Year Follow-up." *JAMA* 268 (1992): 2037–44.

Wynder, E., et al. "High Fiber Intake: Indicator of a Healthy Life-Style." *JAMA* 275, no. 6 (Feb. 14, 1996): 486–87.

Zeevak, G. D., L. P. Bernard, and W. J. Nicklas. "Role of Oxidative Stress and the Glutathione System in Loss of Dopamine Neurons Due to Impairment of Energy Metabolism." *Journal of Neurochemistry* 70, no. 4 (April 1998): 1421–30.

INDEX ~